IgA NEPHROPATHY

TOPICS IN RENAL MEDICINE

Vittorio E. Andreucci, Series Editor

Titles in the Series

Andreucci; *The Kidney in Pregnancy*, 1986.

IgA NEPHROPATHY

EDITED BY

ANTHONY R. CLARKSON

MARTINUS NIJHOFF PUBLISHING
A MEMBER OF THE KLUWER ACADEMIC PUBLISHERS GROUP
BOSTON DORDRECHT LANCASTER

PRINTED IN THE UNITED STATES.

Distributors

for the United States and Canada: Kluwer Academic Publishers, 101 Philip Drive, Assinippi Park, Norwell, MA 02061

for the UK and Ireland: Kluwer Academic Publishers, MTP Press Limited, Falcon House, Queen Square, Lancaster LA1 1RN, UK

for all other countries: Kluwer Academic Publishers Group, Distribution Centre, P.O. Box 322, 3300 AH Dordrecht, The Netherlands

Library of Congress Cataloging-in-Publication Data

IgA nephropathy.

(Topics in renal medicine)
Includes index.
1. IgA glomerulonephritis. I. Clarkson, A. R.
II. Series. [DNLM: 1. Glomerulonephritis, IGA.
WJ 353 I24]
RC918.I35I33 1986 616.6′12 86-28480
ISBN 0-89838-839-2

To my wife, Helen, and children, Andrew, Mary, and Catriona, for their patience, support, understanding, and love.

CONTENTS

CONTRIBUTING AUTHORS

Randall A. Allardyce
Department of Surgery
Christchurch Clinical School of Medicine
Christchurch
New Zealand

Anthony R. Clarkson
Renal Unit
Royal Adelaide Hospital
North Terrace, Adelaide
South Australia 5000
Australia

Giuseppe D'Amico
Division of Nephrology
S. Carlo Hospital
Milan
Italy

Dominique Droz
Département de Néphrologie
Hôpital Necker
161 rue de Sèvres
75742 Paris
France

Jesus Egido
Servicio de Nefrologia
Fundación Jiménez Díaz
Av Reyes Católicos 2
28040 Madrid
Spain

Steven N. Emancipator
Institute of Pathology
Case Western Reserve University
Cleveland, Ohio 44106
USA

Gloria R. Gallo
Department of Pathology
New York University Medical Center
New York, New York 10016
USA

Ronald J. Hogg
Department of Pediatrics
Baylor University Medical Center
3500 Gaston Ave
Dallas, Texas 75246
USA

Michael E. Lamm
Institute of Pathology
Case Western Reserve University
Cleveland, Ohio 44106
USA

Jukka Mustonen
Department of Clinical Sciences
University of Tampere
Teiskontie 35
33520 Tampere 52
Finland

Amos Pasternack
Department of Clinical Sciences
University of Tampere
Teiskontie 35
33520 Tampere 52
Finland

Abdalla Rifai
Department of Pathology and
Laboratory Medicine
University of Texas Medical School
Houston, Texas 77025
USA

Hideto Sakai
Division of Nephrology and Metabolism
Department of Internal Medicine
School of Medicine
Tokai University
Isehara City, Kanagawa-ken
Japan

Fred G. Silva
Department of Pathology
University of Texas Health Science
Center
5323 Harry Hines Boulevard
Dallas, Texas 75235
USA

Rajah Sinniah
Department of Pathology
National University of Singapore
National University Hospital
Lower Kent Ridge Road
Singapore 0511

Judy B. Splawski
University of Tennessee Center for
Health Sciences
956 Court Room 3 B09
Memphis, Tennessee 38163
USA

Yasuhiko Tomino
Department of Internal Medicine
School of Medicine
Tokai University
Isehara City,
Kanagawa-ken 259-11
Japan

Andrew J. Woodroffe
Renal Unit
Royal Adelaide Hospital
North Terrace, Adelaide
South Australia 5000
Australia

Robert J. Wyatt
University of Tennessee Center for
Health Sciences
956 Court Room 3 B09
Memphis, Tennessee 38163
USA

PREFACE

IgA nephropathy has, in the course of two decades, become one of the most important renal diseases. Not only is it the most common form of glomerulonephritis seen in many countries, its increasing recognition by renal biopsy in this time has allowed sufficient study to conclude that it is also one of the most frequent causes of end-stage renal failure.

The clinical features are diverse, and only in a minority do recurrent macroscopic hematuric episodes associated with an upper respiratory tract infection allow a confident clinical diagnosis. All clinicians, from community practitioners to general and specialist internists and surgeons, should be aware of its manifestations in patients of all ages. Its relationship with Henoch-Schönlein purpura is especially interesting.

The discovery of IgA nephropathy has caused an explosion of interest and research. The disease itself (if indeed it can be regarded as a single entity rather than a syndrome) has been studied extensively by many groups and a synopsis is presented by several of the leaders in this clinical field. Parallel with the increased understanding of the renal disease, there has occurred similar incremental knowledge in such diverse fields as the structure and function of the glomerular mesangium, the biology of mucosal immunity, and the IgA immune response. This book has collected essays on these topics that emphasize their importance in the relation to the study of IgA nephropathy.

The contributors have provided up-to-date and clear chapters that have individual merit and yet collectively provide a good reference and comprehensive overview of the subject. I am deeply indebted to them for their time and effort, and hope that their work will stimulate more intensive examination of this most interesting disease.

My sincere thanks is also extended to colleagues who have shared the traumas of this book's gestation. In particular, Drs. Andrew Woodroffe, Ian Aarons, Gerard Hale, Yoshi Hiki, Kym Bannister, Randall Faull, Jane Lomax-Smith, Andrew Wootton, Alan Gormley, Tony Seymour, and Peter McKenzie have made special contributions. Without their help and the close cooperation of many similar units throughout the world working on this subject, this book would not have been possible. To Chris Nagle, Di Paglia, and Anne Filippin, I offer thanks for secretarial assistance and patience. Finally to Dr. Andreucci, the series editor, and to Martinus Nijhoff Publishing, a debt is owed for their persistence and support.

1. IgA NEPHROPATHY: HISTORY, CLASSIFICATION, AND GEOGRAPHIC DISTRIBUTION

ANTHONY R. CLARKSON

Jean Berger, a French pathologist, "discovered" immunoglobulin A (IgA) nephropathy. With Hinglais, he applied fluorescein-conjugated antibodies to IgA to human renal biopsy material for the first time [1, 2]. Approximately 25% of the 300 renal biopsies fluoresced strongly with IgA antisera and, although a few of these biopsies were taken from patients with systemic lupus erythematosus (SLE), Henoch-Schönlein purpura (HSP), and other systemic diseases, the majority were from patients with no overt systemic symptoms. In these latter biopsies, the IgA fluorescence was mesangial in position and accompanied by IgG and C3. IgA was the predominant immunglobulin. The patients suffered recurring bouts of macroscopic hematuria or persistent microscopic hematuria. It is a tribute to Berger's persistence and determination that IgA nephropathy has emerged in a relatively short space of time as the most common form of glomerulonephritis in the world, as at first Berger's observations were greeted with some disbelief. The high incidence of this newly discovered disease prompted nephrologists to regard the entity as uniquely French. In addition, the specificity of IgA antisera used was questioned. In the early 1970s, Berger's disease, an eponym applied to the disease, was frequently couched in tones of skepticism. As immunofluorescence techniques were applied more widely, however, the high incidence of IgA nephropathy described by Berger was confirmed, first in France, then gradually in many other countries. Any skepticism intoned in using the eponym "Berger's disease" has now changed to warmth and respect of deserved recognition. Hail, Jean Berger!

HISTORY

"After a child or adult is affected with acute disease or 'indulged in intemperate use of ardent spirits,' he passes urine tinged with blood or containing albumin." These words of Richard Bright's stated in 1826 may equally apply to IgA nephropathy as any other form of glomerulonephritis. Berger's discovery in 1968 represented therefore the first definition of an old problem. Although descriptive texts of renal pathology were not common before the 1960s, i.e., before the widespread use of percutaneous renal biopsy, some of those existing describe focal and segmental forms of glomerulonephritis as the commonest finding in kidneys from patients dying with end-stage renal failure. Current knowledge clearly suggests that many of these cases were of IgA nephropathy. The lack of any observed mesangial changes may simply reflect inadequate definition of this structure at the time.

While the confirmation of mesangial deposits by electron microscopy dispelled any doubts about Berger's immunofluorescence observations, the greater impetus to study of IgA nephropathy has resulted from advances in understanding of the biology of immunoglobulin A. The roles of IgA in mucosal immunity, secretory component, the enterohepatic circulation, subclasses of the IgA molecule, immune regulation by helper and suppressor T cells of B-cell IgA production, and IgA-containing immune complexes have all attracted wide attention. Recognition of secondary forms of IgA nephropathy has occurred pari passu with the better definition of IgA immunobiology. Associations with such diseases as alcoholic cirrhosis, gluten-sensitive enteropathy, and various cancers are now explicable in terms of immunologic malfunction. Two further observations have provided considerable stimulus to study of the pathogenesis. First, the disease recurs regularly in kidneys transplanted into sufferers of IgA nephropathy [3] and disappears from kidneys housing the disease when transplanted into patients not so afflicted [4]. Second, positive immunofluorescence for IgA is not limited to the glomerular mesangium in IgA nephropathy. It has also been described in capillaries of the dermis [5, 6], lung, liver, and gut. These observations imply that the disease is systemic in nature, an implication strongly supported by finding IgA-containing immune complexes in the serum of patients [7–10]. Further analysis of these complexes and the mesangial IgA deposits has confirmed that both contain macromolecular secretory component-binding IgA1 [11].

The systemic nature of IgA nephropathy also brings into perspective the almost identical immunopathologic features of Henoch-Schönlein purpura (HSP) and begs the question as to whether these conditions are separate entities. Historically, HSP is a much older disease than IgA nephropathy. It is a clinical syndrome readily recognized because of the overt purpura, arthritis, gastrointestinal manifestations, and glomerulonephritis. Like IgA nephropathy, definition of the immunopathology awaited the advent of immunofluorescence of skin [12] and other organs including the glomerular mesangium where IgA deposits are abundant. In HSP, IgA-containing immune complexes are present in the circulation [7, 13, 14], their concentration being related to disease activity, similar aberrations exist in the control of IgA production, there are primary and secondary forms, and the disease recurs in renal transplants. While the clinical features, incidence, and age of onset tend to vary from IgA nephropathy, the many similarities between these conditions suggest strongly that they represent a spectrum of the same systemic disease.

The following chapters cite in more detail important developments in the history of IgA nephropathy, introduce current concepts of pathogenesis, treatment and natural history, and look toward areas that, in the future, may provide the clues needed to solve the mysteries of this most interesting syndrome.

NOMENCLATURE

In this book, the term *IgA nephropathy* is used. It should be recognized that it is a term of convenience and not descriptive. It does not take into account the systemic nature of the disease or the division into primary and secondary forms, nor does it encompass Henoch-Schönlein purpura. It is a term hallowed by common usage, but other alternatives are also frequently found. These include "IgA mesangial nephropathy/glomerulonephritis," "mesangial IgA disease," and "Berger's disease." In like manner, "Henoch-Schönlein purpura" and "Schönlein-Henoch purpura" are used interchangeably with "anaphylactoid purpura," which is a misnomer. In the future, it is hoped that a name will evolve that suitably covers most aspects of the disease.

CLASSIFICATION

IgA nephropathy has a clear association with other disease states, particularly those affecting mucosal surfaces and those where there is a demonstrable immunoglobulin response of the IgA glass. These associations are discussed in chapter 5. Their recognition has enabled the disease to be classified into primary and secondary forms (table 1-1) [15] and emphasizes the clues provided by the associated conditions pointing to potential pathogenetic mechanisms in the primary disease. The decision to include HSP in this classification is perhaps controversial. In a recent review of 91 children in France, Levy et al. [16] chose to split rather than lump the conditions on the basis of their clear clinical differences. We believe, however, that there is more to be gained by studying the numerous similarities and hence have included HSP in this classification. Analysis of our own series of adult

Table 1-1. Classification of the IgA nephropathies

Primary
Isolated or primary IgA nephropathy
Associated with systemic disease: Henoch-Schönlein purpura
Secondary
Alcoholic liver disease
Portal systemic shunts
Celiac disease
Dermatitis herpetiformis
IgA monoclonal gammopathy
Mycosis fungoides
Mucin-secreting and other carcinomas
Leprosy
Pulmonary hemosiderosis
Ankylosing spondylitis and other seronegative spondylarthropathies
Cyclical neutropenia

patients with HSP suggests strongly that primary and secondary forms exist; that pathogenetic factors, immunopathology, natural history, and prognostic factors are extraordinarily similar; and that, like primary IgA nephropathy, the disease recurs in renal transplants. These features are discussed in more detail in chapter 4.

GEOGRAPHIC DISTRIBUTION

After the French, Japanese and Australian nephrologists soon recognized the high frequency and importance of IgA nephropathy, and more recently other Western European and South-East Asian workers have followed suit. Surprisingly, the incidence seems low in North America and the UK although, on the basis of recent reports [17–19], there are pockets in these countries where the frequency approaches 20% of biopsy series. In many countries, IgA nephropathy is the single most common type of primary glomerulonephritis (table 1-2) (reviewed in D'Amico et al. [20] and D'Amico [21]). In France, Italy, Spain, Finland, Singapore, and Australia, the prevalence ranges from 20–25% whereas in Japan it is even higher—30–40%. While the different incidences may reflect real variations in disease occurrence, they may equally be related to differing biopsy policies and use of immunofluorescence examination of biopsy material. In Australia, where the population is heterogeneous and includes many immigrants from Third World countries, all racial groups are affected, although the incidence in Australian Aborigines seems low. It would seem from this evidence that the disease may also be common in underdeveloped countries.

The actual incidence of disease may be even higher than the 20–30% of biopsy populations. IgA nephropathy in many instances is an indolent, slowly progressive disease that may not be manifest clinically until renal failure and/or hypertension develops. Even then, the true renal nature of the problem may remain unrecognized. Moreover, many patients may never come to medical attention unless urinary abnormalities are specifically

Table 1-2. Incidence of IgA nephropathy in biopsy populations in different geographic areas

	No. of patients	% of all biopsied pts with IF	% of all biopsied pts with primary GN
France			
De Werra et al. 1973 [27]	96	—	—
Levy et al. 1972 [28]	36	—	12
Droz 1976 [29]	182	—	22
Simon et al. 1984 [23]	192	—	30.2
Levy et al. 1985 [16]	91	—	12
Italy			
D'Amico et al. 1985 [20]	374	—	23
Mandreoli et al. 1981 [30]	93	15.9	—
Spain			
Egido et al. 1981 [31]	80	—	24
Covarsi et al. 1981 [32]	34	11	17
Guttierez-Millet et al. 1982 [33]	40	—	17
Scandinavia			
Schmekel et al. 1981 [34]	29	7.2	—
Mustonen et al. 1981 [8]	40	14	24
Pettersson et al. 1984 [24]	171	40.9	58.8
The Netherlands			
Van der Peet et al. [35]	27	5	—
Beukhof et al. 1984 [36]	64	—	—
Germany			
Gartner et al. 1979 [25]	153	—	—
Rambausek et al. 1983 [26]	50	—	20
Australia			
Royal Adelaide Hospital series	350	17.5	23.3
Nicholls et al. 1984 [35] [37]	244	—	—
Japan			
Ueda, et al. 1977 [38]	85	28	—
Yokoska et al. 1978 [39]	85	—	30
Nakamoto et al. 1978 [40]	205	—	40
Shirai et al. 1978 [41]	100	35	40
Sakai et al. 1979 [42]	130	—	—
Hiki et al. 1982 [43]	223	—	43
Shigematsu et al. 1982 [44]	65	—	—
Singapore			
Sinniah et al. 1981 [45]	239	33.7	—
Hong Kong			
Ng et al. 1981 [46]	44	—	8
UK			
Sissons et al. 1975 [47]	25	4	—
Davison 1983 [48] (M.R.C. GN study)	229	—	7.9
Power et al. 1985 [19]	26	14.1	21.8
USA			
McCoy et al. 1974 [49]	20	4.3	—
Burkholder et al. 1979 [50]	54	5.0	—
Hood et al. 1981 [51]	37	4.6	—
Lee et al. 1982 [52]	20	1.5	—
SPNSG 1982 [17]	62	—	—
Wyatt et al. 1984 [18]	82	—	—

After D'Amico [16].

sought. Three studies bear strongly on this point. In 200 consecutive autopsies on otherwise healthy victims of trauma in Singapore, Sinniah [22] found mesangial IgA deposits in eight (4%). An epidemiologic survey in France, where routine urinalysis occurs in school and other medical examinations, revealed a high incidence (0.1%) in a confined population [23]. In Finland, where military conscription is compulsory, a similarly high incidence was encountered [24]. We have seen 350 patients with IgA nephropathy over ten years from a draining population of approximately 400,000. Thus an incidence of 1 in 1000 population as seen in France, Finland, and Singapore would also seem to apply to Australia.

SUMMARY

Knowledge concerning IgA nephropathy has expanded greatly in the last 20 years, and its importance as the major form of glomerulonephritis, at least in the Western World, is becoming increasingly apparent. Whether it represents a unified syndrome or simply a marker for many different disease processes remains debatable. With increasing knowledge of the immunobiology of IgA, many of the questions raised in this book may be answered. The most urgent of these refer to finding a reliable serologic marker for the disease, its pathogenesis, and treatment.

REFERENCES

1. Berger J, Hinglais N: Les dépôts intercapillaires d'IgA-IgG. J Urol 74:694–695, 1968.
2. Berger J: IgA glomerular deposits in renal disease. Transplant Proc 1:939–944, 1969.
3. Berger J, Yaneua H, Nabarra B, Barbanel C: Recurrence of mesangial deposition of IgA after renal transplantation. Kidney Int 7:232–241, 1975.
4. Silva FG, Chanda P, Pirani CL, Hardy KA: Disappearance of glomerular IgA deposits after renal allograft transplantation. Transplantation 33:214–216, 1982.
5. Baart de la Faille-Kuyper EH, Kuitjen RH, Kooiker CJ, Wagenaar SS, Van der Zouwen P, Doorhout-Mees EJ: Occurrence of vascular IgA deposits in clinically normal skin of patients with renal disease. Kidney Int 9:424–429, 1976.
6. Thompson AJ, Chan Y-L, Woodroffe AJ, Clarkson AR, Seymour AE: Vascular IgA deposits in clinically normal skin of patients with renal disease. Pathology 12:407–413, 1980.
7. Woodroffe AJ, Gormly AA, McKenzie PE, Wootton AM, Thompson AJ, Seymour AE, Clarkson AR: Immunologic studies in IgA nephropathy. Kidney Int 18:366–374, 1980.
8. Mustonen J, Pasternack A, Helin H, Rilva A, Pentinnen K, Wager O, Harmoinen A: Circulating immune complexes, the concentration of serum IgA and the distribution of HLA antigens in IgA nephropathy. Nephron 29:170–175, 1981.
9. Coppo, R, Basolo B, Martina G, Rollino C, De Marchi M, Giacchino F, Mazzucco G, Messina M, Piccolo G: Circulating immune complexes containing IgA, IgG and IgM in patients with primary IgA nephropathy and with Henoch-Schönlein nephritis: correlation with clinical and histologic signs of activity. Clin Nephrol 18:230–239, 1982.
10. Le Savre PH, Digeon M, Bach JF: Analysis of circulating IgA and detection of immune complexes in primary IgA nephropathy. Clin Exp Immunol 48:61–69, 1982.
11. Valentijn RM, Radl, J, Haaijman JJ, Vermeer BJ, Weening JJ, Kauffmann RH, Daha MR, Vanses LA Circulating and mesangial secretory component-binding IgA_{-1} in primary IgA nephropathy. Kidney Int 26:760–766, 1984.
12. Baart de la Faille-Kuyper EH, Kater L, Kooiker CJ, Doorhovt-Mees EJ: IgA deposits in cutaneous blood vessel walls and mesangium in Henoch-Schönlein syndrome. Lancet 1:892, 1973.

13. Garcia-Fuentes M, Chantler C, Williams DG: Cryoglobulinaemia in Henoch-Schönlein purpura. Br Med J 2:163–165, 1977.
14. Kauffmann RH, Herrmann WA, Meyer CJLM, Daha MR, Van Es LA: Circulating IgA immune complexes in Henoch-Schönlein purpura: a longitudinal study of their relationship to disease activity Am J Med 68:859–864, 1980.
15. Woodroffe AJ, Clarkson AR, Seymour AE, Lomax-Smith JD: Mesangial IgA nephritis. Springer Semin Immunopathol 5:321–332, 1982.
16. Levy M, Gonzalez-Burchard G, Broyer M, Dommergues J-P, Foulard M, Sorez J-P, Habib R: Berger's disease in children: natural history and outcome. Medicine 64:157–180, 1985.
17. Southwest Pediatric Nephrology Study Group: A multicenter study of IgA nephropathy in children: report of the Southwest Pediatric Nephrology Study Group. Kidney Int 22:643–652, 1982.
18. Wyatt RJ, Julian BA, Bhathena DB, Mitchell BL, Holland NH, Malluche HH: IgA nephropathy: presentation, clinical course and prognosis in children and adults. Am J Kidney Dis 4:192–200, 1984.
19. Power DA, Muirhead N, Simpson JG, Nicholls AJ, Horne CHW, Catto GRD, Edward N: IgA nephropathy is not a rare disease in the United Kingdom. Nephron 40:180–184, 1985.
20. D'Amico G, Imbasciati E, Barbiani De Belgioioso G, Bertoli S, Fogazzi G, Ferrario F, Fellin G, Ragni A, Colosanti G, Minetti L, Ponticelli C: Idiopathic IgA mesangial nephropathy: clinical and histological study of 374 patients. Medicine 64:49–60, 1985.
21. D'Amico G: Idiopathic mesangial IgA nephropathy. In: Bertani T, Remuzzi G (eds) Glomerular injury 300 years after Morgagni. Milan: Wichtig Editore, 1983, pp 205–228.
22. Sinniah R: Occurrence of mesangial IgA and IgM deposits in a control necropsy population. J Clin Pathol 36:276–279, 1983.
23. Simon P, Ang K-S, Bavay P, Cloup C, Mignard J-P, Ramee M-P: Glomerulonephrite a immunoglobulines A: épidémiologie dans une population de 250,000 habitants. Presse Med 13:257–260, 1984.
24. Pettersson E, Von Bornsdorf M, Tornroth T, Lindholm, H: Nephritis among young Finnish men. Clin Nephrol 22:217–222, 1984.
25. De Werra P, Morel Maroger L, Leroux-Robert C, Richet G: Glomerulites à dépôts d'IgA diffus dans le mesangium: étude de 96 cas chez l'adulte. Schweiz Med Wochenschr 103:761–803, 1973.
26. Levy M, Beaufils H, Gubler MC, Habib R: Idiopathic recurrent macroscopic hematuria and mesangial IgA-IgG deposits in children (Berger's disease). Clin Nephrol 1:63–69, 1972.
27. Droz D: Natural history of primary glomerulonephritis with mesangial deposits of IgA. Contrib Nephrol 2:150–157, 1976.
28. Mandreoli M, Pasquali S, Donini V, Casanova S, Cagnoli L: Correlazioni anatomo-cliniche in corso di malatti di Berger. Nefrol Dial 1:9–20, 1981.
29. Egido J Rivera Hernandez F, Sancho J, Moreno M, Kriesler M, Hernando L: Estudio del sistema HLA y factores de riesgo para la insuffiencia renal en la glomerulonephritis mesangial IgA. Nefrologia 1:21–27, 1981.
30. Corvasi A, Flores R, Barcelo P, Santaularia JM, Ballarin J, Del Rio G: Glomerulonephritis por depositos mesangiales de IgA (enfermedad de Berger): parametros evolutivos. Nefrologia 1:1–8, 1981.
31. Guttierez Millet V, Navas Palacios JJ, Prieto C, Ruilope LM, Usera G, Barrientos A, Alcazar JM, Peres AJ, Jarillo MD, Rodicio JL: Glomerulonephritis mesangial IgA idiopatica: estudio clinico e immunopatologico de 40 casos y revision de la literatura. Nefrologia 2:21–34, 1982.
32. Schmekel B, Sualander Bucht H, Westberg G: Mesangial IgA glomerulonephritis in adults. Acta Med Scand 210:363–372, 1981.
33. Van der Peet J, Arisz L, Brentjens JRH, Marrink J, Hoedemaker PJ: The clinical course of IgA nephropathy in adults. Clin Nephrol 8:335–340, 1977.
34. Beukhof, JR, Ockhuizen T, Halie LM, Westra J, Beelen JM Donker AJM, Hoedemaker PJ, Van der Hem GK: Subentities within adult primary IgA nephropathy. Clin Nephrol 22:195–199, 1984.
35. Nicholls KM, Fairley KF, Dowling JP, Kincaid-Smith PS: The clinical course of mesangial IgA associated nephropathy in adults. Q J Med 210:227–250, 1984.
36. Ueda Y, Sakai O, Yamagata M, Kitajima T, Kowamwa K: IgA glomerulonephritis in Japan. Contrib Nephrol 4:36–47, 1977.

37. Yokosuka H, Nagase M, Maeda T, Koide K: Mesangial IgA glomerulonephritis: clinicopathological study of 85 cases. Contrib Nephrol 9:111–119, 1978.
38. Nakamoto Y, Asano Y, Dohi K, Fujioka M, Iida H, Kibe Y, Hattori N, Takeuchi J: Primary IgA glomerulonephritis and Schönlein-Henoch purpura nephritis: clinicopathological and immuno-histological characteristics. Q J Med 47:495–516, 1978.
39. Shirai T, Tomino Y, Sato M: IgA nephropathy: clinicopathology and immunopathology. Contrib Nephrol 9:88–100, 1978.
40. Sakai O, Kitajima T, Kawamura K, Ueda Y: Clinicopathological studies on IgA glomerulonephritis In: Yoshitosi Y, Veda Y (eds) Glomerulonephritis. Baltimore: University Park Press, 1979, p 167.
41. Hiki Y, Kobayashi Y, Tateno S, Sada M, Kashiwagi IM: Strong association of HLA-DR4 with benign nephropathy. Nephron 32:222–226, 1982.
42. Shigematsu H, Kobayashi Y, Tateno S, Hiki Y, Kuwao S: Ultra-structural glomerular loop abnormalities in IgA nephritis. Nephron 30:1–7, 1982.
43. Sinniah R, Javier AR, Ku G: The pathology of IgA nephritis with clinical correlation. Histopathology 5:469–490, 1981.
44. Ng WL, Chan CW, Yeung CK, Hua SP: The pathology of primary IgA glomerulonephritis: a renal biopsy study. Pathology 13:137–143, 1981.
45. Sissons JGP, Woodrow DF, Curtis JR: Isolated glomerulonephritis with mesangial IgA deposits. Br Med J 3:611–614, 1975.
46. Davison AM: Data from MRC registry of glomerulonephritis. Personal communication 1983.
47. McCoy RC, Abramowsky CR, Tisher CC: IgA nephropathy. Am J Pathol 76:123–140, 1974.
48. Burkholder PM, Zimmermann SW, Moorthy AV: A clinicopathologic study of the natural history of mesangial IgA nephropathy. In: Yoshitosi Y, Veda Y (eds) Glomerulonephritis. Baltimore: University Park Press, 1979, p 143.
49. Hood SS, Velosa JA, Holley KE, Donadio JV: IgA-IgG nephropathy: predictive indices of progressive disease. Clin Nephrol 16:55–62, 1981.
50. Lee SMK, Rao VM, Franklin WA, Schiffer MS, Aronson AJ, Spargo BH, Katz AI: IgA nephropathy: morphologic predictors of progressive renal disease. Hum Pathol 13:314–322, 1982.

2. CLINICAL AND LABORATORY FEATURES OF IgA NEPHROPATHY

ANTHONY R. CLARKSON

CLINICAL FEATURES

Most clinical features of IgA nephropathy point to a renal problem although it is important to recognize that, on occasions, systemic features may be sufficiently severe to mask a renal presentation. From the nephrologic point of view, the features are diverse. Patients with biopsy-proved IgA nephropathy have been presented to medical attention with nephrotic syndrome, acute nephritis, acute renal failure, malignant hypertension, and chronic renal failure as well as the more frequent recurrent "synpharyngitic" macroscopic hematuria and asymptomatic microscopic hematuria and proteinuria. In our experience, the only reliable symptom pointing to the diagnosis is "synpharyngitic" hematuria although it is pertinent that other forms of glomerulonephritis may behave similarly.

"SYNPHARYNGITIC" HEMATURIA

The passage of bloody urine closely related in time to the development of pharyngitis or tonsillitis has led to use of the term *synpharyngitic* hematuria. In approximately one-third of patients with IgA nephropathy, this will be the presenting feature. Careful history-taking frequently reveals previous episodes and some patients may suffer numerous such attacks during their lifetime. Less frequently, such hematuria will accompany infections of other mucosal surfaces, e.g., pneumonia, gastroenteritis, and urinary tract infections. The hematuria is painless, but often is associated with systemic symptoms such as fever, malaise, fatigue, diffuse muscle aches, and abdominal [1], and loin pain [2]. The macroscopic hematuria frequently lasts for less than one day, but longer episodes (5–7 days) are not unusual.

Resolution usually coincides with disappearance of systemic symptoms and defervescence of the fever. IgA nephropathy is the commonest cause of macroscopic hematuria in children and young adults, but differentiation from other causes is important. In exercise-induced hematuria, the close relationship between onset and vigorous exercise is typical, as is the lack of other physical symptoms. Postinfectious glomerulonephritis causes hematuria some 7–14 days after the infection and usually is accompanied by edema, hypertension, and oliguria. Moreover, the urine in this condition is more commonly smoky grey or dark rather than deep red as in IgA nephropathy. Hereditary nephritis and mesangiocapillary (membranoproliferative) glomerulonephritis may give rise to recurrent macroscopic hematuria, but clinical features help in diagnosis. In the middle-aged and elderly, occurrence of macroscopic hematuria raises the suspicion of urinary tract malignancy although at least in our community it is by no means rare for IgA nephropathy to present in this manner at this age.

Of paramount importance in differential diagnosis of macroscopic hematuria is the examination of the centrifuged urinary sediment by conventional and phase-contrast microscopy. Dysmorphic red blood cells of glomerular origin, granular, and red cell casts typical of a nephritic sediment are not seen in macroscopic hematuria from other causes. Such a simple examination frequently will preclude unnecessary radiographic and urologic investigations, the appropriate next step in most cases being diagnostic renal biopsy.

Macroscopic hematuria was thought initially to be the presenting symptom in the majority of patients with IgA nephropathy. As the disease became more widely studied, however, other presenting features were recognized. Thus, in our series of over 300 patients, only 30–35% of patients presented with obvious urinary blood loss and it occurred subsequently in 10–15% of others.

An equivalent number of patients (30–35%) present for investigation of asymptomatic proteinuria usually accompanied by microscopic hematuria. This observation is commonly made at a routine physical examination as part of a military, superannuation, life insurance, or prework medical examination. The presence of glomerulonephritis in these patients may further be suspected if hypertension is found. Proteinuria and hematuria persist in the majority of cases and certainly are present between episodes of macroscopic hematuria. The reasons why so many patients never suffer macroscopic blood loss are not known. Recognition of this is pertinent to any discussion of the natural history of IgA nephropathy. Accurate timing of disease onset is important in analysis and it is clear in many instances that this is not possible. Dating onset from the first episode of macroscopic hematuria is usual, but it seems likely that many such patients have previously had undetected asymptomatic proteinuria and microscopic hematuria.

The remaining patients present with a variety of symptom complexes. As mentioned previously, it is most unusual for features of the acute nephritic syndrome to be present in IgA nephropathy patients. Very occasionally, however, edema, hypertension, hematuria, and oliguria are present, often with evidence of renal impairment. As a rule, patients with acute exacerbations are not unduly hypertensive and this feature, together with the "synpharyngitic" nature of the hematuria, serves to distinguish the problem from postinfectious glomerulonephritis.

Nephrotic syndrome is seen in two distinct circumstances. In the first, excessive proteinuria results from advanced glomerular disease and, as such, is seen in the context of hypertension and advancing renal failure [3, 4]. In the second, nephrotic syndrome occurs with normal renal function, normotension, and changes in glomeruli similar to those seen in minimal-change nephropathy with the exception of diffuse mesangial proliferation associated with IgA deposits. Whether this represents a distinct subset of IgA nephropathy [5] or the coincidental occurrence of two common diseases is unknown. In these patients, the nephrotic syndrome is reversible, as in minimal-change nephropathy, with corticosteroid therapy.

Increased experience with renal biopsy in patients with advanced renal failure has demonstrated that a significant number of patients with IgA nephropathy will present for the first occasion at this stage. Accompanying severe (and often malignant) hypertension is a feature. Hypertension is such a frequent development in patients with IgA nephropathy that it is surprising more patients do no present at an earlier stage for investigation of hypertension. Routine urinalysis in hypertensive patients is essential for these reasons.

Our original observation [3] that acute reversible renal failure requiring dialysis is a striking presenting feature in 2–3% of patients with IgA nephropathy has recently been confirmed by others [6]. Unlike patients with acute renal failure where trauma, sepsis, or shock are encountered as precipitating factors, no such prodromal events are evident. Save for the presence of macroscopic hematuria, these patients often appear surprisingly healthy considering the absence of renal function. The reasons why acute renal failure occurs in some patients are unknown.

Temporary decrease in renal function is commonly found during exacerbations of "synpharyngitic" hematuria so the finding of a few patients who require dialysis is perhaps not entirely unexpected. Fortunately, these episodes of acute renal failure are reversible with supportive dialytic therapy.

IgA nephropathy may occur in the context of other diseases. In alcoholic cirrhosis, proteinuria and hematuria may be due to a variety of glomerular lesions, the most frequent of which in Australia is mesangial IgA glomerulonephritis. The renal disease tends to be more severe in those patients with portal hypertension although this is by no means an invariable association. In celiac disease, dermatitis herpetiformis, internal malignancies, mycosis fungoides, and in other conditions where IgA nephropathy is thought to be a secondary phenomenon, the renal disease is mild and rarely is a significant factor in the clinical course of the patient. Glomerular disease occurring in the context of seronegative spondylarthropathies is likely to be IgA nephropathy and, in our experience, exacerbates when the arthritis is active and may be progressive.

Unlike systemic lupus erythematosus, there are very few associated clinical features in IgA nephropathy that are of diagnostic importance.

A Japanese group [7] has drawn attention to the association with episcleritis, but this is infrequent. They report up to 8% of patients in their series who have episcleritis in which there are abundant IgA-bearing lymphocytes within the inflammatory focus. Until this report was received, we believed the occurrence in two of our patients was coincidental.

LABORATORY FINDINGS

The importance to the evolution of understanding in systemic lupus erythematosus of discovering the L.E. cell and subsequent evolution of antinuclear antibody and DNA-binding tests cannot be underestimated. In allowing clearer diagnosis, these tests have widened the clinical definition of the disease, provided insight into exacerbations and remissions, and, therefore, natural history, and given the clinician tools whereby therapy may be monitored. There is no such specific serologic test for IgA nephropathy. Positive mesangial immunofluorescence for IgA as the predominant immunoglobulin is the diagnostic hallmark and requires renal biopsy.

Serum concentrations of IgA are elevated in approximately 50% of patients [3, 8, 9]. Intensive recent investigations have been carried out to determine the nature, cause, and specificity of this rise. In particular, effort has concentrated on presence or absence of IgA containing immune complexes, ratios of polymeric to monomeric IgA, IgA1, and IgA2 subclasses, and regulation of IgA production. These topics are discussed in more detail in later chapters; suffice to mention at this juncture that none of this effort has resulted in a specific-sensitive easily reproducible serologic test.

Serum complement components C1q, C2-9 are uniformly normal or elevated as are factor-B properdin, B1H, C3b INA, and C1 esterase inhibitor. Detailed studies indicate the presence occasionally in families of partial deficiencies in single complement components. In these families, it is unclear whether the partial deficiency plays a part in the etiology of IgA nephropathy or is a coincidental finding. In addition to IgA, C3, properdin [10–12], and β1H [13, 14] have been demonstrated in mesangial deposits, suggesting that local activation of the alternative complement pathway occurs. There is also some evidence at least in some patients that the classic pathway may be activated within the mesangium. Miyazaki et al. [14] found mesangial C4-binding protein in 60% of biopsies and C4 in 30% together with elevated serum C4-binding protein concentrations. Despite these observations, there is no specific complement abnormality in IgA nephropathy.

IgA containing immune complexes have been found in the circulation by many workers using a variety of techniques [15–30]. Initially, work in this area was hampered by the lack of specificity for IgA-containing complexes of tests using C1q binding as a basis of detecting IgG-containing complexes. Using a solid-phase C1q assay, Woodroffe et al. [30] were probably the first to demonstrate immune complexes (ICs) by virtue of their IgG content, but it is pertinent that examination of cryoglobulins by Garcia-Fuentes et al. [31] in Henoch-Schönlein purpura had already pointed to this possibility. Recently, assays have become more specific; Raji cell IgA inhibition and conglutinin assays have been utilized to follow the course of disease and treatment. Their use has confirmed reports of raised serum IgA/IC concentrations in the active phase of disease. Perhaps one of the most important clues pointing to a role of IgA-ICs in the pathogenesis of IgA nephropathy is the observation by Le Savre et al. [22] that ICs return in the serum at the time of recurrence of disease in grafts.

The circulating immune complexes contain IgG and IgM in addition to IgA and are intermediate in size [22, 30]. Recent work has detected IgA1-dominant IC phagocytosed by peripheral blood polymorphonuclear leukocytes in IgA nephropathy [28], and studies by Valentijn et al. [32] have confirmed similarity between the circulating macromolecular IgA1 complexes and the mesangial deposits. It is possible that future diagnostic serologic tests may evolve from further elucidating the properties of these complexes.

REFERENCES

1. Walshe JJ, Brentjens JR, Costa GG, Andres GA, Venuto RC: Abdominal pain associated with IgA nephropathy. Am J Med 77:765–767, 1984.
2. MacDonald IM, Fairley KF, Hobbs JB, Kincaid-Smith P: Loin pain as a presenting symptom in idiopathic glomerulonephritis. Clin Nephrol 3:129–133, 1975.
3. Clarkson AR, Seymour AE, Thompson AJ, Haynes WDG, Chan Y-L, Jackson B: IgA nephropathy: a syndrome of uniform morphology, diverse clinical features and uncertain prognosis. Clin Nephrol 8:459–471, 1977.
4. Katz A, Walker JF, Landy PJ: IgA nephritis with nephrotic range proteinuria. Clin Nephrol 20:67–71, 1983.
5. Mustonen J, Pasternack A, Rantala I: The nephrotic syndrome in IgA glomerulonephritis: response to cortico-steroid therapy. Clin Nephrol 20:172–176, 1983.
6. Kincaid-Smith P, Bennett WM, Dowling JP, Ryan GB. Acute renal failure and tubular necrosis associated with haematuria due to glomerulonephritis. Clin Nephrol 19:206–210, 1983.

7. Nomoto Y, Sakai H, Endoh M, Tomino Y: Scleritis and IgA nephropathy. Arch Intern Med 140:783–785, 1980.
8. Lagrue G, Hirbec G, Foornel M, Intrator L: Glomerulonephrite mesangial à dépôts d'IgA: étude des immunoglobulines sérique. J Urol Nephrol (Paris) 80:385–386, 1973.
9. D'Amico G: Idiopathic mesangial IgA nephropathy: In: Bertani T, Remuzzi G (eds) Glomerular injury 300 years after Morgagni. Milan: Wichtig Editore, 1983, pp 205–228.
10. Roy LP, Fish AJ, Vernier RL: Recurrent macroscopic haematuria, focal nephritis and mesangial deposition of immunoglobulin and complement. J Pediat 82:767–774, 1973.
11. Roy LP: Properdin and recurrent macroscopic haematuria. Aust NZJ Med 5:191–194, 1975.
12. Evans DJ, Williams DG, Peters DK, Sissons JGP, Boulton-Jones JM, Ogg CS, Cameron JS, Hoffbrand BI: Glomerular deposition of properdin in Henoch-Schönlein syndrome and idiopathic focal nephritis. Br Med J 3:326–328, 1973.
13. Julian BA, Wyatt RJ, McMorrow RG, Galla JH. Serum complement proteins in IgA nephropathy. Clin Nephrol 20:251–258, 1983.
14. Miyazaki R, Kurda M, Akiyama T, Otani I, Tofuku Y, Takena R: Glomerular deposition and serum levels of complement control proteins in patients with IgA nephropathy. Clin Nephrol 21:335–340, 1984.
15. Coppo R, Basolo B, Martina G, Rollino C, De Marchi M, Giacchino F, Mazzucco G, Messina M, Piccolo G: Circulating immune complexes containing IgA, IgG and IgM in patients with primary IgA nephropathy and with Henoch-Schönlein nephritis: correlation with clinical and histologic signs of activity. Clin Nephrol 18:230–239, 1982.
16. Danielsen H, Eriksen EF, Johansen A, Sølling J: Serum immunoglobulin sedimentation patterns and circulating immune complexes in IgA glomerulonephritis and Schönlein-Henoch nephritis. Acta Med Scand 215:435–438, 1984.
17. Doi T, Kanatsu K, Sekita K, Yoshida H, Nagai H, Hamashima Y: Circulating immune complexes of IgG, IgA and IgM classes in various glomerular diseases. Nephron 32:335–341, 1982.
18. Doi T, Kanatsu K, Sekita K, Yoshida A, Nagai H, Hamashima Y: Detection of IgA-class circulating immune complexes bound to anti-C_3d antibodies in patients with IgA nephropathy. J Immunol Methods 69:95–104, 1984.
19. Egido J, Sancho J, Rivera F, Hernando L: The role of IgA and IgG immune complexes in IgA nephropathy. Nephron 36:52–59, 1984.
20. Gluckman JC, Jacob N, Beaufils H, Baumelau A, Salah H, German A, Legrain M: Clinical significance of circulating immune complexes: detection in chronic glomerulonephritis. Nephron 22:138–145, 1978.
21. Hall RP, Stachura I, Cason J, Whiteside TL, Lawley TJ: IgA containing circulating immune complexes in patients with IgA nephropathy. Am J Med 74:56–63, 1983.
22. Le Savre PH, Digeon M, Bach JF: Analysis of circulating IgA and detection of immune complexes in primary IgA nephropathy. Clin Exp Immunol 48:61–69, 1982.
23. Mustonen J, Pasternack A, Helin H, Rilva A, Penttinen K, Wager O, Harmoinen A: Circulating immune complexes, the concentration of serum IgA and the distribution of HLA antigens in IgA nephropathy. Nephron 29:170–175, 1981.
24. Nagy J, Fust G, Ambrus M, Trinn C, Paal M, Burger T: Circulating immune complexes in patients with IgA glomerulonephritis. Acta Med Acad Sci Hung 39:211–218, 1982.
25. Ooi YM, Ooi BS, Pollak VE: Relationship of levels of circulating immune complexes to histologic patterns of nephritis. J Lab Clin Med 90:891–898, 1977.
26. Sancho J, Egido J, Rivera F, Hernando L: Immune complexes in IgA nephropathy: presence of antibodies against diet antigens and delayed clearance of specific polymeric immune complexes. Clin Exp Immunol 54:194–202, 1983.
27. Tomino Y, Sakai H, Endoh M, Kaneshige H, Nomoto Y: Detection of immune complexes in polymorphonuclear leukocytes by double immunofluorescence in patients with IgA nephropathy. Clin Immunol Immunopathol 24:63–71, 1982.
28. Tomino Y, Miura M, Suga T, Endoh M, Nomoto Y, Sakai H: Detection of IgA_1 dominant immune complexes in peripheral blood polymorphonuclear leukocytes by double immunofluorescence in patients with IgA nephropathy. Nephron 37:137–139, 1984.
29. Valentijn RM, Kauffmann RH, Riviere GB, Daha MR, Van Es L: Presence of circulating macromolecular IgA in patients with haematuria due to primary IgA nephropathy. Am J Med 74:375–381, 1983.

30. Woodroffe AJ, Gormly AA, McKenzie PE, Wootton AM, Thompson AJ, Seymour AE, Clarkson AR: Immunologic studies in IgA nephropathy. Kidney Int 18:366–374, 1980.
31. Garcia-Fuentes M, Chantler C, Williams DG: Cryoglobulinemia in Henoch-Schönlein purpura. Br Med J 2:163–165, 1977.
32. Valentijn RM, Radi J, Haaijman JJ, Vermeer BV, Weening JJ, Kauffmann RH, Daha MR, Van Es LA: Circulating and mesangial secretory component binding IgA-1 in primary IgA nephropathy. Kidney Int 26:760–766, 1984.

3. IgA NEPHROPATHY IN CHILDREN

RONALD J. HOGG and FRED G. SILVA

Reports of IgA nephropathy in children were relatively uncommon prior to 1980 with only one center reporting more than ten patients [1]. The situation has changed dramatically since that time, however, with at least one large pediatric series (and usually more) being reported in each of the last six years. These reports have shown that IgA nephropathy is a very common form of glomerular disease in Japan [26], where it is most often diagnosed following routine urinalysis. Although the disorder appears to be diagnosed less frequently in other parts of the world, there are now many reports implicating IgA nephropathy as an important cause of childhood renal disease in Australia [7, 8], Europe [9–18], and the United States [19–30].

In recent years, there has also been an increasing level of recognition that IgA nephropathy beginning in childhood is not always a benign disorder [5, 10, 12, 29]. Furthermore, it has been pointed out by Croker et al. [31], based on their careful analysis of 81 patients with IgA nephropathy, that this condition "is an indolent disease generally beginning in childhood." This concept, together with the demonstration by Hall et al. [32] that IgA-containing circulating immune complexes are more prevalent in the early stages of the disease, suggests that the initial immunologic insult to the glomerulus occurs most frequently in childhood and adolescence. The corollary to this concept is that therapeutic intervention (if successful therapy were available)—before the phase of glomerular sclerosis and unrelenting progression of glomerular ablation—should probably be attempted during childhood. It is therefore important to evaluate the clinical, serologic, and pathologic features of IgA nephropathy in children and adolescents. It will be even more important to trace into adult life the subsequent course of the patients so identified.

INTERPRETATION OF PEDIATRIC STUDIES OF IgA NEPHROPATHY

It is relevant to note from the outset that indications for performing renal biopsies in children with hematuria or proteinuria vary between countries, between cities, and even between individual nephrologists. Furthermore, the frequency of renal biopsies performed in children with clinical evidence of glomerular disease has tended to decline over the last ten years [33]. This "selection factor" is preeminent in determining the overall frequency of almost every clinical and pathologic feature that is discussed in the sections that follow.

FREQUENCY OF IgA NEPHROPATHY IN CHILDREN WITH HEMATURIA

There have been a number of studies evaluating the overall frequency of IgA nephropathy in children with hematuria [5, 29, 30, 34–37]. Some recent insight into the question was provided by Piel et al. [34] in their report of renal biopsy findings in 61 children with unexplained hematuria. These authors indicated that findings characteristic of IgA nephropathy were present in 18 (30%) of the biopsies. Of these 18 children, 12 had episodes of gross hematuria (five with fever or physical activity and seven without any associated event). In a similar study [35], the International Study of Kidney Disease in Children reported that IgA nephropathy occurred in 12 (16%) of 75 children who were biopsied because of recurrent or persistent hematuria. These children had no family history of nephritis. It was noted that focal global or segmental glomerular sclerosis was present in the biopsies of ten, and tubular atrophy in nine, of these children. When taken together, these two studies showed the presence of IgA nephropathy in approximately 22% (30 out of 136) of the children with hematuria who were studied. This figure is remarkably similar to the worldwide frequency of IgA nephropathy in patients with primary glomerular diseases that has been estimated as 20%.

Epidemiologic surveys of children with hematuria and/or proteinuria conducted in Japan suggest that IgA nephropathy accounts for a similar percentage of primary glomerulopathies in that country. Kitajima et al. [5] conducted a survey of 26 departments of pediatrics and found IgA nephropathy in 19.2% of children with primary glomerular disease. Most of the patients were detected by "chance" proteinuria and/or hematuria. In another Japanese survey [36], IgA nephropathy was found in 33.3% of children (46 of 138) presenting with "chance" proteinuria and/or hematuria. It is noteworthy that this high figure was still considerably less than the frequency of IgA nephropathy found in adults in the same study (62.9%). It is of interest that, prior to the description of IgA nephropathy by Berger, a relatively high frequency of the biopsies performed in children with recurrent hematuria revealed focal glomerulonephritis [38, 39].

STUDIES OF IMMUNOREGULATION IN CHILDREN WITH IgA NEPHROPATHY

Although there have been numerous adult patient protocols designed to unravel the pathogenesis of this disorder, there have been very few reports of similar studies in children. As discussed in chapter 12, the balance of evidence in the adult series favors the concept that a disorder of immunoregulation exists in which peripheral lymphocyte immunoglobulin production is abnormal, with excess IgA production being present. In a recent study oriented primarily toward children and young adults with IgA nephropathy, however, Linne and Wasserman [40] studied peripheral lymphocyte subpopulations and immunoglobulin production following pokeweed antigen stimulation during an infection-free period. This study, which differed from most previous reports in that the "infection state" of the patients was well defined, revealed that there was no significant disturbance in stimulated immunoglobulin production during infection-free periods in these patients.

CLINICAL FEATURES

Children with IgA nephropathy may show many diverse clinical features, and the relative frequency of each often differs from that seen in adults. This variance with adult series is observed in both the mode of presentation and in the subsequent clinical course. The most striking difference concerns the higher frequency of episodes of gross hematuria that is observed in pediatric centers—at least those outside Japan. In this regard, we have summarized pertinent clinical features described in all pediatric series of IgA nephropathy that we have identified in terms of the country of origin of each series (table 3-1). It should be noted, however, that such data were only taken from series where authors identified the frequency of specific clinical features in patients less than 18 years—the age that we have used as the criterion for patient selection in this chapter. In later sections of the chapter, we consider the prognostic relevance of some of these features and their correlation with pathologic lesions found on renal biopsy.

RAPIDLY PROGRESSIVE (CRESCENTIC) IgA NEPHROPATHY IN CHILDREN

There have been a number of papers in recent years that have documented clearly a subset of patients with IgA nephropathy that have a rapidly progressive course [10, 41–43]. It is important to note that many of these patients were less than 18 years of age at the time end-stage renal disease (ESRD) supervened. In a recent review of published cases of crescentic IgA nephropathy, Abuelo et al. [42] showed that 41% of patients with this rapidly progressive form of IgA nephropathy were aged 16 years or less (range 9–16 years). In the patients observed by Abuelo personally, the percentage of such patients was even higher (60%—three of five patients).

Table 3-1. IgA nephropathy in children: clinical features at presentation

Country/ continent	Total no. Patients	Boys	Mean age	Presenting features (% total)							$\bar{x}$ Duration s/s prebiopsy (mos)
				GH	U/A	Other	GFR ↓	Prot	BP ↑	NS	
Japan [2–6]	629	61%	10.4	14.5%	74.2%	11.3%	10.4%	73%	3.7%	8%	11.5
n		629	94	629	629	629	567	594	561	629	94
Australia [7, 8]	9	78%	14.3	100%	0	0	0	0	12%	0	54
n		9	9	9	9	9	9	4	9	9	5
Europe [9–18]	160	75%	10.3	76%	19%	5%	17.9%	44%	4.3%	4.4%	22
n		157	160	160	160	160	78	101	70	160	147
USA [19–30]	216	75%	10.5	84%	16%	0	13.2%	42.8%	5.1%	5.1%	17
n		193	198	191	191	191	144	144	137	216	195
Total	1014	66%	10.5	38.6%	53.4%	8.0%	11.5%	64%	4.1%	6.7%	17.9
n		988	461	989	989	989	798	843	777	1014	441

n, number of patients from which each set of data was derived; GH, gross hematuria as presenting feature; U/A, urinary abnormality identified during routine urinalysis; Other, patient identified on basis of abnormality other than GH or U/A; GFR, decreased GFR documented during initial presentation; BP, hypertension; NS, nephrotic syndrome; and S/S, symptoms or signs of renal disease.

PATHOLOGIC FEATURES OF IgA NEPHROPATHY IN CHILDREN

The following sections, by necessity, cover only a small fraction of the pathologic features that have been described in the renal biopsies of children with IgA nephropathy. However, a comprehensive guide to references that cover each feature is given in table 3-3 [1–76].

Immunofluorescence studies

By definition, children with IgA nephropathy have either dominant or codominant IgA deposition in the glomerular mesangial regions. In most pediatric reports, IgA is present only in the glomerular mesangial regions. This is sometimes along the paramesangial regions just under the overlying glomerular basement membrane (GBM), giving an almost linear pseudocapillary wall appearance by immunofluorescence [44]. A recent report by Andreoli et al. [29], however, showed definite evidence of both glomerular mesangial and peripheral capillary wall staining for IgA in seven (41%) of 17 patients (figure 3-1). In this study, patients with peripheral glomerular capillary wall distribution of IgA had other indications of more severe glomerular disease (crescents, severe proteinuria) and a poor prognosis [29]. Kitajima et al. also described IgA deposits in glomerular capillary walls in a relatively high percentage (23.7%) of 500 children with IgA nephropathy [5]. These latter authors noted the controversy that exists with regard to the inclusion of patients with glomerular capillary wall deposits of IgA within the diagnostic entity of "IgA nephropathy." For example, in the series reported by Kogoshi et al. [3], a clear distinction was made between 14 children who had a pure mesangial pattern of IgA deposition as opposed to 14 children who had a mesangial *and* a peripheral capillary wall pattern of distribution. These authors found that patients with this latter pattern of IgA deposition were more likely to have proteinuria ≥2+ (ten of 13 vs four of 14

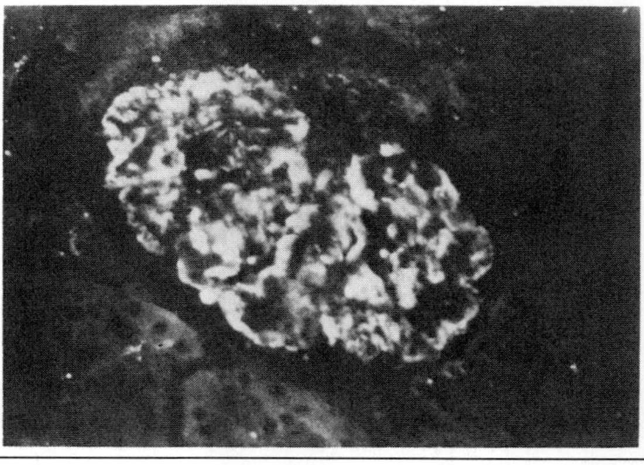

Figure 3-1. Immunofluorescence of a glomerulus showing mesangial and peripheral capillary wall staining for IgA. Immunofluorescence, anti-IgA, ×400. From Andreoli et al. [29].

in the group with mesangial IgA alone) and that "fixed low renal function" was present only in the patients with peripheral capillary wall IgA deposition (two of 13 patients). These results are very similar to the subsequent findings by Andreoli et al. [29]. Whether the copresence of glomerular peripheral capillary wall IgA deposition denotes a variant within the spectrum of Berger's description of IgA nephropathy remains to be clarified. Extra-glomerular staining for IgA has been noted rarely.

Other immunoreactants are often present in the biopsies from children with IgA nephropathy (table 3-2). In a review of the literature of pediatric cases (where the information was available and extractable), we found that 60% of biopsies showed IgG deposition, 32% showed IgM deposition, and 75% showed deposition of C3. However, it should be noted that, in a number of series, specific information regarding the frequency of individual immunoreactants was not given. For example, in the study of 500 children reported by Kitajima et al. [5], it was reported that almost 60% of the biopsies contained IgA and/or IgG and/or IgM and complement. Since specific details regarding each of these immunoreactants were not given, information from this large multicenter study could not be incorporated into table 3-2. Very few reports include data for IgE or IgD. Early complement pathway components (C1 and C4) were each present in less than 10% of biopsies studied, whereas properdin was identified in 50% of the biopsies tested. Fibrin-related antigens were also found in half of the cases. These figures are similar to those obtained in studies of IgA nephropathy in adult patients; they did not appear to differ much in frequency from country to country.

Light microscopy

In children, as in adults, deposition of IgA in the glomerular mesangium may be associated with a variety of glomerular changes by light microscopy, ranging from essentially normal glomeruli to severe proliferative and crescentic glomerulonephritis. Many classifications have evolved in order to organize the diverse types of glomerular patterns that are seen with IgA nephropathy in patients of all ages, including children. This discordance or nonuniformity in classification makes a comparative review between series very difficult, if not impossible. There are at least three basic requirements for the acceptance of a histologic classification: (a) that the classification be *clinically significant*, (b) that it be *morphologically reproducible*, and (c) that it be based on fact and, as far as possible, *scientifically correct*. That several morphological classifications have been suggested attest to the fact that no classification is yet final, perfect, or globally accepted. However, three appear to be the most commonly used in the descriptive "pigeon-holing" of the glomerular pattern in pediatric IgA nephropathy. These will now be discussed briefly.

The World Health Organization (WHO) Classification of Glomerular Disease [45] subdivided glomerular lesions in a variety of renal diseases into

Table 3-2. Immunofluorescence findings in children with IgA nephropathy

Continent/country	IgA	IgM	IgG	IgE	C3	C1	C4	FRA	Properdin
Japan[2, 3, 6]	94/94 (100%)	18/94 (19%)	36/94 (38%)	0/22 (0%)	65/94 (69%)	0/27 (0%)	1/58 (2%)	31/48 (65%)	—
Australia[7, 8]	9/9 (100%)	0/5 (0%)	4/9 (44%)	—	0/5 (0%)	—	—	2/5 (40%)	—
Europe[9–11, 14, 15, 17, 61]	76/76 (100%)	6/43 (14%)	58/67 (87%)	0/12 (0%)	62/76 (82%)	2/34 (6%)	1/25 (4%)	10/41 (25%)	6/10 (60%)
USA[20–27, 30]	167/167 (100%)	48/100 (48%)	100/162 (62%)	1/5 (20%)	126/162 (78%)	9/76 (12%)	12/77 (16%)	64/128 (50%)	28/58 (48%)
Total	346/346 (100%)	78/242 (32%)	198/332 (60%)	1/39 (2%)	253/337 (75%)	11/137 (8%)	14/160 (9%)	107/222 (48%)	34/68 (50%)

a series of basic groups. Although there is no official WHO classification of IgA nephropathy per se [46], a few authors [5, 47] have recently utilized the WHO classification of glomerular diseases to provide the following light-microscopic classification of IgA nephropathy: (WHO-A) minor glomerular lesions, (WHO-B) focal glomerulonephritis, and (WHO-C) diffuse mesangial proliferative glomerulonephritis. This modified classification was used in the large multicenter study of Japanese children reported by Kitajima et al. [5]. In this huge study of 500 children from 26 departments of pediatrics, 109 patients (22%) were in WHO-A, 137 (28%) were in WHO-B, and 239 (50%) were in WHO-C. However, other large series have used somewhat different classifications. For example, the Southwest Pediatric Nephrology Study Group (SPNSG), in their report of 82 patients from the USA [26], classified the glomerular patterns into three broad morphologic groups: (I) normal or essentially normal glomeruli (25 patients), (II) pure mesangial [focal/segmental or diffuse] hypercellularity (28 patients) (figure 3-2), and (III) focal and segmental proliferative and/or sclerosing glomerulonephritis or more severe and diffuse glomerulonephritis (with closure or effacement of glomerular capillary loops) with/without crescents (30 patients) (figure 3-3). In contrast, Levy et al. [10] separated their 91 pediatric patients into five groups: (I) minimal glomerular changes (26 patients), (II) focal and segmental glomerulonephritis (41 patients), (III) pure diffuse proliferative glomerulonephritis (three patients), and (IV) proliferative glomerulonephritis with focal (20 patients) or diffuse (V) (one patient) crescents.

It is evident from these diverse classifications that comparisons between studies are difficult to interpret. In addition, when some authors refer to "diffuse proliferative glomerulonephritis," it is often difficult to determine whether they were referring to pure mesangial hypercellularity (figure 3-2) or to a more severe, active proliferative lesion with closure of the glomerular capillary loops, necrosis, and crescent formation. Although many reports do not indicate clearly either the type of lesion that is present or its distribution pattern, we have attempted to extract from the literature the most common glomerular patterns that have been described in children with IgA nephropathy. These limitations in our attempts to extract information from the literature must be acknowledged before proceeding on to a discussion of light-microscopic findings that have been observed around the world in children with IgA nephropathy.

When the Japanese [6], Australian [7, 8], European [6, 10–12, 14, 17, 18, 48, 49] and United States [19–27] published experience of pediatric cases is collated together, it appears that about one-third of renal biopsies show a more severe active glomerulonephritis with closure of the glomerular capillary loops, necrosis, severe sclerosis, or crescent formation. When the four geographic regions are compared, there does not appear to be any major differences in the frequency of these various glomerular patterns, nor does there appear to be much difference in glomerular pattern from country to

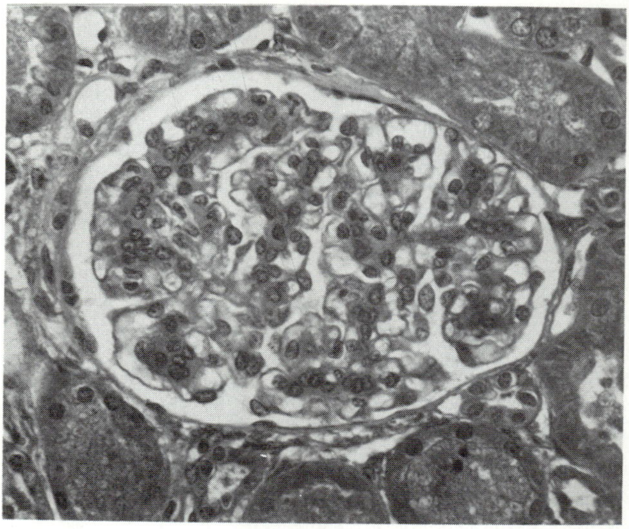

Figure 3-2. Diffuse mesangial hypercellularity in a pediatric patient with IgA nephropathy. There are more than three cells in glomerular mesangial regions away from the vascular pole in this 2- to 3-micron section. However, we do not regard this as diffuse proliferative glomerulo*nephritis* (although authors in some other series have made this interpretation).

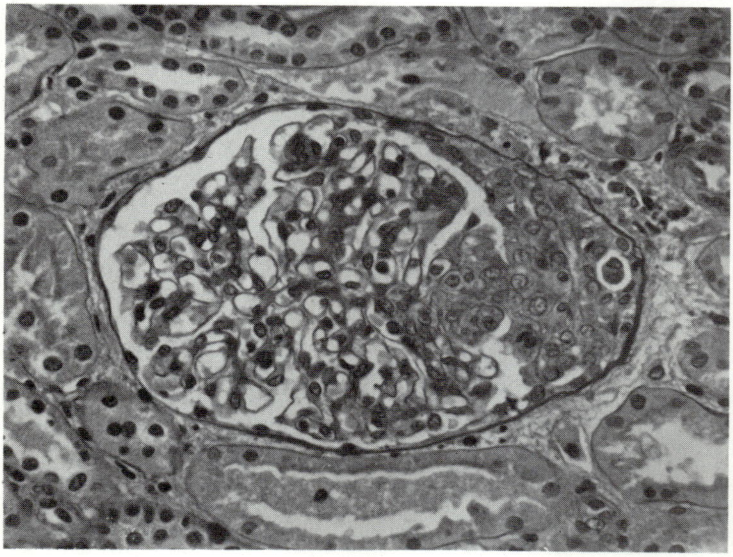

Figure 3-3. Crescentic glomerulonephritis in a pediatric patient with IgA nephropathy. The biopsy from this patient with IgA nephropathy contained several glomeruli with segmental regions of glomerular extracapillary hypercellularity (crescent formation). Periodic acid–Schiff, ×350. From SPNSG [44].

country within Europe. Although there are many different and varied selection biases in which patients come to renal biopsy (within the same institutions, much less the same region, country, or continent, as indicated before), and we therefore do not know the *true* incidence in the population, the percentage of *reported* pediatric patients with active focal segmental proliferative, necrotizing, or sclerosing glomerulonephritis seems to be present in slightly over one-half of the biopsies from European pediatric patients as a whole (with the larger German and French series having the highest frequency of severe glomerulonephritic changes), as compared with approximately 30% in Japan and the USA, and approximately 40% in Australia (the latter with a very small number of pediatric patients identified with specific information). A large number of different glomerular changes have been noted in renal biopsies from pediatric patients with IgA nephropathy, and these are listed in table 3-3. Glomerular patterns resembling, if not identical to, minimal-change glomerulonephropathy (nil disease) [26, 50–53], focal sclerosis [6, 8, 11, 26, 54], membranoproliferative (mesangiocapillary) glomerulonephritis [6, 44, 55, 56], and crescentic glomerulonephritis (as noted above) [10, 41–43, 57] have all been described. These patterns have also been seen in adults with IgA nephropathy. Other glomerular patterns, such as membranous glomerulonephropathy, though seen rarely in adults with IgA nephropathy, have not been described in children at the time of writing. In addition, "dual glomerulonephropathies" are being described in the same patient's biopsy (i.e., two different glomerular diseases in the same patient), and IgA nephropathy has been noted in a pediatric patient with diabetic glomerulosclerosis [60]. Whether IgA nephropathy (with features of nil disease) in nephrotic syndrome represents one disease or two is uncertain [50].

Tubulointerstitial changes, such as tubular atrophy, interstitial fibrosis, and inflammation, have been noted in over one-half of patients from the large pediatric series we collated (59% of 61 patients in the Japanese study [6], 53% of 115 patients in the US studies [19, 20, 22, 25, 26], and 38% of 39 patients in the European studies [11, 12, 14, 61]). Vascular disease (i.e., arterial or arteriolar sclerosis) is very unusual in the pediatric age group and has only been noted in a few renal biopsies from pediatric patients in Australia [8]. Europe [11], and the United States [24]. Vascular disease was found in less than 4% of the 80+ biopsies in which the presence or absence of vascular disease was indicated in the publications. We did not find it in our study of 83 pediatric patients [26], although Feiner et al. found it in three of 12 children in their study [24]. These vascular changes are probably much more common in adults, where they may play an important role in the progression of the renal disease [24].

Electron microscopy

Electron-microscopic studies of biopsies showing IgA nephropathy in children are not numerous, as evidenced by the fact that no information regarding electron-microscopic findings was provided in two of the three

Table 3-3. Renal pathologic changes in children with IgA nephropathy

I. Light-microscopic changes: glomerular
- Normal/essentially normal[1, 6, 11, 12, 16–18, 24, 26, 44]
- Diffuse mesangial hypercellularity only[1, 6–8, 10–12, 14, 17, 19, 20, 22–27, 44] (or mesangial hypercellularity unspecified)
- Focal/segmental mesangial hypercellularity[1, 6, 8, 10, 20, 22, 24, 26, 27, 44]
- Glomerular adhesions[12, 17, 22, 49, 61]
- Capillary wall thickening[12, 22, 25]
- Focal glomerulonephritis[1, 6, 8, 10, 11, 17, 20, 23, 24, 26, 27, 43, 44, 65, 66]
- Crescentic glomerulonephritis or presence of crescents[1, 6, 7, 10, 11, 17, 20, 24, 26, 41–44, 57, 61, 65]
- Minimal-change glomerulonephropathy[26, 50–53] (nil disease)
- Membranoproliferative (mesangiocapillary) pattern[6, 55, 56]
- Focal segmental sclerosis[6, 8, 11, 26, 54] (focal sclerosis)
- Global sclerosis[12, 19, 20, 24, 26, 44, 61]

II. Light-microscopic changes: nonglomerular
- Tubulointerstitial disease[6, 11, 12, 14, 19, 20, 22, 25, 26, 42, 44, 61, 68]
- Vascular changes[8, 11, 24, 62]

III. Electron-microscopic changes: glomerular
- Mesangial deposits[6, 8–9, 11, 16–17, 19, 24, 26, 42, 44, 51, 65, 69]
- Absence of mesangial deposits[26, 44, 69]
- Subendothelial deposits[1, 6, 10, 11, 22, 24–26, 42, 44]
- Subepithelial deposits[1, 6, 8, 10, 11, 26, 42, 44]
- Intramembranous deposits[22, 26, 44]
- Glomerular basement membrane gaps[11]
- Thinning/thickening/rarefaction/splitting of glomerular basement membrane[8, 26, 42, 44]
- Circumferential mesangial interposition[26, 44, 55]
- Myxo-virus-like microtubular structures in glomerular endothelium[26, 44]
- Widespread "fusion" or effacement of visceral epithelial cell foot processes[26, 50–53]
- Disruption of the basal lamina of Bowman's capsule[42, 57]

IV. Immunofluorescence: glomeruli
- IgA in all studies quoted (by definition)
- IgA in afferent arterioles[45, 69]
- IgM[1, 2, 6, 10, 11, 15, 17, 20–22, 25, 26, 44, 49, 51, 61, 65, 76]
- IgG[1, 2, 6–8, 10, 11, 15–18, 20–27, 44, 49, 65]
- C3[1, 2, 6, 10, 11, 15–18, 21–27, 44, 51, 61, 65, 76]
- C1[11, 20, 26, 27, 44]
- C4[6, 11, 20, 25–27, 44]
- Late C5 to C9 components[11]
- Secretory component (noted to be absent)[15]
- Properdin[11, 20, 26–27, 44]
- Fibrin-related antigens[2, 6, 7, 11, 15, 17, 20–27, 44, 65]
- Loss of IgA in repeat biopsy/transplant[56, 72–75]
- Recurrence of IgA in transplant[66]
- Immunoelectron microscopy[70]
- Absence of IgA in incidental autopsies in children[71]

Table 3-4. Electron-microscopic findings in children with IgA nephropathy

	Glomerular changes			
Continent/country	Mesangial deposits	Subendothelial deposits	Subepithelial deposits	[a]Structural changes in GBM
Japan[6]	49/51 (98%)	20/51 (40%)	15/51 (30%)	—
Australia[8]	4/4 (100%)	0/4 (0%)	2/4 (50%)	1/4 (25%)
Europe[1, 9, 11]	45/45 (100%)	15/45 (33%)	8/45 (18%)	0/10
USA[25, 26]	82/82 (100%)	11/82 (13%)	7/77 (10%)	26/77 (34%)
Total	180/182 (99%)	46/182 (25%)	32/177 (18%)	27/91 (30%)

[a]GBM structural changes, one or more of the following: thinning, thickening, splitting, rarefaction.

large series of children with IgA nephropathy (table 3-4). As in adult patients, the predominant finding in the vast majority of biopsies in children features glomerular mesangial/paramesangial discrete electron-dense "immune-type" deposits (figure 3-4). These mesangial deposits vary in electron density and size. The quantity of mesangial deposits varies from region to region, even within the same glomerulus. We have seen a few biopsies in which the enlarged mesangial regions show only severe mesangial sclerosis in some regions with no obvious osmiophilic deposits, whereas other less sclerotic mesangial regions contain identifiable discrete deposits. In our SPNSG series, we occasionally noted the *arc de cercle* or elevation of the GBM over large paramesangial deposits, but this was not a common finding [26]. Collagen was not detected in the mesangial regions.

Glomerular capillary wall electron-dense deposits have been reported infrequently in children. In the SPNSG study, we found extramesangial glomerular deposits in 14 (18%) of 77 patients (figure 3-5) [26]. These glomerular subendothelial, intramembranous, or subepithelial glomerular deposits were small, infrequent, and usually were noted near the mesangial regions. Review of the literature suggests that approximately one-fourth of pediatric patients have small subendothelial deposits and even fewer have subepithelial or intramembranous deposits.

A more common electron-microscopic finding in our experience is segmental rarefaction, thinning, and splitting of the GBM: we found this in one-third of our patients (figure 3-6) [26]. Similar findings in children have been noted by others [8, 42, 44]. This segmental glomerular capillary wall lesion does not represent hereditary nephropathy [62–64], but the etiology and relationship to clinical findings and prognosis are unclear. We have not identified discrete "immune-type" electron-dense deposits in Bowman's

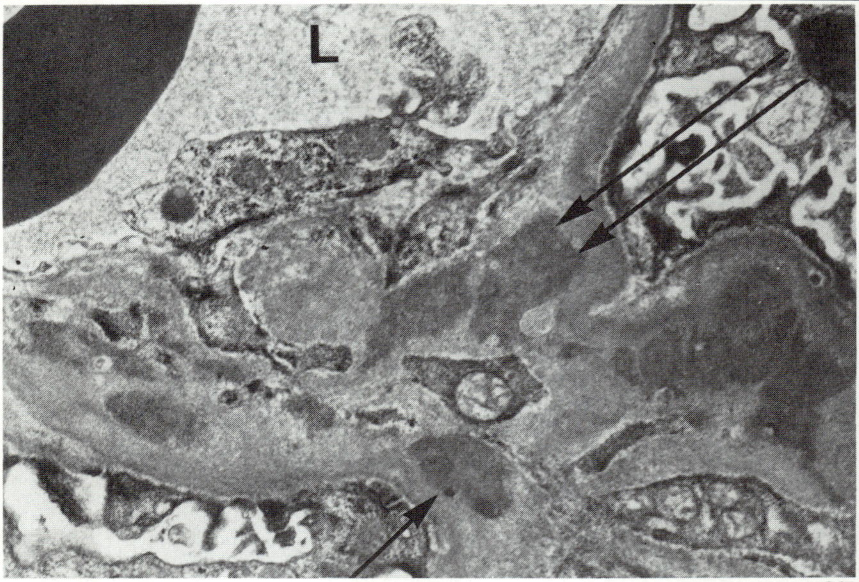

Figure 3-4. A segment of a glomerulus showing discrete electron-dense "immune-type" deposits in the mesangial region (*arrows*). Note that the mesangial deposits are not within the mesangial cells themselves per se, but instead in the nearby mesangial matrix. *L*, glomerular capillary lumen. Electron microscopy, ×20,000.

capsule or in extraglomerular sites [26]. Diffuse widespread effacement of visceral epithelial cell foot processes in conjunction with essentially normal glomeruli by light microscopy and the nephrotic syndrome (as seen in nil disease) has been noted (figure 3-7) [26, 50–53].

CLINICOPATHOLOGIC CORRELATIONS

Proteinuria

Levy et al. [1], in the first large pediatric series of patients with IgA nephropathy, documented an association between diffuse proliferation of glomeruli (seen in six children) and persistent proteinuria (in four of the six). These observations have been confirmed in a recent larger series from the same authors [10]. In the patients studied by Andreoli et al. [29] and Kogoshi et al. [3], proteinuria (>1 g/24 h or ≥2+) was associated with peripheral glomerular capillary wall IgA, and in Andreoli's series was also associated with crescentic glomerulonephritis. In the SPNSG series of patients [26, 44], a significant correlation was found between proteinuria (≥2+) and more severe glomerular lesions on light microscopy and, although not statistically significant, our group also found that peripheral GBM changes on electron microscopy (including thinning, thickening, splitting, and splintering, as

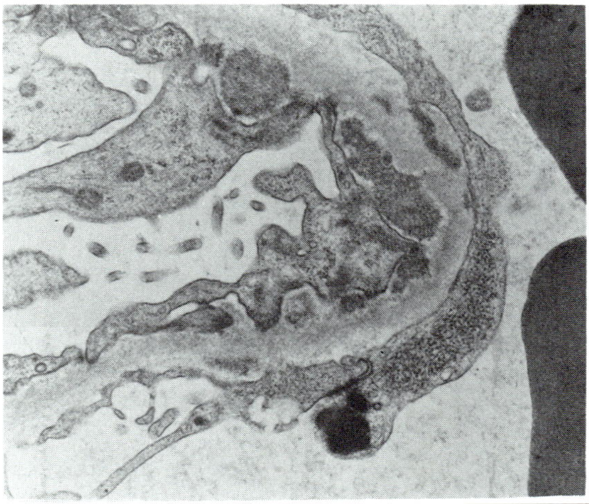

Figure 3-5. A peripheral segment of a glomerular capillary wall showing discrete "immune-type" electron-dense deposits in both subendothelial and subepithelial regions. Note that the glomerular endothelial cells contain microtubular "myxo-virus-like particles" (a feature that is frequenty seen in patients with systemic lupus erythematosus). Electron microscopy, ×18,000.

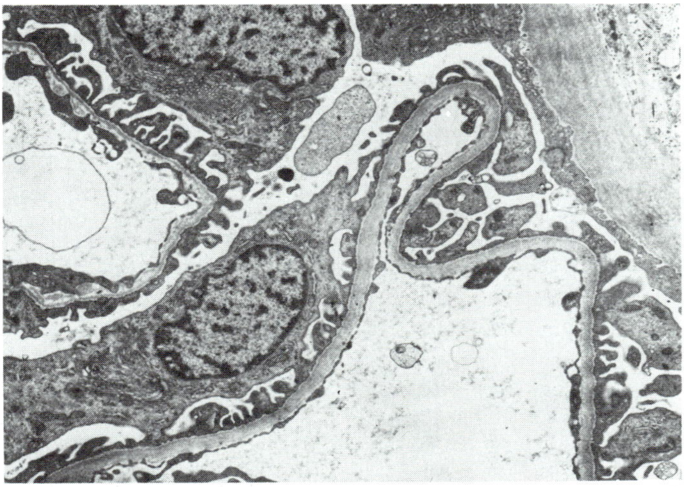

Figure 3-6. A segment of two glomerular capillaries, one of which shows extreme thinning of the glomerular basement membrane. Electron microscopy, ×6000. From SPNSG [44].

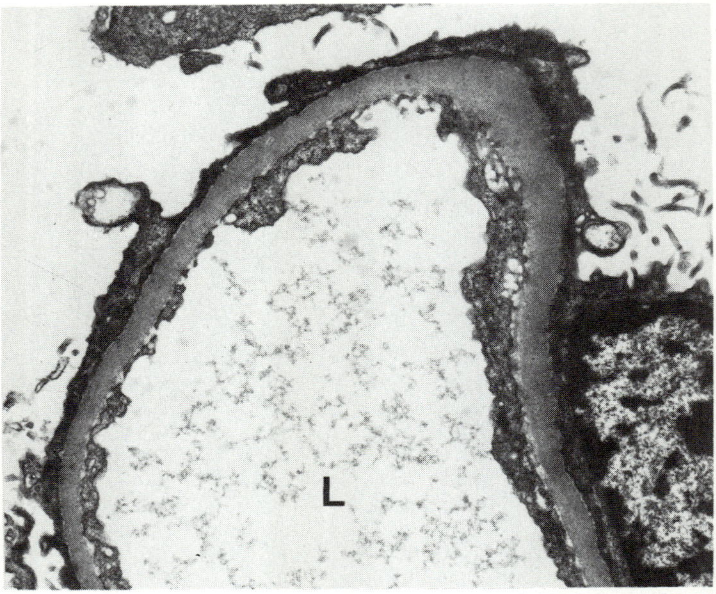

Figure 3-7. A segment of glomerular capillary wall showing diffuse effacement ("fusion") of visceral epithelial cell foot processes in a pediatric patient with IgA nephropathy and the nephrotic syndrome. There is also villous transformation of the visceral epithelium. The glomeruli were normal by light microscopy. *L*, glomerular capillary lumen: and *S* Bowman's space. Electron micrograph, ×12,000.

well as the presence of electron-dense deposits) were associated with increased proteinuria. These studies are all compatible with the concept that, in most patients, persistent proteinuria of moderate-to-severe degree is associated with more pronounced morphologic evidence of glomerular damage.

It should be noted, however, that a number of recent reports have indicated the existence of a subset of patients in whom "nephrotic range" proteinuria may be associated with mild glomerular lesions, a favorable long-term clinical outcome, and often a good response to corticosteroid therapy [26, 50–53]. We have suggested previously that the apparent disparity existing between this group of patients and the majority of IgA nephropathy patients with moderate-to-severe proteinuria is best explained by the coexistence of two separate glomerulopathies, i.e., IgA nephropathy and minimal-change nephrotic syndrome [50]. This proposal was supported by the observation that two of the four patients reported by the SPNSG had early biopsies performed when the patients presented with nephrotic syndrome that showed no evidence of mesangial IgA deposition, followed by later biopsies (performed because of an episode of gross hematuria) that showed diffuse mesangial IgA deposition [50].

Gross hematuria

The clinicopathologic implications of gross hematuria in IgA nephropathy is a matter for continued debate. In *pediatric* series outside Japan, the number of patients who *do not* experience at least one episode of gross hematuria is so few that attempts to correlate this with renal pathology have been very difficult. In the SPNSG series, only 18% of children did not have gross hematuria; however, the relatively large patient population under study made it possible to draw some conclusions [26]. A *history* of gross hematuria (most children did not have gross hematuria at the time of biopsy) was associated with increased severity of glomerular changes by light microscopy. Although not statistically significant, patients with gross hematuria were also more likely to have ultrastructural abnormalities of the GBM (thinning, splitting, or rarefaction) [26, 44].

Although it appears that gross hematuria is associated with more severe pathologic lesions in some pediatric patients, the question that has not been resolved pertains to the permanency of these changes. For example, in the 17 children with IgA nephropathy described by Linne et al. [12], gross hematuria was observed as a presenting symptom in 14 (82%) of the 17 and glomerular filtration rate (GFR) was initially depressed in nine of 16 patients—all of these patients had gross hematuria. The authors also demonstrated in eight patients (one of whom had not presented with gross hematuria) that subsequent episodes of gross hematuria were associated with a fall in GFR. They observed, however, that depression of GFR associated with bouts of macroscopic hematuria during early stages of the disease was usually transient. Furthermore, repeat renal biopsies performed in two of their patients during such episodes did not show additional acute proliferative changes; they concluded that depression of GFR in the early stages of IgA nephropathy may be largely functional.

The transient nature of many episodes of decreased GFR and macroscopic hematuria was also emphasized by Talwalkar et al. [77] in a case report involving an 11-year-old boy who had three such episodes in 13 months. One of these "attacks" was particularly striking, with the patient requiring a short period of dialysis after developing acute renal failure (serum creatinine 22.5 mg/dl; BUN 297 mg/dl) and hypertensive encephalopathy. Significant improvement in renal function was observed subsequently—without any specific therapy—and the patient had a serum creatinine of 0.9 mg/dl four weeks after discharge from hospital.

The clinicopathologic relevance of gross hematuria in children with IgA nephropathy is further confused when one examines this feature in Japanese children [5]. In the large multicenter series reported by Kitajima et al. [5], gross hematuria was the presenting sign in only 14% of the patients. However, the distribution of glomerular lesions in the patients that were classified showed that almost 50% (239 of 485) had evidence of relatively severe glomerular disease—defined as WHO-C. This is a higher percentage of "severe" lesions than has been reported in most of the pediatric series in which gross hematuria is present in 80–90% of patients.

The study of Yoshikawa and Matsuo [6] is very pertinent to the question of the low apparent frequency of gross hematuria in Japanese children with IgA nephropathy. In their series of 61 children, only 14 (23%) of 61 children had clinical evidence of renal disease at presentation (gross hematuria in 11 [18%] and edema in three), whereas 77% were identified following routine urinalysis. In a mean follow-up period of only two years, however, 37 (61%) of their 61 children had one or more episodes of gross hematuria. This figure is much closer to the frequency observed in series of the Western world. It is also relevant to note that these episodes "were often associated with febrile illnesses, especially upper respiratory infection"—a feature that is also noted frequently in Western series. This particular study is compatible with the concept that the difference in frequency of gross hematuria that appears to exist between Western and Eastern series may be spurious, with the apparent differences resulting from the fact that many pediatric patients in Japan are diagnosed prior to the time of their first episode of gross hematuria.

Duration of disease prior to diagnostic renal biopsy

Patients with a longer history of clinical renal disease were more likely to have evidence of focal global sclerosis (>10% of glomeruli involved) in the SPNSG experience [26, 44]. However, there was no evidence of more severe interstitial disease in patients with a longer history of clinical symptoms. Since, in most series, children are biopsied within 1–2 years of clinical presentation, the relevance of this factor is difficult to analyze.

Sex

In pediatric series, there has been little attention paid to the relative severity of glomerular lesions in males and females—since most of the series have included so few female patients. In some large adult series, it appears that males have a worse prognosis than females [28]. The SPNSG [26, 44] reported that girls were more likely to show a mild lesion on light microscopy; this occurred in 50% of girls but in only 22% of boys. However, the follow-up evaluation of these children is too short to allow conclusions regarding prognosis.

Another series that provided data compatible with the concept that IgA nephropathy may be more severe in males was published by Kogoshi et al. [3]. When these authors distinguished between patients in whom IgA was deposited in mesangial areas alone versus those who had a glomerular capillary wall distribution of IgA, a significant difference emerged in the apparent severity of glomerular damage between the two groups—as assessed by the frequency of proteinuria ≥2+ (four of 14 in the first group versus ten of 13 in the second). It is of interest to note that the "milder" group of 14 children was composed of an equal number of boys and girls whereas the latter, more severely affected group was made up predominantly of boys (ten out of 13). However, these patient numbers are insufficient to draw firm conclusions regarding the influence of the sex of the patient on the severity of disease.

PROGNOSIS OF CHILDREN WITH IgA NEPHROPATHY

Interpretation of renal function in children with IgA nephropathy

When considering clinical outcomes and prognostic indicators, it is relevant to underline the importance of age-related differences in normal serum creatinine values when comparing reports of renal functional status in papers dealing with children and adults with IgA nephropathy. Some authors have considered "evidence of impaired renal function" or "chronic renal insufficiency" to be present when serum creatinine values are above 1.3 or 1.5 mg/dl. For many children, these "high normal" values would only be reached after the patient has suffered 50% or more impairment of GFR. This point is particularly important when dealing with IgA nephropathy, since patients afflicted with this disorder may show an insidious, yet relentless, deterioration of GFR. Early detection and, hopefully, successful therapy (yet to be realized) will be one of the major goals of physicians caring for patients with IgA nephropathy.

Of the pediatric series dealing with IgA nephropathy, Andreoli et al. [29] and Linne et al. [12] have observed a relatively high frequency of progressive renal insufficiency whereas most other studies have suggested that this condition is usually benign in children. In Andreoli's study [29], 17 patients were followed for periods ranging from one month to six years (mean, two years); four (23.5%) of the 17 showed decreased renal function and three (18%) progressed to dialysis. The most helpful prognostic indicators in their patients were proteinuria >1 g at the time of biopsy, crescents in the glomeruli, and evidence of GBM involvement—based on the pattern of IgA staining (mesangial and glomerular capillary wall deposition).

Linne et al. [12] described clinical information for 17 children with IgA nephropathy who had been followed for 5–23 years. Of 12 patients with follow-up greater than nine years, three (25%) had hypertension and advanced renal failure and two others had hypertension but normal GFR.

Prognostic implications of episodes of gross hematuria in children

Linne et al. [12], in their study of 17 children with IgA nephropathy, reported that frequent and intensive episodes of macroscopic hematuria seemed to be associated with the development of permanent renal damage. However, it should be noted that no pediatric series has documented conclusively that episodes of gross hematuria are associated with a worse prognosis. In fact the Japanese series reported by Kogoshi et al. [3] would seem to provide evidence that this may not be the case—at least in that country. Although no specific analysis of the prognostic importance of gross hematuria was provided, it is noteworthy that, after an average follow-up of only 29 months, 62 (13%) of 481 children showed either chronic renal failure or evidence of progressive disease despite the fact that gross hematuria was present at presentation in only 14% of the entire group of patients.

Relationship between pediatric and adult cases of IgA nephropathy

Although IgA nephropathy appears to carry a more ominous prognosis with increasing age, it is apparent from a number of reports of IgA nephropathy in adults that evidence of renal disease was present since childhood in many such patients. Berger [75] reported that some of his adult patients who progressed to chronic renal failure had a history of hematuria that dated back to their childhood. Belton et al. [13] demonstrated this point even more clearly in their description of 32 patients with IgA nephropathy. Although only eight (25%) of their patients were less than 18 years at the time of diagnosis, almost half of the patients (14 of 31) reported symptoms of renal disease first appearing at 18 years of age or less. Finally, in a recent comparison of 24 children and 58 adults with IgA nephropathy, Wyatt et al. reported that five of the patients presenting as adults had an onset with macroscopic hematuria in childhood [28]. Three of these patients progressed to end-stage renal disease.

TREATMENT

Steroids

There have been no controlled studies demonstrating benefit from the use of steroids in childhood IgA nephropathy. In an early report, McEnery et al. [23] reported that some of their patients showed at least transient benefit from alternate-day prednisone. However, these authors have not subsequently found such treatment to be of benefit (McEnery, personal communication). Anecdotal experience with daily prednisone therapy has been reported by Bergstein [72] in a seven-year-old boy with IgA nephropathy and a rapid decline in GFR. This patient showed an excellent recovery of renal function after being placed on steroid treatment. The patient was very unusual, however, in that a repeat renal biopsy performed immediately before starting prednisone showed no evidence of mesangial IgA deposits, despite the presence of a more severe histologic pattern—including crescents. In addition, caution must be exercised in interpreting such anecdotal reports of "response" to treatment in view of the spontaneous resolution of severe episodes of acute renal failure that are sometimes observed in this condition. High-dose ("pulse") steroids have also been used recently in an attempt to reverse the "rapidly progressive" form of IgA nephropathy in both children and adults [42]. Although there is no conclusive evidence of permanent benefit with this therapy, final conclusions are not warranted from the limited uncontrolled data available at the present time.

Dilantin (phenytoin)

Specific studies of children have not been included in any prospective studies of phenytoin in IgA nephropathy. Although specific information regarding pediatric patients has not been available, the overall conclusion is that phenytoin does not confer any long-lasting benefit for patients with this condition (reviewed in chapter 15). However, it is possible that agents (such as phenytoin) which may alter the immunologic injury that appears in early phases of IgA nephropathy may have little or no benefit in patients with chronic sclerosing lesions. The results in such patients may therefore cloud any benefit that this agent may have no patients with the "early lesions."

COMPARISON BETWEEN HSP AND IgA NEPHROPATHY

Although recent articles have differed in their evaluation of the relationship between these two "conditions," Meadow and Scott have advanced the point that the two conditions represent different expressions of a single disease [49]. They reported two siblings with IgA nephropathy: one child had classic symptoms of HSP whereas the sibling presented with no such evidence of "concomitant systemic disease." Although it is possible that the two siblings developed two different conditions at the same time, it appears more likely that they displayed different clinical expressions of the same disease. This controversial issue is covered more extensively in chapter 4.

REFERENCES

1. Levy M, Beaufils H, Gubler MC, Habib R: Idiopathic recurrent macroscopic hematuria and mesangial IgA-IgG deposits in children (Berger's disease). Clin Nephrol 1:63–69, 1973.
2. Nomoto Y, Sakai H: Cold-reacting antinuclear factor in sera from patients with IgA nephropathy. J Lab Clin Med 94:76–87, 1979.
3. Kogoshi T, Sawaguchi H, Murakami M, Yamamoto H, Ueda Y, Sugisaki Y, Ishizaka M, Masugi Y: Clinico-pathological studies of immunoglobulin A associated idiopathic glomerulonephritis in childhood. Nippon Jimzo Gakkai Shi 22:1463–1475, 1980.
4. Nakahara C, Aosai F, Hasegawa O, Ito H, Matsuo N, Hajikano H, Sakaguchi H: IgA nephropathy in children: a modified view of clinico-pathological characteristics. Pediatr Res 14:995(a), 1980.
5. Kitajima T, Murakami M, Sakai O: Clinicopathological features in the Japanese patients with IgA nephropathy, Jpn J Med 22:219–222, 1983.
6. Yoshikawa N, Matsuo T: IgA nephropathy in children. Comp Ther 10:35–41, 1984.
7. Woodroffe AJ, Thomson NM, Meadows R, Lawrence JR: IgA-associated glomerulonephritis. Aust NZ J Med 5:97–100, 1975.
8. Clarkson AR, Seymour AE, Thompson AJ, Haynes WDG, Chan Y-L, Jackson B: IgA nephropathy: a syndrome of uniform morphology, diverse clinical features and uncertain prognosis. Clin Nephrol 8:549–471, 1977.
9. Navas-Palacios JJ, Gutierrez-Millet V, Usera-Sarraga G, Garzon-Martin A: IgA nephropathy: an ultrastructural study. Ultrastruct Pathol 2:151–161, 1981.
10. Levy M, Gonzalez-Burchard G, Broyer M, Dommergues J-P, Foulard M, Sorez J-P, Habib R: Berger's disease in children: natural history and outcome. Medicine 64:157–180, 1985.

11. Michalk D, Waldherr R, Seelig HP, Weber HP, Scharer K: Idiopathic mesangial IgA-glomerulonephritis in childhood: description of 19 pediatric cases and review of the literature. Eur J Pediatr 134:13–22, 1980.
12. Linne T, Aperia A, Broberger O, Bergstrand A, Bohman S-O, Rekola S: Course of renal function in IgA glomerulonephritis in children and adolescents. Acta Paediatr Scand 71:735–743, 1982.
13. Belton P, Carmondy M, Donohue J, O'Dwyer WF: IgA nephropathy (Berger's disease): a clinical study of 32 cases. Irish J Med Sci 310–314, 1976.
14. Van der Peet J, Arisz L, Brentjens JRH, Marrink J, Hoedemaeker PhJ: The clinical course of IgA nephropathy in adults. Clin Nephrol 8:335–340, 1977.
15. Nagy J, Brasch H, Sule T, Hamori A, Deak G, Ambrus M: IgA glomerulonephritis: mesangial IgA deposition without systemic signs (Berger's disease). Int Urol Nephrol 11:367–375, 1979.
16. Joshua H, Sharon Z, Gutglas E, Rosenfeld J, Ben-Bassat M: IgA-IgG nephropathy: a clinicopathologic entity with slow evolution and favorable prognosis. Am J Clin Pathol 67:289–295, 1977.
17. Sissons JGP, Woodrow DF, Curtis JR, Evans DJ, Gower PE, Sloper JC, Peters DK: Isolated glomerulonephritis with mesangial IgA deposits. Br Med J 3:611–614, 1975.
18. Davies DR, Tighe JR, Jones NF, Brown GW: Recurrent haematuria and mesangial IgA deposition. J Clin Pathol 26:672–677, 1973.
19. Hood SA, Velosa JA, Holley KE, Donadio JV Jr: IgA-IgG nephropathy: predictive indices of progressive disease. Clin Nephrol 16:55–62, 1981.
20. McCoy RC, Abramowsky Cr, Tisher CC: IgA nephropathy. Am J Pathol 76:123–140, 1974.
21. Zimmerman SW, Burkholder PM: Immunoglobulin A nephropathy. Arch Intern Med 135:1217–1223, 1975.
22. Finlayson G, Alexander R, Juncos L, Schlein E, Teague P, Waldman R, Cade R: Immunoglobulin A glomerulonephritis: a clinicopathologic study. Lab Invest 32:140–148, 1975.
23. McEnery PT, McAdams AJ, West CD: Glomerular morphology, natural history and treatment of children with IgA-IgG mesangial nephropathy. In: Kincaid-Smith P, Mathew TH, Becker EL (eds) *Glomerulonephritis*. New York: John Wiley and Sons, 1973, pp 305–320.
24. Feiner HD, Cabili S, Baldwin DS, Schacht RG, Gallo GR: Intrarenal vascular sclerosis in IgA nephropathy. Clin Nephrol 18:183–192, 1982.
25. Lee S-M K, Rao VM, Franklin WA, Schiffer MS, Aronson AJ, Spargo BH, Katz AI: IgA nephropathy: morphologic predictors of progressive renal disease. Hum Pathol 13:314–322, 1982.
26. Hogg RJ, Silva FG: IgA nephropathy: natural history and prognostic indices in children. Contrib Nephrol 40:214–221, 1984.
27. Kher KK, Makker SP, Moorthy B: IgA nephropathy (Berger's disease): a clinicopathologic study in children. Int J Pediatr Nephrol 4:11–18, 1983.
28. Wyatt RJ, Julian BA, Bhathena DB, Mitchell BL, Holland NH, Malluche HH: IgA nephropathy: presentation, clinical course, and prognosis in children and adults. Am J Kidney Dis 4:192–200, 1984.
29. Andreoli SP, Yum MN, Bergstein JM: IgA nephropathy in children: significance of glomerular basement membrane deposition of IgA. Am J Nephrol 6:28–33, 1986.
30. Weiss RA, Jodorkovsky R, Bennett B, Greifer I: Clinical and histologic spectrum of IgA nephropathy in children and adolescents. (Personal communication)
31. Croker BP, Dawson DV, Sanfilippo F: IgA nephropathy: correlation of clinical and histologic features. Lab Invest 48:19–24, 1983.
32. Hall RP, Stachura I, Cason J, Whiteside TL, Lawley TJ: IgA-containing circulating immune complexes in patients with IgA nephropathy. Am J Med 74:56–63, 1983.
33. Hogg RJ: Diagnostic, prognostic and therapeutic implications of renal biopsies in children with renal disease. In: Kurtzman NA (ed) *Seminars in nephrology*. New York: Grune and Stratton 5:240–254, 1985.
34. Piel CF, Biava CG, Goodman JR: Unexplained hematuria: histologic diagnosis in 61 children. Pediatr Res 18:367A, 1984.
35. International Study of Kidney Disease in Children: Clinical pathological correlations in recurrent and persistent hematuria syndromes. Pediatr Res 14:995A, 1980.

36. Ohno J: Discussion p 134. In: Glassock RJ, Kurokawa K: IgA nephropathy in Japan. Am J Nephrol 5:127–137, 1985.
37. Pardo V, Berian MG, Levi DF, Strauss J: Benign primary hematuria: clinicopathologic study of 65 patients. Am J Med 65:817–822, 1979.
38. Bodian M, Black JA, Kobayashi N, Lake BD, Shuler SE: Recurrent haematuria in childhood. Q J Med 34:359–382, 1965.
39. Singer DB, Hill LL, Rosenberg HS, Marshall J, Swenson R: Recurrent hematuria in childhood. N Engl J Med 279:7–12, 1968.
40. Linne T, Wasserman J: Lymphocyte subpopulations and immunoglobulin production in IgA nephropathy. Clin Nephrol 23:109–111, 1985.
41. Martini A, Magrini U, Scelsi M, Capelli V, Barberis L: Chronic mesangioproliferative IgA glomerulonephritis complicated by a rapidly progressive course in a 14-year-old boy: a case report. Nephron 29:164–166, 1981.
42. Abuelo JG, Esparza AR, Matarese RA, Endreny RG, Carvalho JS, Allergra SR: Crescentic IgA nephropathy. Medicine 63:396–406, 1984.
43. Nicholls K, Walker RG, Dowling JP, Kincaid-Smith P: "Malignant" IgA nephropathy. Am J Kidney Dis 5:42–46, 1985.
44. Southwest Pediatric Nephrology Study Group: A multicenter study of IgA nephropathy in children. Kidney Int 22:643–652, 1982.
45. Churg J, Sobin LH: WHO classification and atlas of glomerular diseases. Tokyo: Igaku-Shoin, 1982.
46. Churg J: Personal communication.
47. Sinniah RK: Clinicopathologic correlations in IgA nephropathy. In: Robinson RR (ed) *Nephrology*, vol 1. New York: Springer-Verlag, 1984, pp 665–685.
48. Yoshikawa N, Cameron AH, White RHR: Glomerular morphometry. II. Familial and nonfamilial haematuria. Histopathology 5:251–256, 1981.
49. Meadow SR, Scott DG: Berger disease: Henoch-Schönlein syndrome without the rash. J Pediatr 106:27–32, 1985.
50. Southwest Pediatric Nephrology Study Group: Association of IgA nephropathy with steroid-responsive nephrotic syndrome. Am J Kidney Dis 5:157–164, 1985.
51. Mustonen J, Pasternak A, Rantala I: The nephrotic syndrome in IgA glomerulonephritis: response to corticosteroid therapy. Clin Nephrol 20:172–176, 1983.
52. St-André JP, Simard CL, Spiesser R, et al.: Syndrome néphrotique de l'enfant à lesions glomérularies minimes, avec dépôts mesangiaux. Nouv Presse Med 9:531–532, 1980.
53. Sinnassamy P, O'Regan S: Mesangial IgA deposits with steroid responsive nephrotic syndrome: probable minimal lesion nephrosis. Am J Kidney Dis 5:267–269, 1985.
54. Hawkins E, Silva F, Hogg R (for the Southwest Pediatric Nephrology Study Group): Multicenter collaborative study of IgA nephropathy with focal sclerosis. Kidney Int 25:223A, 1984.
55. Hawkins E, Berry PH: Membranoproliferative glomerulonephritis with significant IgA deposits. Lab Invest 46:6P(A), 1982.
56. Nakamoto Y, Asano Y, Dohi K, et al.: Primary IgA glomerulonephritis and Schönlein-Henoch purpura nephritis: clinicopathological and immunohistological characteristics. Q J Med 47:495–516, 1978.
57. Southwest Pediatric Nephrology Study Group: A clinico-pathologic study of crescentic glomerulonephritis in 50 children. Kidney Int 27:450–458, 1985.
58. Bertani T, Appel GB, D'Agati V, et al.: Focal segmental membranous glomerulonephropathy associated with other glomerular diseases. Am J Kidney Dis 2:439–448, 1983.
59. Bertani T, Olesnicky L, Abu-Regiaha S, et al.: Concomitant presence of three different glomerular diseases in the same patient. Nephron 34:260–266, 1983.
60. O'Neill WM Jr, Wallin JD, Walker PD: Hematuria and red cell casts in typical diabetic nephropathy. Am J Med 74:389–395, 1983.
61. Doyle GD, O'Dwyer WF, Carmody M, Campbell E, Browne O: IgA nephropathy: an immunopathological study. Irish J Med Sci 292–303, 1976.
62. Hill GS, Jenis EH, Goodloe S: The nonspecificity of the ultrastructural alteration in hereditary nephritis. Lab Invest 31:516–532, 1974.
63. Kohaut EC, Singer DB, Nevels BK, Hill LL: The specificity of split renal membranes in hereditary nephritis. Arch Pathol Lab Med 100:475–479, 1976.
64. Rumpelt HJ: Hereditary nephropathy (Alport's syndrome): spectrum and development of

glomerular lesions. In: Rosen S (ed) *Pathology of glomerular disease.* New York: Churchill Livingstone, 1983, pp 225–238.
65. Sinniah R, Churg J: Effect of IgA deposits on the glomerular mesangium in Berger's disease. Ultrastruct Pathol 4:9–22, 1983.
66. Berger J, Yaneva H, Nabarra B, Barbanel C: Recurrence of mesangial deposition of IgA after renal transplantation. Kidney Int 7:232–241, 1975.
67. Shigematsu H, Kobayashi Y, Tateno S, Tsukada M: Ultrastructure of acute glomerular injury in IgA nephritis. Arch Pathol Lab Med 104:303–307, 1980.
68. Frasca GM, Vangelista A, Biagini G, Bonomini V: Immunological tubulo-interstitial deposits in IgA nephropathy. Kidney Int 22:184–191, 1982.
69. Katz A, Underdown BJ, Minta JO, Lepow IH: Glomerulonephritis with mesangial deposits of IgA unassociated with systemic disease. CMA J 114:209–215, 1976.
70. Doi T, Kanatsu K, Nagai H, Kohrogi N, Kuwahara T, Hamashima Y: Immunoelectron microscopic studies of IgA nephropathy. Nephron 36:246–251, 1984.
71. Sinniah R: Occurrence of mesangial IgA and IgM deposits in a control necropsy population. J Clin Pathol 36:276–179, 1983.
72. Bergstein J: IgA nephropathy [letter to the editor]. Clin Nephrol 9:258–259, 1978.
73. Silva FG, Chander P, Pirani CL, Hardy MA: Disappearance of glomerular mesangial IgA deposits after renal allogroft transplantation [letter to the editor]. Transplantation 33:214–216, 1982.
74. Sanfilippo F, Croker BP, Bollinger RR: Fate of four cadaveric donor renal allografts with mesangial IgA deposits. Transplantation 33:370–376, 1982.
75. Berger J: Idiopathic mesangial deposition of IgA. In: Hamburger J. Crosnier J, Brunfeld JP (eds) *Nephrology.* New York: John Wiley and Sons, 1979, pp 535–541.
76. Sabatier JC, Genin C, Assenat H, Colon S, Ducret F, Berthoux FC: Mesangial IgA glomerulonephritis in HLA-identical brothers. Clin Nephrol 11:35–38, 1979.
77. Talwalkar YB, Price WH, Musgrave JE: Recurrent resolving renal failure in IgA nephropathy. J Pediatr 92:596–597, 1978.

4. HENOCH-SCHÖNLEIN PURPURA AND IgA NEPHROPATHY: TO SEPARATE OR UNIFY?

ANTHONY R. CLARKSON

Henoch-Schönlein purpura (HSP) is a readily recognizable clinical syndrome familiar to most physicians and characterized by the appearance of a vasculitic rash especially on the legs and buttocks, flitting arthropathy, gastrointestinal problems, and glomerulonephritis. The introduction of immunofluorescence studies of renal biopsies brought confirmation of the immunologic nature of the pathologic lesions and the remarkable similarity between the renal lesion of HSP and IgA nephropathy. This chapter explores the differences and similarities between the two conditions and points strongly to a concept of unity. To this time, however, this concept is not proved; proof probably awaits a specific diagnostic test similar to the L.E. cell or antinuclear antibody test in systemic lupus erythematosus.

CLINICAL PRESENTATION

HSP clearly is a systemic disease and the characteristic skin, joint, gut, and renal involvement usually makes it easily identifiable in children and adults. In some cases, however, some of the features are mild or evanescent and detected only by careful search or questioning. In others, one or more facet of the disease may be absent. In patients with HSP and glomerulonephritis, skin, gut, or joint involvement serve to separate these subjects from those with idiopathic IgA nephropathy where such clearly defined systemic symptoms are not usually a feature. In a significant but small proportion of cases, this distinction is blurred, especially in cases where systemic manifestations of HSP are mild and during exacerbations of IgA nephropathy. Here intermittent and occasionally severe abdominal pain, generalized muscle aches, loin pain, and fever are often associated with synpharyngitic macroscopic hematuria, but fall short of the extent, severity, and clarity of the systemic features of HSP. Rarely, transitions between the two diseases have been reported [1, 2] and, more commonly, episodes of synpharyngitic hematuria appear in patients whose initial presentation was with classic HSP. Furthermore, in our experience, many patients with HSP have persistent proteinuria, microscopic hematuria, and an "active" urinary sediment years after the initial episode. Renal biopsy in these patients reveals mesangial proliferative glomerulonephritis with positive immunofluorescence for IgA and C3. The simultaneous appearance of HSP and "Berger's disease" in identical twins [3] strengthens further the impression that primary IgA nephropathy is a monosymptomatic form of HSP.

Estimates of the incidence of glomerulonephritis in HSP vary considerably from 20% to 100% and probably depend on the vigor for which evidence of it is sought. Renal involvement is usually apparent early in the course of disease although many cases are described where the overt features of glomerulonephritis develop only after several weeks or months. Microscopic hematuria with minor degrees of proteinuria are frequent accompanying signs in early disease, however, and in a large number of patients may be the only indication of renal disease. Most of these patients are not investigated as it is clear that, at least in the short term, the majority have a benign, self-limiting episode of glomerulonephritis. Long-term follow-up studies of a large cohort of such patients into adult life are few, although the report by Counahen et al. [4] suggests that progressive disease may occur in about 20%.

Greater attention has been paid to the study of patients with more severe or relapsing forms of glomerulonephritis. As with IgA nephropathy, intermittent macroscopic hematuria with persistent microscopic hematuria between episodes are observed. These exacerbations in some patients are quite frequent and may or may not be accompanied by the vasculitic rash. Patients with more severe renal disease develop significant proteinuria, nephrotic syndrome, hypertension, and renal impairment. While these features are more likely to develop during the initial phases of the disease or within the first few months, their occurrence after several years is not unusual. Even when renal impairment occurs early in the course of HSP, the prognosis is not necessarily bad. As in patients with IgA nephropathy, temporary reduction in renal function is not unusual during acute exacerbations, renal function improving gradually as systemic symptoms subside. When initial renal damage is severe and when renal impairment develops gradually over the course of several years, end-stage renal failure can be predicted confidently. Our experience suggests that this occurs in from 2–5% of patients and is more frequent in adults.

The clinical similarity between the glomerulonephritis of HSP and IgA nephropathy can be extended when factors provoking acute disease are considered. For many years, HSP was thought to result from hypersensitivity to various allergens, infecting organisms [5], food [6], or drugs [7]. It is now recognized, however, that the majority of cases occur following nonspecific upper respiratory or gastrointestinal infections. Like IgA nephropathy, exacerbations in HSP may be frequent and usually are manifest by macroscopic hematuria. To further the comparison, HSP occurs in relation to liver disease, especially alcoholic cirrhosis, cancer [8] and lymphoma (Clarkson, unpublished) and, like IgA nephropathy, recurs in renal transplants [9].

DEMOGRAPHY

While the high worldwide incidence of IgA nephropathy is becoming increasingly recognized, the same information is not available for HSP. It is common knowledge, however, that HSP is a relatively frequent disease of young children in the Western world, the majority of cases occurring between the ages of two and 11 years [10]. Distinctly uncommon before the age of two years, it becomes progressively uncommon again after adolescence. IgA nephropathy, on the other hand, has a peak incidence in the second and third decades of life and, like HSP, affects males more frequently than females. In a preliminary study of disease incidence over a ten-year period at the Adelaide Children's Hospital, 220 cases of HSP were seen whereas only 25 of primary IgA nephropathy were encountered (K.F. Jureidini, personal communication). Over the same period at the nearby Royal Adelaide Hospital catering only to adults, 31 patients between 15 and 81 years were registered with HSP, whereas there were 352 cases of primary IgA nephropathy. There is thus a strikingly clear difference between peak age incidences of these conditions, which together with the overt dissimilarities in clinical expression, has kept them as separate entities in the minds of most physicians. Conceivably, however, the differences are simply quantitative and based on abnormalities or aberrations in development of the mucosal immune system.

PATHOLOGY

The overlap of pathologic features in primary IgA nephropathy and HSP is now widely recognized. "Since the differences appear more quantitative than qualitative...the nephritic component of Henoch-Schönlein purpura and primary IgA nephropathy [are] similar and suggest that the same pathogenetic mechanisms underlie both diseases, albeit to different extents" [11]. Responsible investigators such as Levy at al. [12] still prefer to separate the entities on clinical and pathologic grounds although, apart from the obvious leukocytoclastic vasculitis that affects skin and other organs in HSP, there are few renal pathologic differences.

The immunopathology is qualitatively identical with predominant mesangial deposition of IgA and C3 and variable deposition of IgG, IgM, and fibrinogen. There tends, in cases with more severe renal pathology, to be increased deposition of fibrinogen and IgA along peripheral glomerular capillary loops. Based on the grading criteria of Counahan et al. [4] for HSP, we have found no major differences in the light-microscopic features of 45 cases of HSP and 350 patients with primary IgA nephropathy. While there is a tendency for the HSP patient with acute decline in renal function to show more marked glomerular endocapillary and extracapillary changes, such features are also seen in patients with IgA nephropathy. Of course, such histologic gradings are arbitrary and take little account of the likelihood of many, if not all, histologic grades being present in the one biopsy. Electron-microscopic studies also fail to clarify any differences. A careful analysis of biopsies from 35 patients with HSP and 48 with IgA nephropathy by Mihatsch et al. [13] demonstrated in HSP more subepithelial and subendothelial deposits and a greater degree of glomerular capillary basement membrane change in response to these deposits. Mesangial deposits tended to be less in quantity than in IgA nephropathy. Once again, however, the differences were quantitative as similar abnormal features were seen in both entities.

Positive IgA immunofluorescence is seen consistently in the vasculitic skin lesions and in the subdermal capillaries of normal skin in patients with HSP. Our experience [14] like that of others suggests that IgA is found frequently in dermal capillaries in adults with IgA nephropathy [15, 16].

On the other hand, Levy et al. [12] report that IgA is frequently absent from skin of children with IgA nephropathy, and other workers suggest it is not a universal finding [17–19]. Disparities such as these may be used to emphasize differences between the conditions, although they equally could represent the same quantitative problem as discussed with the renal pathology.

Although histopathologic, immunopathologic, and ultrastructural changes are almost identical in both conditions, inflammatory changes in extrarenal vessels (vasculitis) is the exclusive preserve of HSP. This has given rise to the suggestion that HSP is a diffuse vascular form of IgA nephropathy [20].

IMMUNOPATHOGENESIS

Nature of glomerular deposits

Despite the observation by André et al. [21] that IgA2 was the main IgA subclass in the immune deposits of HSP, this subsequently has not been confirmed. As with IgA nephropathy, most workers now agree that IgA1 predominates. Using monoclonal antisera to IgA1 and IgA2, Tomino et al.

[20] identified only IgA1 in patients with HSP and further domonstrated the presence of J chain in these deposits. Additional evidence supporting the presence of IgA1 polymers in glomeruli is their affinity for secretory component [22]. It must be assumed that the greater degrees of acute damage seen in some patients with HSP result from a higher proportion of glomerular capillary basement membrane deposits, thus inferring a possible disparity in size and/or charge of immune complexes between the conditions. However, the mechanisms of glomerular injury are otherwise unclear. Properdin as well as C3 is deposited in both conditions, suggesting that activation of complement via the alternative pathway plays a role.

Immune complexes

The finding of cryoglobulinemia in patients with HSP by Garcia-Fuentes et al. [23], was the first direct confirmation that the glomerular deposits may be derived from the circulation. Their presence occurred during acute episodes and in those with chronic glomerulonephritis, but could not be demonstrated in patients who had recovered. In this study, cryoglobulins contained IgA, C4, C3, and properdin, suggesting strongly their immune complex nature. Despite initial methodologic problems, the finding of circulating immune complexes in HSP has now been widely confirmed with various techniques, [36, 37, 38]. Analysis of IgA subclasses in the IgA-containing immune complexes showed both IgA1 and IgA2 to be present and these related to phases of clinical activity [24]. All these observations are similar to those in IgA nephropathy.

IMMUNOREGULATION

Total serum IgA concentrations in HSP are elevated in approximately 50% of patients, the elevation tending to be greater during disease activity [25, 26]. As with IgA nephropathy, considerable work has been performed to determine the cause of this rise. In particular, efforts have concentrated on defects in regulation of IgA production by peripheral blood and mucosally sited lymphocytes. The information for HSP is not as complete as in IgA nephropathy, although that existing suggests similar abnormalities. IgA is the major immunoglobulin produced in unstimulated cultures of peripheral blood mononuclear cells [27, 28] from patients with HSP; this disturbance was present whether or not the disease was active. On the other hand, Casanueva et al. [29] have demonstrated a selective increase in the number of circulating IgA-producing cells during disease activity.

Stimulation of peripheral blood mononuclear cells from patients with HSP with pokeweed mitogen has resulted in decreased synthesis of IgA in the hands of Beale et al. [28] and Bannister et al. [27]. This is in sharp contrast to the further stimulation of IgA synthesis observed in patients with IgA nephropathy and more in keeping with results obtained with cells from SLE patients. It has not been determined whether this discrepancy represents a significant difference in pathogenesis between HSP and IgA nephropathy or simply is related to disease activity or the systemic nature of the condition.

B-cell hyperactivity seems to be a feature of both conditions, but whether in HSP it is IgA specific as demonstrated by Hale et al. [30] for IgA nephropathy is not yet known. In the latter case, it is tempting to speculate that antigen preactivation of B cells in vivo may be more intense for IgA-producing cells because the antigens are encountered at mucosal surfaces. Defective Fc-specific reticuloendothelial clearance exists in both conditions [31, 32]. It is unclear whether the clearance defects represent a primary event or result from saturation of receptor sites by IgA-containing immune complexes. The same question applies to the B-cell hyperactivity which indeed may be associated with the defective clearance. Current evidence points to a basic abnormality of mucosal immunity in both conditions. No antigen has been found that is specific in either condition and it seems likely that non-specific or ubiquitous antigens, whether bacterial, viral, food or other, may be capable of engendering a similar high IgA antibody response in both.

ANIMAL MODELS

Recently, several animal models of IgA nephropathy have been developed and the disease occurs spontaneously in others. None has been manipualted with the intention of producing symptoms akin to HSP for which no animal model currently is available. Perhaps attention should be paid to this in the future.

TREATMENT

The presence of skin rash, arthritis, and gastrointestinal disturbances together with nephritis frequently evokes a more alarmist response from the physician than when nephritis occurs as an isolated problem. In this context, corticosteroids have been used widely in patients with florid HSP. However, their administration does not seem to influence the course of arthritis, rash, or nephritis. Response of the gastrointestinal lesion may be dramatic, on the other hand, due presumably to reduction of local inflammation and edema. Recently, plasma-exchange treatment has had a vogue in severe cases although once again there is no objective evidence of benefit despite decrease in circulating concentrations of IgA immune complexes [33–35].

No specific therapy therefore exists and, as in IgA nephropathy, this will probably await clarification of basic pathogenetic mechanisms.

REFERENCES

1. Nakamoto Y, Asano Y, Dahi K, Fujioka M, Ida H, Keda H, Kibe Y, Hattori N, Takeuchi S: Primary IgA glomerulonephritis and Schönlein-Henoch purpura nephritis: clinicopathological and immunohistological characteristics. Q J Med 47:495–516, 1978.

2. Weiss JH, Bhathena DB, Curtis JJ: A possible relationship between Henoch-Schönlein syndrome and IgA nephropathy (Berger's disease). Lancet 1:347, 1975.
3. Meadow, SR, Scott DG: Berger's disease: Henoch-Schönlein syndrome without the rash. J Pediatr 106:27–32, 1985.
4. Counahan R, Winterborn MH, White RHR, Heaton JM, Meadow SR, Bluett NH, Swetschin H, Cameron JS, Chantler C: Prognosis of Henoch-Schönlein nephritis in children. Br Med J 2:11–14, 1977.
5. Bywaters EGL, Isdale I, Kempton JJ: Schönlein-Henoch purpura evidence for a group A, beta-haemolytic streptococcal infection. Q J Med 26:261–274, 1957.
6. Ackroyd JF: Allergic purpura, including purpura due to food, drugs and infections. Am J Med 14:605–610, 1953.
7. McCombs RP, Patterson JF, MacMahon HE: Syndromes associated with "allergic" vasculitis. N Engl J Med 255:251–261, 1956.
8. Cairns SA, Mallick NP, Lawler W, Williams G: Squamous cell carcinoma of the bronchus presenting with Henoch-Schönlein purpura. Br Med J 3:474–475, 1978.
9. Levy M, Moussa RA, Habib R, Gagnadoux MF, Broyer M: Anaphylactoid purpura nephritis and transplantation [abstr]. Kidney Int 22:326, 1982.
10. Meadow SR, Glasgow EF, White RHR, Moncrieff MW, Cameron JS, Ogg CS: Schönlein-Henoch nephritis. Q J Med 41:241–258, 1972.
11. Emancipator SN, Gallo GR, Lamm ME: IgA nephropathy: perspectives on pathogenesis and classification. Clin Nephrol 24:161–179, 1985.
12. Levy M, Gonzalez-Burchard G, Broyer M, Dommergues J-P, Foulard M, Sorez J-P Habib R: Berger's disease in children: natural history and outcome. Medicine 64:157–180, 1985.
13. Mihatsch MJ, Imbasciati E, Fogazzi G, Giani M, Ghio L, Gaboardi F: Ultrastructural lesions of Henoch-Schönlein syndrome and of IgA nephropathy: similarities and differences. Contrib Nephrol 40:255–263, 1984.
14. Thompson AJ, Chan Y-L, Woodroffe AJ, Clarkson AR, Seymour AE: Vascular IgA deposits in clinically normal skin of patients with renal disease. Pathology 12:407–413, 1980.
15. Baart de la Faille Kuyper EH, Kater L, Kuitjen RH, Kooiker CJ, Wagenaar SS, Van der Zowen P, Doorhaut Mees EJ: Occurrence of vascular IgA deposits in clinically normal skin of patients with renal disease. Kidney Int 9:424–429, 1976.
16. Waldherr R, Rambauser M, Rauterberg W, Andrassy K, Ritz E: Immunohistochemical features of mesangial IgA glomerulonephritis. Contrib Nephrol 40:99–106, 1984.
17. D'Amico G, Ferrario F, Colasanti G, Ragni A, Bestetti-Bosisio, M: IgA mesangial nephropathy (Berger's disease) with rapid decline in renal function. Clin Nephrol 16:251–257, 1981.
18. Hasbargen JA, Copley JB: Utility of skin biopsy in the diagnosis of IgA nephropathy. Am J Kidney Dis 6:100–102, 1985.
19. Tomino Y, Endoh M, Miura M, Nomoto Y, Sakai H: Immunopathological similarities between IgA nephropathy and Henoch-Schönlein purpura nephritis. Acta Pathol Jpn 33:113–122, 1983.
20. Tomino Y, Endoh M, Suga T, Miura M, Kaneschige H, Nomoto Y, Sakai H: Prevalence of IgA_1 deposits in Henoch-Schönlein purpura (HSP) nephritis. Toka J Exp Clin Med 7:527–532, 1982.
21. Andre C, Berthous FC, Andre F, Gillon G, Genin C, Sabatier JC: Prevalence of IgA_2 deposits in IgA nephropathies: a clue to their pathogenesis. N Engl J Med 303:1343–1346, 1980.
22. Egido J, Sancho J, Mampaso F, Lopez-Trascasa M, Sanchez Crespo M, Blasco R, Hernando L: A possible common pathogenesis of the mesangial IgA glomerulonephritis in patients with Berger's disease, and Schönlein-Henoch syndrome. Proc Eur Dial Transplant Assoc 17:660–666, 1980.
23. Garcia-Fuentes M, Chantler C, Williams DG: Cryoglobulinaemia in Henoch-Schönlein purpura. Br Med J 2:163–165, 1977.
24. Coppo R, Basolo B, Piccoli G, Mazzucco G, Bulzomi MR, Roccatello D, Di Marchi M, Carbonara AO, Barbiano Di Belgiojoso G: IgA_1 and IgA_2 immune complexes in primary IgA nephropathy and Henoch-Schönlein nephritis. Clin Exp Immunol 57:583–590, 1984.
25. Levinsky RJ, Barratt TM: IgA immune complexes in Henoch-Schönlein purpura. Lancet 2:1100–1102, 1979.

26. Woodroffe AJ, Gormly AA, McKenzie PE, Wootton AM, Thompson AJ, Seymour AE, Clarkson AR: Immunologic studies in IgA nephropathy. Kidney Int 18:366–374, 1980.
27. Bannister KM, Drew PA, Clarkson AR, Woodroffe AJ: Immunoregulation in glomerulonephritis, Henoch-Schönlein purpura and lupus nephritis. Clin Exp Immunol 53:384–390, 1983.
28. Beale MG, Nash GS, Bertovich MJ, McDermott P: Similar disturbances of B-cell activity and regulatory T-cell function in Henoch-Schönlein purpura and systemic lupus erythematosus. J Immunol 128:486–491, 1982.
29. Casanueva B, Rodriguez-Valverde V, Merino J, Arias M, Garcia-Fuentes M: Increased IgA producing cells in the blood of patients with active Henoch-Schönlein purpura. Arthritis Rheum 26:854–860, 1983.
30. Hale GM, McIntosh SL, Hiki Y, Clarkson AR, Woodroffe AJ: Evidence for IgA-specific B-cell hyperactivity in patients with IgA nephropathy. Kidney Int 29:718–724, 1986.
31. Bannister KM, Hay J, Clarkson AR, Woodroffe AJ: Fc-specific reticulo-endothelial clearance in systemic lupus erythematosus and glomerulonephritis. Am J Kidney Dis 3:287–292, 1984.
32. Lawrence S, Pussell BA, Charlesworth JA: Mesangial IgA nephropathy: detection of defective reticulo-phagocytic function in vivo. Clin Nephrol 16:280–283, 1983.
33. Hene RJ, Kater L: Plasmapheresis in nephritis associated with Henoch-Schönlein purpura and in primary IgA-nephropathy. Plasma Ther Transfus Technol 4:165–173, 1983.
34. Kauffmann RH, Houwert DA: Plasmapheresis in rapidly progressive Henoch-Schönlein glomerulonephritis and the effect on circulating immune complexes. Clin Nephrol 16:155–160, 1981.
35. McKenzie PE, Taylor AE, Woodroffe AJ, Seymour AE, Chan Y-L, Clarkson AR: Plasmapheresis in glomerulonephritis. Clin Nephrol 12:97–108, 1979.
36. Coppo R, Basolo B, Martina G, Rollino C, Di Marchi M, Giacchino F, Mazzucco G, Messina M, Piccoli G: Circulating immune complexes containing IgA, IgG and IgM in patients with primary IgA nephropathy and with Henoch-Schönlein nephritis: correlation with clinical and histologic signs of activity. Clin Nephrol 18:230–239, 1982.
37. Danielsen H, Eriksen EF, Johansen A, Sølling J: Serum immunoglobulin sedimentation patterns and circulating immune complexes in IgA glomerulonephritis and Schönlein-Henoch nephritis. Acta Med Scand 215:435–441, 1984.
38. Kauffmann, RH, Herrmann WA, Meyer CJLM, Daha MR, Van Es LS: Circulating IgA immune complexes in Henoch-Schönlein purpura: a longitudinal study of their relationship to disease activity Am J Med 68:859–866, 1980.

5. ASSOCIATED DISEASES IN IgA NEPHROPATHY

JUKKA MUSTONEN and AMOS PASTERNACK

In the original study by Berger [1], IgA nephropathy was described as a primary glomerulonephritis and also in patients with Henoch-Schönlein purpura. Soon thereafter, Manigand et al. [2] found that glomerular IgA deposits were often present in association with alcoholic liver cirrhosis. During the 1970s and 1980s, IgA nephropathy has been found to coexist with several types of diseases as presented in table 5-1 [1–38].

The systemic nature of IgA nephropathy has recently been stressed by many authors [18, 39, 40]. Battle [39] considered that the clinical spectrum of IgA nephropathy includes systemic disease in an undetermined number of patients. According to Cameron's view, the presence of IgA immune complexes, raised serum levels of IgA and polymeric IgA, as well as IgA deposition at extrarenal vasculature point to IgA nephropathy as a systemic disease [40]. Clarkson et al. [18] have suggested that IgA nephropathy should be regarded as a syndrome, and they divide IgA nephropathy into primary and secondary forms. In a new international classification and atlas of glomerular diseases, Berger's disease is classified as a glomerulonephritis of systemic diseases [41].

The present review is a presentation of these associations. Moreover, the results of our own material of 230 patients with IgA nephropathy are reported.

Table 5-1. Diseases that have previously been described in association with IgA nephropathy

Diseases group	References
Rheumatic	
Henoch-Schönlein purpura	1, 3, 4
Seronegative spondylarthropathies	5–10
Rheumatoid arthritis	11
Mixed connective tissue disease	12
Postinfectious arthritis	13, 14
Systemic lupus erythematosus	15
Gastrointestinal	
Celiac disease	16
Ulcerative colitis	17
Crohn's disease	17, 18
Hepatic	
Cirrhosis	2, 19–21
Steatosis	22
Chronic active hepatitis	17
Dermatologic	
Dermatitis herpetiformis	16, 23
Psoriasis	5, 7, 9, 10, 17
Ophthalmologic	
Scleritis	24–26
Hematologic	
Cyclical neutropaenia	27
Mixed cryoglobulinemia	17, 28
Immunothrombocytopenia	29
Polycythemia	17
Neoplastic	
Bronchial carcinoma	30, 31
Laryngeal carcinoma	11
IgA monoclonal gammopathy	17, 32
Mycosis fungoides	33
Mucin-secreting adenocarcinomas	34
Non-Hodgkin lymphoma	17
Unclassified	
Idiopathic pulmonary hemosiderosis	35
Retroperitoneal sclerosis	17
Sarcoidosis	17
Amyloidosis	17
Myasthenia gravis	25
Leprosy	36
Familial properdin deficiency	37
Portal systemic shunts	38

CHRONIC LIVER DISEASES

Morphology and clinical features

For some decades, glomerular changes have been known to exist in patients with cirrhosis of the liver. The changes have mostly consisted of thickening of the mesangial stalk, and they have been defined as hepatic glomerulosclerosis [42]. Manigand et al. [2] were the first to demonstrate the presence of IgG, IgA, and C3 deposits in the glomeruli from three of their four cirrhotic patients. Callard et al. [19] studied cirrhotic patients who had portacaval hypertension. They found glomerular lesions in nine of ten patients; glomerulosclerosis was the main histologic finding. Immunofluorescence microscopy showed massive or limited mesangial, and occasionally capillary, distribution of IgA. The staining with other immunoglobulins was less intense. Electron-microscopic study disclosed the presence of electron-dense granular deposits usually mesangial in location [19]. In some cases, the findings of cirrhotic glomerulosclerosis resembled those of membranoproliferative glomerulonephritis. Notable was that only one patient had clinical symptoms of renal disease [19].

Nochy et al. [22] studied patients with overt glomerulonephritis and liver disease. They had 34 patients, 22 of whom had cirrhosis and 12 sclerosis and/or steatosis. All patients had proteinuria, and microscopic hematuria was a nearly constant finding. The most usual renal morphologic finding was glomerulosclerosis associated with mesangial IgA deposition, this combination being present in 15 patients. Membranoproliferative glomerulonephritis was found in 11 patients, ten of whom had glomerular IgA deposits. Glomerulosclerosis without immune deposits was present in three patients, endocapillary proliferative glomerulonephritis also in three patients, and membranous glomerulonephritis in two patients. All the patients of this series had had a chronic alcoholic excess, and alcohol ingestion always preceded the appearance of the renal disease [22]. Most patients did not have significant portacaval hypertension. Some patients were rebiopsied, and it was found that glomerular IgA deposits, but not glomerular sclerosis, were able to disappear.

In a large study by Berger et al. [20], 100 patients with cirrhosis of the liver were examined postmortem. In 61 cases, granular deposits with IgA as the main immunoglobulin were found in the glomeruli. The amount and the pattern of deposits were not related to the cause of cirrhosis, the presence of Australia antigen, or the existence of portacaval shunt. Even in this group, the glomerular changes did not usually induce urinary abnormalities.

Japanese investigators have demonstrated that the more chronic the course that the liver disease followed, the more frequently a significant glomerular IgA deposition emerged, occurring in 60% of their cirrhotic patients [21]. They observed that the incidence of urinary abnormalities in chronic hepatitis and liver cirrhosis was 1% and 9%, respectively. The type of cirrhosis, alcohol intake, and the presence of hepatoma and HbsAg did not show any relation to the light-microscopic or immunofluorescence findings of the renal biopsies [21].

In a recent report by Sinniah [43], mesangial IgA as the predominant immunoglobulin was found in 36% of the patients with liver cirrhosis. There were no direct correlations between the history of alcoholism and HBs antigen or orceinpositivity in liver cells and the deposition of IgA in the glomerulus in this series, either. In many cases with mesangial IgA deposits, the glomerular light-microscopic finding was normal or only minor changes were present.

Many studies have thus documented the presence of structural abnormalities of glomeruli in patients with various types of chronic liver diseases. The most common histologic picture consists of an increase in mesangial matrix or cellularity. Extracapillary proliferative lesions are very uncommon in this type of IgA nephropathy. Mesangial and sometimes subendothelial IgA deposits are the most common immunofluorescence findings. The immunofluorescence picture is similar to that found in primary IgA nephropathy, except that glomerular IgG and C1q deposits are more often present in patients with hepatic disease [44]. The incidence of IgA nephropathy in patients with liver diseases is uncertain. Recently, Bene et al. [45] presented the view that there is only a very low frequency of renal disease in alcoholic liver cirrhosis. They found mesangial IgA nephropathy in only one patient out of 20 with alcoholic liver cirrhosis and clinical signs of glomerular disease.

Most patients with chronic liver disease are clinically silent. In symptomatic patients, microscopic hematuria and proteinuria are most commonly found, whereas visible hematuria and the nephrotic syndrome are more rare [22]. Renal function impairment is usually associated with membranoproliferative glomerulopathy [22].

Immunopathogenesis

The pathogenetic mechanisms that contribute to renal IgA deposition in chronic liver diseases are not clear yet. It is known that serum IgA concentration is elevated in patients with chronic alcoholic liver disease [46]. This high serum IgA has been related to the glomerular IgA deposition [19], although the relationship between these findings has not been resolved [47]. A general abnormality in IgA metabolism is suggested by the finding of IgA deposition in addition to glomeruli in hepatic sinusoids and capillaries of the gut [48] as well as in superficial dermal capillaries and in choroid plexus [38, 48, 49].

In liver cirrhosis in man, an increase in the proportion of serum polymeric IgA has been observed [44, 50]. According to Kalsi et al. [51], these individuals show significant elevations of the serum levels of both monomeric and polymeric IgA. The results of a Spanish group showed the presence of high amounts of monomeric and polymeric IgA in the serum and also in the kidneys of patients with alcoholic liver disease and IgA nephropathy [52]. According to Delacroix et al. [53], the high serum IgA does not represent immune complexes, whereas Sancho et al. [52] have reported high amounts of IgA to exist partially as immune complexes.

It is possible that alcohol causes injury to the intestinal mucosa that might lead to the absorption of materials normally not absorbed from the intestine.

The presence of antibodies against dietary antigens and intestinal bacterial antigens in the serum of patients with alcoholic liver disease has previously been documented [44, 54, 55]. These findings may be associated with abnormal local IgA immune response and an excessive delivery of IgA presented to the liver via the portal venous system. In this state of hyperimmunization, depending on the metabolic capacity of the liver, elevated serum IgA levels might occur [47]. It is also possible that IgA-containing immune complexes from the intestine might bypass the liver via collateral shunts and induce an IgA response that may lead to glomerular IgA deposition [43].

The elevation of serum IgA in patients with liver diseases is also considered to reflect failure of normal hepatic clearance and/or increased synthesis of polymeric IgA [56]. In experimental works, high levels of serum IgA are known to result in rats with ligated bile ducts [57] and with parenchymal liver damage [58]. Experimental IgA nephropathy has also been observed in rats rendered cirrhotic by carbon tetrachloride [59] or by bile duct ligitation [60]. These findings suggest a central role of liver in IgA clearance in animals; the same is possibly true also in human IgA metabolism. According to Delacroix et al. [53], biliary obstruction in man does not result in significant increase in serum polymeric IgA whereas, in parenchymal liver disease, serum polymeric IgA increases, which in cirrhosis patients correlates with a reduction of the fractional catabolic rates of polymeric IgA. In cirrhotics, the presence or absence of surgical portacaval shunt does not influence the levels of serum polymeric IgA [53].

A third explanation for the elevated serum IgA in cirrhotic patients is enchanced synthesis. Kalsi et al. [51] found that greater amounts of monomeric and polymeric IgA were formed by peripheral blood lymphocytes from patients with cirrhosis compared with normal controls. Recently, McKeever et al. [61] also reported a significant increase in spontaneous IgA synthesis by circulating mononuclear cells in patients with alcoholic liver disease.

An additional mechanism that might lead to mesangial IgA deposits in alcoholic cirrhosis has recently been suggested. Australian investigators have detected antibody reactivity to alcoholic Mallory hyaline in glomerular suspensions from kidneys containing IgA deposit in cirrhotic patients [62].

In addition to the abnormalities in IgA metabolism mentioned above, some other immunologic investigations have shown abnormal findings in patients with IgA nephropathy associated with chronic liver diseases. Serum C3 level has been low in many patients [19, 44] and mixed cryoglobulins have also been detected in several of these patients [20, 22]. The presence of cryoglobulins is usually considered as evidence for circulating immune complexes [22]. The low C3 level that is unusual in primary IgA nephropathy is probably due to increased catabolism and/or decreased synthesis of C3. The presence of circulating C3d has been confirmed in these patients, which suggests increased catabolism and complement activation [63].

GASTROINTESTINAL DISEASES

Celiac disease

A possible pathogenetic relationship between celiac disease and IgA nephropathy is very interesting. It is well known that celiac disease often occurs in association with diseases of immunologic origin [64]. A theory has been suggested that these associated diseases might be related to the immune complexes originating from immunologic reactions in gluten-damaged small-intestinal mucosa [65]. Significant increases in serum IgA have been found in celiac disease, and they are related to the quantity of gluten ingested [66]. IgA-class immune complexes are often present in these patients [67]. These complexes were also detectable in all the three patients with celiac disease and IgA nephropathy previously described by us [16].

In dermatitis herpetiformis, a blistering skin disease characterized by gluten-sensitive enteropathy, IgA deposits found in the skin have recently been shown to be dimeric, since they contain J chain and are able to bind a secretory component [68]. This finding supports the concept that they originate from plasma cells in the small intestine. Further, it is known that the dermal IgA deposits in dermatitis herpetiformis disappear after a gluten-free diet [69]. No data is available at present on the fate of renal IgA during the diet in patients with celiac disease and IgA nephropathy.

It is, however, to be noted that there is probably no uniform abnormality in the mucosal immune system of the small intestine in IgA nephropathy. Westberg et al. [70] performed intestinal biopsies in five IgA nephropathy patients with no history of gastrointestinal disease. They observed that the mean immunocyte number and the mean percentages of cells producing IgA, IgM, and IgG were within normal limits [70].

In a previous article, we reported on a patient with IgA nephropathy and celiac disease who showed no clinical or laboratory evidence of renal disease [16]. We have since performed, systemically, renal fine-needle aspiration biopsies [71] in patients with celiac disease and processed the specimens for immunofluorescence microscopy [72]. We have found asymptomatic glomerular immune deposits in several patients, including some cases with typical findings of IgA nephropathy (manuscript in preparation). In this respect, there seems to be a similarity to IgA nephropathies associated with chronic liver diseases; most patients are asymptomatic. Further studies are needed to explore the association between celiac disease and IgA nephropathy. These should include studies on the effects of gluten-free diet on the clinical and morphologic findings of IgA nephropathy.

Other diseases

Other gastrointestinal diseases have only rarely been reported in IgA nephropathy patients (table 5-1). Our biopsy material includes ten such patients (table 5-2). A previous analysis has, however, showed that gastro-

Table 5-2. Associated diseases found in 125 out of 230 patients with IgA nephropathy

Disease group	Total no. of patients	No. of cases in different disease	Diseases
Dermatologic	35	8	Allergic eczema
		6	Purpura (without other symptoms of Henoch-Schönlein purpura)
		4	Acne rosacea, chronic urticaria, erythema nodosum.
		3	Psoriasis (without arthritis)
		2	Dermatitis herpetiformis, chronic folliculitis, seborrheic dermatitis
Endocrinologic	10	7	Diabetes mellitus
		3	Primary hypothyroidism
Gastrointestinal	10	5	Celiac disease
		2	Ulcerative colitis
		1	Atrophic gastritis, chronic pancreatitis, Menetrier's disease
Hepatic	4	4	Steatosis
Ophthalmologic	14	7	Iritis
		3	Scleritis
		3	Keratoconjunctivitis sicca
Otorhinolaryngologic	17	12	Allergic rhinitis
		3	Chronic maxillary sinuitis
		2	Chronic otitis media
Pulmonary	21	6	Bronchial asthma, pulmonary fibrosis
		3	Chronic bronchitis
		2	Bronchiectasias
		1	Chronic hydrothorax, idiopathic pulmonary hemosiderosis
Rheumatic	31	7	Henoch-Schönlein purpura
		4	Postinfectious arthritis, rheumatoid arthritis
		3	Gout, systemic lupus erythematosus
		2	Polymyalgia rheumatica, psoriatic arthritis, unclassified collagenosis
		1	Ankylosing spondylitis, juvenile rheumatoid arthritis, Reiter's syndrome, sacroilitis, scleroderma
Neoplastic	8	3	Bronchial carcinoma
		1	Carcinoma of the tongue, nasopharyngeal papilloma, pancreatic carcinoma, renal adenocarcinoma, retroperitoneal liposarcoma
Unclassified	8	2	Paroxysmal angioedema
		1	Amyloidosis, chronic osteomyelitis, porphyria, primary pulmonary hypertension, retroperitoneal fibrosis, thrombocytopenia.

intestinal diseases are statistically significantly more often present in patients with IgA nephropathy than in those with other mesangial glomerulonephritis [73].

RHEUMATIC DISEASES

Henoch-Schönlein purpura

In addition to the description of a new primary glomerulonephritis, IgA nephropathy, Berger also demonstrated that, in Henoch-Schönlein purpura, the glomerular immune deposits contain mainly IgA [1]. A close relationship between primary IgA nephropathy and Henoch-Schönlein purpura nephritis has since been documented by many authors, and these diseases are often held to be parts of a spectrum of diseases, with IgA nephritis on one side and purpura nephritis on the other side with more systemic manifestations [3, 4, 74, 75]. A certain clinical spectrum can be also seen in our own material, as seven patients had a fully developed Henoch-Schönlein purpura and six had only a purpuric rash in addition to IgA nephropathy (table 5-2). A detailed analysis of the relationship between Henoch-Schönlein purpura and IgA nephropathy is presented in chapter 4 of this book.

Seronegative spondylarthropathies

In 1975, Sissons et al. [5] described a group of 25 IgA nephropathy patients, of whom one patient had ankylosing spondylitis. This rheumatic disease has since been found by several authors to coexist with IgA nephropathy [6–10]. Both the reports by Bailey et al. [6] and Jennette et al. [7] included two patients with ankylosing spondylitis and, in the latter one, there was a third patient with "incomplete Reiter's syndrome."

The exact incidence of IgA nephropathy in association with ankylosing spondylitis is unknown [9]. In a previous Finnish study by Linder and Pasternack [76], glomerular immunoglobulin and C3 deposits were found in all of nine patients with ankylosing spondylitis. Unfortunately, the specimens were not examined with an antiserum against IgA, so a possible finding of IgA nephropathy in these cases remained obscure. A pathogenetic relationship between ankylosing spondylitis and IgA nephropathy is possibly suggested by the finding of raised levels of serum IgA in patients with ankylosing spondylitis [77–79]. Further, increased IgA has been found to associate with active inflammatory disease [78]. These observations have been considered to suggest that a microbial triggering agent acting across an IgA-secreting organ (gut) is involved in the pathogenesis of ankylosing spondylitis [78], as is also possible in IgA nephropathy.

According to our own experience, it seems that, in addition to ankylosing spondylitis, even other types of seronegative spondylarthropathies are associated with IgA nephropathy. Three of our four IgA nephropathy patients with postinfectious arthritis had post-*Yersinia* arthropathy (table 5-2).

This postenteric arthropathy has been previously described in two reports to associate with IgA nephropathy [13, 14]. Interesting in this connection is the finding by Granfors [80] of a prolonged IgA response in those patients with *Yersinia* infection who develop arthritis, compared with those who do not.

In addition to the diseases mentioned above, there are some other representatives of seronegative spondylarthropathies [81] among our IgA nephropathy patients (table 5-2): two cases of psoriatic arthritis, one of Reiter's disease, one of sacroilitis, and one of juvenile rheumatoid arthritis (Still's disease). It has been suggested that the association of seronegative spondylarthropathies with IgA nephropathy could be due to the fact that both diseases result from abnormal mucosal immune response [7]. Interesting also was a recent report by Lagrue et al. [10] where the therapy of seronegative spondylarthritis was shown to be benefical also for symptoms of IgA nephropathy.

It is noteworthy, however, that not all patients with seronegative spondylarthropathies and renal abnormalities have IgA nephropathy. Recently a case with mesangial IgM nephropathy was described in a patient with spondylarthropathy [82].

Systemic lupus erythematosus

Renal biopsy specimens of lupus nephropathy patients often contain IgA deposits [1]. Some authors consider that, in systemic lupus erythematosus, glomerular IgG and C1q are always present in greater amounts than IgA [3, 83]. Among our patients with IgA nephropathy (table 5-2), however, there were three patients whose rheumatic disease fulfilled the diagnostic criteria of systemic lupus erythematosus, which suggests that, in some cases, lupus nephritis can have the morphologic features of IgA nephropathy. The same has previously been noted by Spargo et al. [15]. This renal morphologic finding is, however, unusual also in our total renal biopsy material, which contains about 30 cases of lupus nephritis. It has previously been found that histologic and ultrastructural findings and the polyclonal deposition of immunoglobulins suggest a certain similarity between IgA nephropathy and autoimmune collagen diseases [84, 85]. Interesting was the finding of Japanese workers of the presence of a cold-reacting antinuclear antibody, mainly of IgM class, in patients with IgA nephropathy [85]. This finding was considered to suggest that some autoimmune factors play a role in IgA nephropathy [85]. It is also known that the serum IgA level is sometimes very high in patients with lupus nephritis and glomerular IgA deposits [86]. The occurrence of IgA nephropathy in systemic lupus has been thought to reflect the heterogeneity of mesangial IgA nephropathy [87].

Other rheumatic diseases

Four patients with rheumatoid arthritis (two definite and two classic) and IgA nephropathy were included among our patients (table 5-2). We do not know, of course, if the association between IgA nephropathy and rheumatoid arthritis is real or only fortuitous. It is also possible that IgA nephropathy could in some cases represent some form of gold-induced glomerular disease. In two of our four patients, the renal disease manifested itself during the treatment of parenteral gold therapy.

It is interesting that in our series (table 5-2) there were two cases of polymylalgia rheumatica and one with scleroderma, whose renal biopsy showed typical features of IgA nephropathy. These diseases have not previously been described in association with IgA nephropathy.

In summary, the data from the literature and our own experience suggest that there is an association of many types of autoimmune collagen diseases with IgA nephropathy. Further studies are necessary to examine, e.g., how the therapy of these systemic diseases influences the clinical manifestations and the course of IgA nephropathy.

DISEASES OF THE EYE

The first report on an association between IgA nephropathy and ophthalmologic diseases was presented in 1980 [24]. A group of 113 patients with various types of primary glomerular diseases was described and, among these, six patients exhibited deep scleritis or episcleritis. All six of these patients were found to have IgA nephropathy. Nomoto et al. [24] found that the patients with scleritis were significantly older than those without scleritis; the reason for this remained obscure. The authors suggested that IgA nephropathy is associated with some autoimmune alterations.

Recently the above findings were confirmed by French workers [26]. In their material, scleritis was present in 18% of IgA nephropathy patients. It was found in 15% of those of Nomoto et al. [24]. Also in the French series other causes of scleritis were not found in the patients. The same authors have since described a patient with Berger's disease and frequent episodes of episcleritis, in whom numerous dimeric IgA-secreting cells were demonstrated in the episcleral inflammatory infiltrate [88]. They also found a clear association between episodes of episcleritis and hematuria in this patient. The hypothesis was presented that a generalized abnormality of mucosal response may exist in some patients with IgA nephropathy.

In our material, there were six nephropathy patients with scleritis (table 5-2). Our findings thus agree with those of Nomoto et al. [24] and De Ligny et al. [26], even though the prevalence of scleritis in our series was lower than in the other two.

We have seen in the literature no previous reports on the coexistence of IgA nephropathy and iritis. Our present group included seven patients with iritis (table 5-2). Interestingly enough, four of these patients had no other systemic diseases known to be associated with iritis. Three patients with keratoconjunctivitis sicca and IgA nephropathy were observed in our series.

A high serum level of polymeric IgA has recently been found in the sicca syndrome [53].

Episcleritis is known to occur often in patients with various autoimmune collagen diseases such as rheumatoid arthritis, periarteritis nodosa, and Wegener's granulomatosis or with infectious and/or allergic disorders [89]. The association of iritis with various rheumatic diseases is also well known. The finding of scleritis, iritis, and keratoconjunctivitis sicca in several patients with IgA nephropathy clearly suggests the systemic nature of IgA nephropathy.

NEOPLASTIC DISEASES

The original report of paraneoplastic glomerulonephritis was published 20 years ago [90]. Since then, many authors have found that the most common clinical manifestation of paraneoplastic glomerulonephritis is the nephrotic syndrome. The histopathologic finding in patients with carcinoma has usually been membranous glomerulonephritis, whereas the minimal-change lesion has been most common when lymphomas have been associated with the nephrotic syndrome [91–93]. Other morphologic pictures, e.g., focal or diffuse proliferative glomerulonephritis, have been found only exceptionally in patients with neoplasms [94].

The first documentation of a relationship between IgA nephropathy and a malignant disease was that by Cairns et al. [30], who described two patients with bronchial squamous cell carcinoma and Henoch-Schönlein purpura. It was notable that, in one of their patients, the renal symptoms resolved rapidly after the operative therapy of the tumor. Various other tumors have since been found in association with IgA nephropathy. In a series described by Burkholder et al. [11], there was a patient with IgA nephropathy who also had laryngeal carcinoma. Dosa et al. [32] have described a patient with relapsing Henoch-Schönlein purpura and IgA monoclonal gammopathy. During therapy, all clinical manifestations including those of IgA nephropathy resolved simultaneously with the disappearance of the light chains. This suggested that there was one underlying mechanism common to the development of all manifestations [32]. Ramirez et al. [33] described two IgA nephropathy patients who also had mycosis fungoides, a malignancy that primarily affects the skin, and in which T-cell helper activity is increased. In 1982, Sinniah [34] reported subclinical IgA nephropathy in several patients with mucin-secreting adenocarcinomas of lung, stomach, large intestine, and pancreas. At autopsy, eight out of 11 patients with mucin-secreting cancers had heavy glomerular IgA deposits, whereas 35 of those with non-mucin-secreting cancers were negative for IgA deposits [34]. A recent series published by Makdassy et al. [17] contained a patient with IgA nephropathy and non-Hodgkin lymphoma.

Our own renal biopsy material includes eight patients with IgA nephropathy and a neoplastic disease (table 5-2). These neoplasms are histogenetically different but, with respect to their location, it is interesting that most of them affect mucosal membranes. Moreover, the neoplasms are such as have earlier been shown to associate with high serum IgA levels [95–97]. It is possible that increased IgA production in these patients represents a non-specific response to chronic mucosal irritation or a response to a specific tumor antigen. Neoplastic diseases affecting mucosal membranes and IgA nephropathy may thus be pathogenetically related. We have previously calculated that, among old patients with IgA nephropathy, neoplastic diseases are found clearly more often than expected [94]. There is probably an analogy to membranous glomerulonephritis, which, in adults over 60 years of age, has been found to be associated with a neoplastic disease in 22% of the cases [98]. We thus regard it as important to take into account the possibility of a neoplastic disease when IgA nephropathy is diagnosed in an elderly patient. Especially neoplasms that affect the respiratory tract should be noted in this respect.

Most of the previous studies on paraneoplastic glomerulonephritides deal with patients with the nephrotic syndrome. Because in IgA nephropathy the nephrotic syndrome is present only rarely [99], the potential cases with paraneoplastic IgA nephropathy should be sought among patients with hematuria and slight proteinuria, the clinical findings typical of IgA nephropathy. It must also be remembered that previous studies have often shown paraneoplastic glomerular immune deposits in patients with no clinical renal abnormalities [100, 101] as was also seen in the cases with glomerular IgA deposits reported by Sinniah [34].

PULMONARY DISEASES

Acute infectious respiratory diseases often induce clinical exacerbations in IgA nephropathy patients. Chronic pulmonary diseases, however, have only exceptionally been connected to IgA nephropathy (table 5-1). Yum et al. [35] have described IgA nephropathy in a patient with idiopathic pulmonary hemosiderosis. A similar patient was included in our own material (table 5-2). In addition to this patient, there were 20 other patients with various chronic pulmonary diseases and IgA nephropathy among our patients (table 5-2). A pathologic serum IgA level has previously been found in at least chronic bronchitis [102], pulmonary fibrosis [103], sarcoidosis [104], and idiopathic pulmonary hemosiderosis [105], findings that may speak in favor of a pathogenetic relationship between these diseases and IgA nephropathy. Further, in our previous analysis, we found that pulmonary diseases were quite often present in IgA nephropathy patients [73].

OUR OWN MATERIAL

Patients were selected from the renal biopsy material of Tampere University Central Hospital during the years 1976–1985. Biopsy specimens were processed as previously described [99]. In 230 specimens, IgA was the sole or main glomerular immunofluorescence finding, the IgA being granular in nature and distributed totally or mainly in mesangial regions. The 230 patients with IgA nephropathy included 148 males and 82 females aged 10–76 years (mean, 40 years) at the time of renal biopsy.

In table 5-2, the diseases found in 125 (54%) out of 230 IgA nephropathy patients are presented. These diseases do not include various infectious diseases that were often found to provoke the clinical manifestations of IgA nephropathy.

DISCUSSION

IgA nephropathy exists as a primary glomerulonephritis (Berger's disease), and is quite often associated with various other diseases. Henoch-Schönlein purpura is a syndrome in which IgA nephropathy is so regular that it has been suggested that only those patients who have IgA in their mesangium really have Henoch-Schönlein purpura [106]. Other well-known associations are chronic liver diseases, both alcoholic and nonalcoholic, in which, however, even types of glomerular damage other than IgA nephropathy can be seen. And finally there is a large group of diseases which, according to more or less sporadic case reports, have been associated with IgA nephropathy. In this last group, the associations have not yet been clarified and, in some cases, they may be merely a chance occurrence of IgA nephropathy as a common disease in many countries [107]. It should be noted, however, that, both in the material of Makdassy et al. [17] and in ours (table 5-2), more than half of the IgA nephropathy patients had one or more associated disease. In a previous analysis, we observed that the patients with IgA nephropathy have significantly more coexisting diseases than do patients with mesangial glomerulonephritis of other types [73]. In the following disease groups, the prevalence of diseases found in IgA nephropathy patients was statistically higher than that in control glomerulonephritic patients: gastrointestinal, pulmonary, and unclassified diseases [73].

In another study, we examined whether there are any differences in the clinical, histopathologic, and immunologic features of IgA nephropathy between the patient groups with associated diseases and those without any extrarenal diseases [108]. The only differences were higher prevalence of renal interstitial cell infiltrates and IgA deposited along glomerular capillary walls in patients with associated diseases. No differences were observed in the severity or prognosis of IgA nephropathy between these two groups of patients [108].

The presence of IgA deposits in dermal and skeletal muscle vessels and in the capillaries of the gut in IgA nephropathy patients has been documented in several studies [109–113]. These findings, as well as raised serum IgA levels, have been considered to point to IgA nephropathy as a systemic disease [40]. High serum IgA is often found in patients with primary IgA nephropathy

[114] and also in several of the diseases found to be associated with IgA nephropathy (tables 5-1 and 5-2): Henoch-Schönlein purpura [3], alcoholic liver diseases [46], celiac disease [66], ankylosing spondylitis [78], psoriatic arthritis [115], scleroderma [116], systemic lupus erythematosus [86], rheumatoid arthritis [53], sicca syndrome [53], idiopathic pulmonary hemosiderosis [105], chronic bronchitis [102], pulmonary fibrosis [103], bronchial carcinoma [96], and oral cancer [95]. These findings can be an expression of generally disturbed IgA metabolism present in some patients with these associated diseases and IgA nephropathy. Egido et al. [117] have shown that mitogen-stimulated peripheral blood lymphocytes from patients with IgA nephropathy produce in vitro increased amounts of IgA. The results of an investigation made by Endoh et al. [118] suggested that these patients might also in vivo be high responders of IgA antibody production. In our own vaccination study with mumps virus vaccine, it emerged that IgA nephropathy patients reacted with a higher and more long-lasting IgA response than did patients with IgM glomerulonephritis and the controls [119]. Further, we observed a correlation between the specific IgA response and the original serum IgA level in IgA nephropathy [119]. At present, however, the possible causal relationships between associated diseases and IgA nephropathy are largely undefined. They have been studied most extensively in patients with IgA nephropathy associated with chronic liver diseases, but are still far from resolved even in this type of IgA nephropathy.

Further, it is probable that there are differences in the characteristics (size and subclass) of IgA itself in the different forms of IgA nephropathies. In chronic parenchymal liver diseases, a significant increase in the proportion of serum polymeric IgA has been found [44, 50, 53] whereas, in primary IgA nephropathy, the results have been rather conflicting. In IgA subclasses, a predominance of IgA2 has been observed in the serum and mesangium of patients with alcoholic cirrhosis [53, 120] whereas, in primary IgA nephropathy, Henoch-Schönlein purpura, and systemic lupus erythematosus, the serum and tissue IgA has been identified to be mainly IgA1 [53, 121, 122]. Further studies may lead to exact distinctions between different IgA nephropathies and IgA-associated diseases [47]. It is likewise possible that different IgA nephropathies may have different pathogenetic mechanisms. Australian investigators have divided secondary forms of IgA nephropathy into those with increased antigen uptake (celiac disease, dermatitis herpetiformis), decreased clearance of immune complexes (alcoholic cirrhosis), and increased production of IgA (IgA paraproteinemia) [18, 123]. In addition to primary IgA nephropathy (Berger's disease) and the secondary forms of IgA nephropathy mentioned above, there may exist a large group of syndromes in which IgA nephropathy and various extrarenal clinical manifestations are present together as a reaction to some (unknown) antigenic stimulus.

REFERENCES

1. Berger J: IgA glomerular deposits in renal disease. Transplant Proc: 1:939–944, 1969.
2. Manigand G, Morel-Maroger L, Simon J, Deparis M: Lésions rénales glomérulaires et cirrhose du foie: note préliminaire sur les lésions histologiques de rein au cours des cirrhoses hépatiques, d'après 20 prélevements biopsiques. Rev Eur Etud Clin Biol 15:989–996, 1970.
3. Nakamoto Y, Hattori N, Yakeuchi J: Primary IgA glomerulonephritis and Schönlein-Henoch purpura nephritis: clinicopathological and immunohistological characteristics. Q J Med 48:495–516, 1978.
4. Weiss JH, Bhathena DB, Curtis JJ, Lucas BA, Luke RG: A possible relationship between Henoch-Schönlein syndrome and IgA nephropathy (Berger's disease). Nephron 22:582–591, 1978.
5. Sissons JGP, Woodrow DF, Curtis JR, Evans DJ, Gower PE, Sloper JC, Peters DK: Isolated glomerulonephritis with mesangial IgA deposits. Br Med J 3:611–614, 1975.
6. Bailey RR, Burry AF, McGiven AR, Kirk JA, Laing JK, Moller P: A renal lesion in ankylosing spondylitis. Nephron 26:171–173, 1980.
7. Jennette JC, Ferguson AL, Moore MA, Freeman DG. IgA nephropathy associated with seronegative spondylarthopathies. Arthritis Rheum 25:144–149, 1982.
8. Dard S, Kenouch S, Mery JPh, Baumelou A, Beaufils H: Une nouvelle association: spondylarthrite ankylosante et maladie de Berger. Néphrologie 3:183, 1982.
9. Krothapalli R, Neeland B, Small S, Duffy WB, Gyorkey F, Senekjian HO. IgA nephropathy in a patient with ankylosing spondylitis and a solitary kidney. Clin Nephrol 21:134–137, 1984.
10. Lagrue G, Bruneau C, Intrator L, Laurent J: IgA nephropathy associated with seronegative spondylarthropathies: efficacy of non steroidal anti-inflammatory drugs (NSAIDs). Clin Nephrol 23:107–108, 1985.
11. Burkholder PM, Zimmermann SW, Moorthy AV: A clinicopathologic study of the natural history of mesangial IgA nephropathy. In: Yoshitoshiy, Ueda (eds) Glomerulonephritis. Baltimore: University Park Press, 1979.
12. Brun C, Olsen S: Atlas of renal biopsy. Copenhagen: Munksgaard, 1981, p 110.
13. Forsström J, Viander M, Lehtonen A, Ekfors T: *Yersinia enterocolitica* infection complicated by glomerulonephritis. Scand J Infect Dis 9:253–256, 1977.
14. Cusack D, Martin P, Schinittger T, McCafferky M, Keane C, Keogh B: IgA nephropathy in association with *Yersinia enterocolitica*. Irish J Med Sci 152:311–312, 1983.
15. Spargo BH, Seymour AE, Ordonez NG: Mesangial proliferative glomerulonephritis. In: Renal biopsy pathology with diagnostic and therapeutic implications, New York: John Wiley and Sons, 1980, pp 71–82.
16. Helin H, Mustonen J, Reunala T, Pasternack A: IgA nephropathy associated with celiac disease and dermatitis herpetiformis. Arch Pathol Lab Med 107:324–327, 1983.
17. Makdassy R, Beaufils M, Meyrier A, Mignon F, Molonguet-Doleris L, Richet G: Pathologic conditions associated with IgA mesangial nephropathy: preliminary results. Contrib Nephrol 40:292–295, 1984.
18. Clarkson AR, Woodroffe AJ, Bannister KM, Lomax-Smith JD, Aarons I: The syndrome of IgA nephropathy. Clin Nephrol 21:7–14, 1984.
19. Callard P, Feldmann G, Prandi D, Belair MF, Mandet C, Weiss Y, Druet P, Benhamou JP, Bariety J: Immune complex type glomerulonephritis in cirrhosis of the liver. Am J Pathol 80:329–340, 1975.
20. Berger J, Yaneva H, Nabarra B: Glomerular changes in patients with cirrhosis of the liver. Adv Nephrol 7:3–14, 1978.
21. Nakamoto Y, Iida H, Kobayashi K, Dohi K, Kida H, Hattori N, Takeuchi J: Hepatic glomerulonephritis: characteristics of hepatic IgA glomerulonephritis as the major part. Virchows Archiv [Pathol Anat] 392:45–54, 1981.
22. Nochy D, Callard P, Bellon B, Bariety J, Druet P: Association of overt glomerulonephritis and liver disease: a study of 34 patients. Clin Nephrol 6:422–427, 1976.
23. Pape JF, Mellbye OJ, Oystese B, Browall EK: Glomerulonephritis in dermatitis herpetiformis. Acta Med Scand 203:445–448, 1978.
24. Nomoto Y, Sakai H, Endoh M, Tomino Y: Scleritis and IgA nephropathy. Arch Intern Med 140:783–785, 1980.

25. Endoh M, Kaneshige H, Tomino Y, Nomoto Y, Sakai H, Arimori S, Shinbo T, Ishihara T: IgA nephropathy associated with myasthenia gravis and scleritis. Tokai J Exp Clin Med 6:421–425, 1981.
26. De Ligny BH, Sirbat D, Bene MC, Faure G, Kessler M: Scleritis associated with glomerulonephritis. Nephron 35:207, 1983.
27. Nash H, Binns GF, Clarkson AR, Beare TH: Concomitant IgA nephropathy and cyclical neutropaenia. Aust NZ J Med 8:184–188, 1978.
28. Hookerjee BK, Maddison PJ, Reichlin M: Mesangial IgA-IgG deposition in mixed cryoglobulinemia. Am J Med Sci 276:221–225, 1978.
29. Spichtin HP, Truniger B, Mihatsch MJ, Bucher U, Gudat F, Zollinger HU: Immunothrombocytopenia and IgA nephritis. Clin Nephrol 14:304–308, 1980.
30. Cairns SA, Mallick NP, Lawler W, Williams G: Squamous cell carcinoma of bronchus presenting with Henoch-Schönlein purpura. Br Med J 2:474–475, 1978.
31. Mustonen J, Helin H, Pasternack A: IgA nephropathy associated with bronchial small-cell carcinoma. Am J Clin Pathal 76:652–656, 1981.
32. Dosa S, Cairns SA, Mallick NP, Lawler W, Willians G: Relapsing Henoch-Schönlein syndrome with renal involvement in a patient with IgA monoclonal gammopathy. Nephron 26:145–148, 1980.
33. Ramirez G, Stinson JB, Zawada ET, Moatamed F: IgA nephritis associated with mycosis fungoides. Arch Intern Med 141:1287–1291, 1981.
34. Sinniah R: Mucin-secreting cancer with mesangial IgA deposits. Pathology 14:303–308, 1982.
35. Yum MN, Lampton LM, Bloom PM, Edwards JL: Asymptomatic IgA nephropathy associated with pulmonary hemosiderosis. Am J Med 64:1056–1060, 1978.
36. Valles M, Cantarell C, Fort J, Carrera M: IgA nephropathy in leprosy. Arch Intern Med 142:1238, 1982.
37. Wyatt RJ, Julian BA, Galla JH: Properdin deficiency with IgA nephropathy. N Engl J Med 305:1097, 1981.
38. Woodroffe AJ: IgA, glomerulonephritis and liver disease. Aust NZ J Med [Suppl 1] 11:109–111, 1981.
39. Battle DC: IgA glomerulonephritis, asymptomatic hematuria, and systemic disease. Arch Intern Med 141:1264–1265, 1981.
40. Cameron JS: Glomerulonephritis in renal transplants. Transplantation 34:237–245, 1982.
41. Churg J, Sobin LH: Classification and atlas of glomerular diseases Tokyo: Igaku-Shoin, 1982.
42. Bloodworth JBM, Sommers SC: Cirrhotic glomerulosclerosis: a renal lesion associated with hepatic cirrhosis. Lab Invest 8:962–978, 1959.
43. Sinniah R: Heterogenous IgA glomerulonephropathy in liver cirrhosis. Histopathology 8:947–962, 1984.
44. Woodroffe AJ, Gormly AA, McKenzie PE, Wootton AM, Thompson AJ, Seymour AE, Clarkson AR: Immunologic studies in IgA nephropathy. Kidney Int 18:366–374, 1980.
45. Bene MC, Faure G, De Korvin J, De Ligny B, Kessler M, Gaucher P, Duheille J: Renal and hepatic immunohistopathology of cirrhosis [abstr] Kidney Int 26:227, 1984.
46. Lee FJ: Immunoglobulins in viral hepatitis and active alcoholic liver disease. Lancet 2:1043–1046, 1965.
47. Van de Wiel A, Schurrman HJ, Kater L: Immunoglobulin A in alcoholic liver disease. Contrib Nephrol 40:276–282, 1984.
48. Kater L, Jöbsis AC, Baart de la Faille-Kuyper EH, Vogten AJM, Grijm R: Alcoholic hepatic disease: specificity of IgA deposits in liver. Am J Clin Pathol 71:51–57, 1979.
49. Swerdlow MA, Chowdhury LN, Mishra V, Kavin H: IgA deposits in skin in alocholic liver disease. J Am Acad Dermatol 9:232–236, 1983.
50. Kutteh WH, Prince SJ, Phillips JO, Spenney JG, Mestecky J: Properties of immunoglobulin A in serum of individuals with liver diseases and in hepatic bile. Gastroenterology 82:184–193, 1982.
51. Kalsi J, Delacroix DL, Hodgson HJF: IgA in alcoholic cirrhoisis. Clin Exp Immunol 52:499–504, 1983.
52. Sancho J, Egido J, Sanchez-Crespo M, Blasco R: Detection of monomeric and polymeric IgA containing immune complexes in serum and kidney from patients with alcoholic liver disease. Clin Exp Immunol 47:327–335, 1981.

53. Delacroix DL, Elkon KB, Geubel AP, Hodgson HF, Dive C, Vaerman JP: Changes in size, subclass, and metabolic properties of serum immunoglobulin A in liver diseases and in other diseases with high serum immunoglobulin A. J Clin Invest 71:358–367, 1983.
54. Bjørneboe M, Prytz H, Ørskov F: Antibodies to intestinal microbes in serum of patients with cirrhosis of the liver. Lancet 1:58–63, 1972.
55. Triger DR, Alp MH, Wright R: Bacterial and dietary antibodies in liver diseases. Lancet 1:60–63, 1972.
56. Chandy KG, Hubscher SG, Elias E, Berg J, Khan M: Dual role of the liver in regulating circulating polymeric IgA in man: studies on patients with liver disease. Clin Exp Immunol 52:207–218, 1983.
57. Orlans E, Peppard J, Reynolds J, Hall JG: Rapid active transport of IgA from blood to bile in rats. J Exp Med 147:588–602, 1978.
58. Kaartinen M: Liver damage in mice and rats causes ten-fold increase of blood immunoglobulin A. Scand J Immunol 7:519–522, 1978.
59. Gormly AA, Smith PS, Seymour AE, Clarkson AR, Woodroffe AJ: IgA glomerular deposits in experimental cirrhosis. Am J Pathol 104:50–54, 1981.
60. Melvin T, Burke B, Michael AF, Kim Y: Experimental IgA nephropathy in bile duct ligated rats. Clin Immunol Immunopathol 27:369–377, 1983.
61. McKeever U, O'Mahony C, Whelan CA, Weir DG: Helper and suppressor T-lymphocyte function in severe alcoholic liver disease. Clin Exp Immunol 60:39–48, 1985.
62. Woodroffe AJ: Discussion. Contrib Nephrol 40:296–301, 1984.
63. Nochy D, Druet P, Bariety J: IgA nephropathy in chronic liver disease. Contrib Nephrol 40:268–275, 1984.
64. Cooper BT, Holmes GKT, Cooke WT: Coeliac disease and immunologic disorders. Br Med J 1:537–539, 1978.
65. Scott BR, Losowsky MS: Celiac disease: a cause of various associated diseases? Lancet 2:596–957, 1975.
66. Asquith P, Thompson RA, Cooke WT: Serum-immunoglobulins in adult coeliac disease. Lancet 2:129–131, 1969.
67. Hall RP, Strober W, Katz SI, Lawley TJ: IgA-containing circulating immune complexes in gluten-sensitive enteropathy. Clin Exp Immunol 45:234–239, 1981.
68. Unsworth DJ, Payne AW, Leonard JN, Fry L, Holborow EJ: IgA in dermatitis-herpetiformis skin is dimeric. Lancet 1:478–480, 1982.
69. Leonard J, Halffenden G, Tucker W, Unsworth J, Swain F, McMinn R, Holborow J, Fry L: Gluten challenge in dermatitis herpetiformis. N Engl J Med 308:816–819, 1983.
70. Westberg NG, Baklien K, Schmekel B, Gillberg R, Brandtzaeg P: Quantitation of immunoglobulin-producing cells in small intestinal mucosa of patients with IgA nephropathy. Clin Immunol Immunopathol 26:442–445, 1983.
71. Pasternack A, Helin H, Törnroth T, Rantala I, Väisänen J, Rahka R: Aspiration biopsy of the kidney with a new fine needle: a way to obtain glomeruli for morphological study. Clin Nephrol 10:79–84, 1978.
72. Rantala I, Laasonen A, Pasternack A, Mustonen J: Immunofluorescence microscopy of paraffin-embedded human kidney specimens obtained by fine-needle aspiration biopsy. Am J Clin Pathol 79:489–492, 1983.
73. Mustonen J: IgA glomerulonephritis and associated diseases. Ann Clin Res 16:161–166, 1984.
74. Glassock RJ, Cohen AH, Bennett CM, Martinez-Maldonado M: In: Brenner BM, Rector FC (eds) The kidney. Philadelphia: WB Saunders, 1981, pp 1400–1401.
75. Meadow SR, Scott DG: Berger disease: Henoch-Schönlein syndrome without the rash. J Pediatr 106:27–32, 1985.
76. Linder E, Pasternack A: Immunofluorescence studies on kidney biopsies in ankylosing spondylitis. Acta Pathol Microbiol Scand [B] 78:517–525, 1970.
77. Kinsella TD, Espinoza L, Vasey FB: Serum complement and immunoglobulin levels in sporadic and familial ankylosing spondylitis. J Rheumatol 2:308–313, 1975.
78. Cowling P, Ebringer R, Ebringer A: Association of inflammation with raised serum IgA in ankylosing spondylitis. Ann Rheum Dis 39:545–549, 1980.
79. Calguneri M, Swinburne L, Shinebaum R, Cooke EM, Wright V: Secretory IgA: immune defence pattern in ankylosing spondylitis and klebsiella. Ann Rheum Dis 40:600–604, 1981.
80. Granfors K: Measurement of immunoglobulin M (IgM), IgG, and IgA antibodies against

Yersinia enterocolitica by enzyme-linked immunosorbent assay: persistence of serum antibodies during disease. J Clin Microbiol 9:336–341, 1979.
81. Wright V: A unifying concept for the spondylarthropathies. Clin Orthop 143:8–14, 1979.
82. Steinsson K, Hirszel P, Weinstein A: Mesangial IgM nephropathy in a patient with HLA-B27 spondylarthropathy. Arthritis Rheum 26:1056, 1983.
83. Baldwin DS, Gluck MC, Lowenstein J, Gallo GR: Lupus nephritis: clinical course as related to morphologic forms and their transitions. Am J Med 62:12–30, 1977.
84. Burkholder PM: Nephritis associated with systemic lupus erythematosus. In: Atlas of human glomerular pathology. New York: Harper and Row, 1974.
85. Nomoto Y, Sakai H: Cold-reacting antinuclear factor in sera from patients with IgA nephropathy. J Lab Clin Med 94:76–87, 1979.
86. Whitworth JA, Leibowitz S, Kennedy MC, Cameron JS, Chantler C: IgA and glomerular disease. Clin Nephrol 5:33–36, 1976.
87. Cameron JS: Discussion. Contrib Nephrol 40:296–301, 1984.
88. Bene MC, De Ligny BH, Sirbat D, Faure G, Kessler M, Duheille J: IgA nephropathy: dimeric IgA-secreting cells are present in episcleral infiltrate. Am J Clin Pathol 82:608–611, 1984.
89. McGavin DDM, Williamson J, Forrester FV: Episcleritis and scleritis. Br J Ophthalmol 60:192–226, 1976.
90. Lee JC, Yamauchi H, Hopper J: The association of cancer and the nephrotic syndrome. Ann Intern Med 64:41–51, 1966.
91. Eagen JW, Lewis EJ: Glomerulopathies of neoplasia. Kidney Int 11:297–306, 1977.
92. Gagliano RG, Costanzi JJ, Beathard GA, Sarles HE, Bell JD: The nephrotic syndrome associated with neoplasia: an unusual paraneoplastic syndrome. Am J Med 60:1026–1031, 1976.
93. Glassock RJ, Friedler RM, Massry SG: Kidney and electrolytic disturbances in neoplastic diseases. Contrib Nephrol 7:2–41, 1977.
94. Mustonen J, Pasternack A, Helin H: IgA mesangial nephropathy in neoplastic diseases. Contrib Nephrol 40:283–291, 1984.
95. Brown AM, Lally ET, Frankel A, Harwick R, Davis LW, Rominger CJ: The association of the IgA levels of serum and whole saliva with the progression of oral cancer. Cancer 35:1154–1162, 1975.
96. Krant MJ, Manskopf GM, Brandrup CS, Madoff MA: Immunologic alterations in bronchogenic cancer. Cancer 21:623–631, 1968.
97. Wara WM, Ammann AJ, Wara DW, Phillips TL: Serum IgA in the diagnosis of nasopharyngeal and paranasal sinus carcinoma. Radiology 116:409–411, 1975.
98. Zech P, Colon S, Pointet P, Deteix P, Labeeuw M, Leitienne P: The nephrotic syndrome in adults aged over 60: etiology, evolution and treatment of 76 cases. Clin Nephrol 18:232–236, 1982.
99. Mustonen J, Pasternack A, Rantala I: The nephrotic syndrome in IgA glomerulonephritis: response to corticosteroid therapy. Clin Nephrol 20:172–176, 1983.
100. Pascal RR, Innaccone PM, Rollwagen FM, Harding TA, Bennet SJ: Electron microscopy and immunofluorescence of glomerular immune deposits in cancer patients. Cancer Res 36:43–47, 1976.
101. Helin H, Pasternack A, Hakala T, Penttinen K, Wager O: Glomerular electron-dense deposits and circulating immune complexes in patients with malignant tumours. Clin Nephrol 14:23–30, 1980.
102. Falk GA, Siskind GW, Smith JP: Immunoglobulin elevations in the serum of patients with chronic bronchitis and emphysema. J Immunol 105:1559–1562, 1970.
103. Schwartz RH: Serum immunoglobulin levels in cystic fibrosis. Am J Dis Child 111:408–411, 1966.
104. Daniele RP, Daubert JH, Rossman MD: Immunologic abnormalities in sarcoidosis. Ann Intern Med 92:406–416, 1980.
105. Valassi-Adam H, Rouska A, Karpouzas J, Matsaniotis N: Raised IgA in idiopathic pulmonary haemosiderosis. Arch Dis Child 50:320–323, 1975.
106. Habib R: Discussion. Contrib Nephrol 40:264–267, 1984.
107. Kincaid-Smith P, Nicholls K: Mesangial IgA nephropathy. Am J Kidney Dis 3:90–102, 1983.

108. Mustonen J, Pasternack A, Helin H, Nikkilä M: Clinicopathologic correlations in a series of 143 patients with IgA glomerulonephritis. Am J Nephrol 5:150–157, 1985.
109. Tsai CC, Giangiacomo J, Zuckner J: Dermal IgA deposits in Henoch-Schönlein purpura and Berger's nephritis. Lancet 1:342–343, 1975.
110. Baart de la Faille-Kuyper EH, Kater L, Kuijten RH, Kooiker CJ, Wagenaar SS, Van der Zouwen P, Mees EJD: Occurrence of vascular IgA deposits in clinically normal skin of patients with renal disease. Kidney Int 9:424–429, 1976.
111. Clarkson AR, Seymour AE, Chan Y-L, Thompson AJ, Woodroffe AJ: Clinical, pathological, and therapeutic aspects of IgA nephropathy. In: Kincaid-Smith P, Apice AJF, Atkins RC (eds) Progress of glomerulonephritis. New York: John Wiley and Sons, 1979, pp 247–259.
112. Lamperi S, Carozzi S: Skin-muscle biopsy in patients with various nephropathies. Nephron 24:46–50, 1979.
113. Tomino Y, Nomoto Y, Endoh M, Sakai H: Deposition of IgA-dominant immune-complexes in muscular vessels from patients with IgA nephropathy. Acta Pathol Jpn 31:361–365, 1981.
114. Mustonen J, Pasternack A, Helin H, Rilva A, Penttinen K, Wager O, Harmoinen A: Circulating immune complexes, the concentration of serum IgA and the distribution of HLA antigens in IgA nephropathy. Nephron 29:170–175, 1981.
115. Kammer GM, Soter NA, Gibson DF, Schur PH: Psoriatic arthritis: a clinical, immunologic and HLA study of 100 patients. Semin Arthritis Rheum 9:75–97, 1979.
116. Rodnan GP: Progressive systemic sclerosis (scleroderma). In: McCarty DJ (ed) Arthritis and allied conditions. Philadelphia: Lea and Febiger, 1979, p 762.
117. Egido J, Blasco R, Sancho J, Lozano L, Sanchez-Crespo M: Increased rates of polymeric IgA synthesis by circulating lymphoid cells in IgA mesangial glomerulonephritis. Clin Exp Immunol 47:309–316, 1982.
118. Endoh M, Suga T, Miura M, Tomino Y, Nomoto Y, Sakai H: In vivo alteration of antibody production in patients with IgA nephropathy. Clin Exp Immunol 57:564–570, 1984.
119. Pasternack A, Mustonen J, Leinikki P: Humoral immune response in patients with IgA and IgM glomerulonephritis. Clin Exp Immunol 63:228–223, 1986.
120. Andre C, Berthoux FC, Andre F, Gillon J, Genin C, Sabatier J-C: Prevalence of IgA2 deposits in IgA nephropathies. N Engl J Med 303:1343–1346, 1980.
121. Conley ME, Cooper MD, Michael AF: Selective deposition of immunoglobulin A1 in immunoglobulin A nephropathy, anaphylactoid purpura nephritis, and systemic lupus erythematosus. J Clin Invest 66:1432–1436, 1980.
122. Conley ME, Koopman WJ: Serum IgA1 and IgA2 in normal adults and patients with systemic lupus erythematosus and hepatic disease. Clin Immunol Immunopathol 26:390–397, 1983.
123. Woodroffe AJ, Clarkson AR, Seymour AE, Lomax-Smith JD: Mesangial IgA nephritis. Springer Semin Immunopathol 5:321–332, 1982.

6. THE PATHOLOGY OF IgA NEPHROPATHY

RAJA SINNIAH

Mesangial IgA nephropathy was first identified in France by Berger in 1968 [1, 2], and has been referred to as Berger's disease. The lesion is characterized by diffuse mesangial deposition of immunoglobulins, with IgA predominating. There should be no systemic manifestations, and secondary diseases of systemic lupus erythematosus [3], Henoch-Schönlein purpura [4, 5], liver cirrhosis [6–8], and cancer, especially mucin-secreting adenocarcinomas [9, 10] should be excluded, as they are also known to have IgA deposits in the glomerular mesangium. The glomerular immunopathology of IgA nephropathy is identical with that of Henoch-Schönlein purpura, and some authors believe that IgA nephropathy is a forme fruste of Henoch-Schönlein purpura.

IgA nephropathy is now recognized as one of the most common, if not the most frequent, form of primary glomerulonephritis in many parts of the world, including France [11, 12], Italy [13–15], Japan [16, 17], Australia [4], and Singapore [18, 19], accounting for 20–40% of the reported cases. The pathology and immunopathology of this important type of kidney disease have been extensively studied.

PATHOLOGY OF IgA NEPHROPATHY

Immunofluorescence microscopy

The initial descriptions of this lesion were derived from France, where the preliminary observations were diffuse mesangial deposits of IgA-IgG and C3,

Table 6-1. Combinations of immunoglobulins, complements, and fibrinogen in IgA nephropathy

Reference	No. of cases	% Positive cases IgG	IgM	C3	C4	C1q	Fibrinogen
Europe							
Druet et al. 1970 [29]	52	>70	17	80	—	—	15
Davies et al. 1973 [30]	6	16.6	50	83	—	—	33.3
Sissons et al. 1975 [23]	25	74	42	88	—	0	79
Covarsi et al. 1981 [31]	34	27	9	82	—	16	15
Mandreoli et al. 1981 [32]	93	28	30	100	0	0	12
D'Amico 1983 [28]	149	48.6	30.1	88.5	9.9	4.7	23.1
Vangelista et al. 1984 [33]	142	15	51	100	—	8	39
Waldherr et al. 1984 [34]	75	65	64	100	7	7	60
North America							
McCoy et al. 1974 [22]	20	60	60	85	0	0	50
Zimmerman and Burkholder 1975 [35]	78	78	66.6	100	20	—	61.1
Katz et al. 1976 [36]	61	<50	12	70	0	—	20
Burkholder et al. 1979 [37]	54	73	67	94	36	—	78
Australia							
Woodroffe et al. 1980 [38]	78	22	43	82	14	14	50
Asia							
Ueda et al. 1977 [39]	85	70	10.6	88	—	—	—
Yokoska et al. 1978 [40]	85	80	47	78	—	7	36
Nakamoto et al. 1978 [41]	205	51	22	61	—	15	49
Shirai et al. 1978 [16]	100	38	35	82	0	21	30
Sakai et al. 1979 [17]	130	75	16	99	19	5	—
Ng et al. 1981 [42]	44	50	41	79	—	—	27
Sinniah et al. 1981 [19]	239	50.1	21.4	82.5	2.4	2.4	37.2
Sinniah and Ku 1984 [43]	268	47.7	25.3	82.8	3.7	3.7	72[a]

[a]Includes grade 1+ positive fluorescence for fibrinogen.

but not IgM [1, 2, 11, 20]. Several earlier studies also supported Berger's original report [21–23]. However, experiences drawn from larger numbers of patients and studies from many separate centers revealed that an IgA-IgG combination was found in only approximately 50% of cases [18, 19, 24–27], and Berger's disease has now been accepted by the term *IgA nephropathy*. Various combinations of immunoglobulins accompanying the predominant IgA immunoproteins have been reported. Table 6-1 (modified from D'Amico [28]) shows the combinations of immunoglobulins and complements in idiopathic IgA nephropathy.

Patterns of immunoprotein deposits

The IgA is deposited diffusely in all glomeruli as confluent masses or as discrete granules in the mesangium in an arborized pattern (figure 6-1). In approximately 65% of cases, the IgA and other proteins were confined to the mesangium, and in the remaining 35% there were extensions of deposits in the paramesangium–subendothelium along the peripheral capillary loops

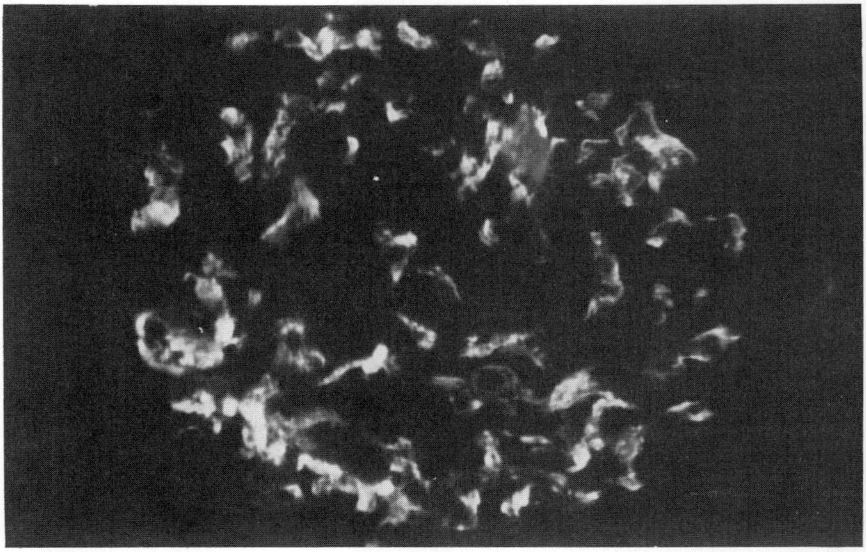

Figure 6-1. Immunofluorescence microscopy shows localization of immunoprotein A predominantly in the glomerular mesangium. ×300.

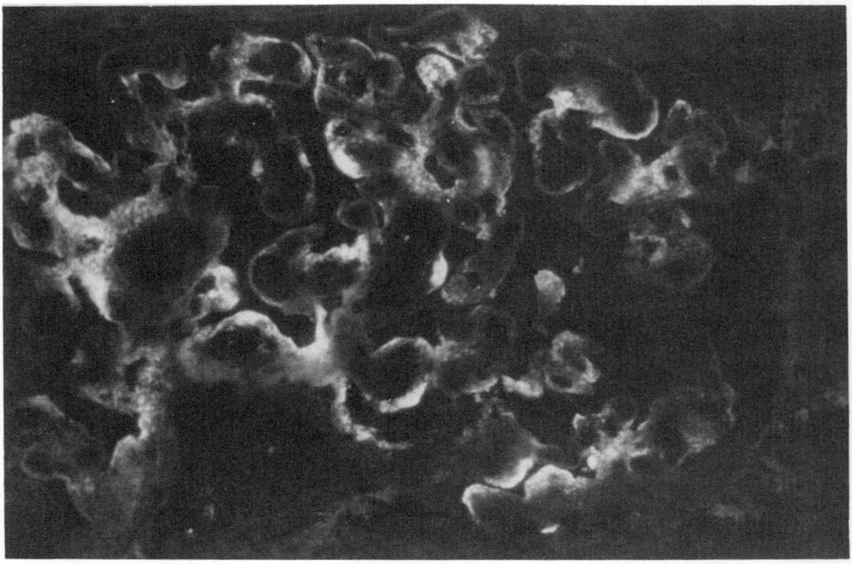

Figure 6-2. Immunofluorescence microscopy shows localization of immunoprotein A predominantly in the subendothelium of the peripheral glomerular capillaries. ×350.

[19] (figure 6-2). Similar observations were made in a number of studies. D'Amico [28] observed IgA deposits confined to the mesangial area in 44% of 149 patients, while the remainder showed definite extension to some of the peripheral capillary loops in a subendothelial parietal position. The sites of depositions had some predictive value, as a purely mesangial location was less frequently associated with hypertension than those with subendothelial extensions. Extensive capillary wall involvement was uniformly associated with a more severe clinical course. Mesangial and capillary deposits indicated more severe glomerular disease. The extension of the deposits to the adjacent capillary loops correlated with the severity of the mesangial proliferation at light microscopy [17, 28, 34, 43, 44]. There was a good correlation between the presence of crescents and IgA on capillary walls: 56% of the biopsies with crescents at light microscopy, compared with 20% in cases without crescents $p < 0.001$. Peripheral capillary wall deposits of IgA were found in 26%, IgG in 10%, and IgM in 31% of the 142 cases of IgA nephropathy [33].

The *type and intensity of associated immunoglobulins* did not show any relationship with light-microscopic findings or clinical course [16, 19, 33, 43]. There was no relation to the known duration of disease, presence or absence of elevated serum creatinine, and absence or presence of elevated blood pressure [34]. IgM was found in more than 60% of cases by many workers from the United States, whereas, in reports from Southern Europe, Asia, and Australia, there was a lower prevalence. Sakai et al. [17] observed severe histologic lesions demonstrated by light microscopy in many of the group with IgM.

Complement activation

Early-acting complement components C4 and C1q were invariably reported as absent or present in a very small number of cases, indicating, in conjunction with the frequently reported presence of properdin, complement activation via the alternative pathway [36, 45, 46]. IgA and C3 in extraglomerular contiguous arterioles and tubules have been described in a limited number of patients [4, 19, 47]. Others have found the immunoglobulin localization in extraglomerular vessels to be rare [16]. Arteriolar hyalinosis, and deposits of C3, with or without IgM are frequent findings. However, IgA deposits were not detected [19, 34]. The IgA deposits persisted unchanged in all patients who had repeat biopsies [34, 48], and the IgA deposits reacted with both kappa and lambda antibodies in all cases examined.

Nature of the IgA

No IgA secretory piece (SC) could be found deposited in the glomeruli by a number of studies [16, 19, 22, 40, 49–51]. IgA-SC localization was observed occasionally in tubular epithelial cells and in tubular lumen [22, 34, 36, 43,

53]. There has recently been some controversy as to the *subclass of IgA* deposited in the mesangium. IgA is the main active immunoglobulin at the mucus membrane. There, IgA is dimerized and transformed into secretory IgA by an SC and J chain. The presence of predominant IgA2 would point to a mucosal origin, whereas the presence of IgA1, the major circulating IgA subclass, would point to a systemic origin. André et al. [54], and Bene et al. [55], using polyclonal antisera, found predominantly IgA2 in all patients, as well as IgA1. However, others [56–61] using monoclonal antibodies found predominantly IgA1 and polymeric. Some other studies also using monoclonal antibodies showed that, though IgA1 was deposited in all cases, it was identical in distribution to that of IgA common; in addition, IgA2 was also found in some cases at a weaker intensity. Vangelista et al. [33] found IgA2 in 12 of 25 cases, and Waldherr et al. [34] in three of 18 cases.

Of the 15 cases with idiopathic IgA nephropathy studied by us, using monoclonal antibodies to human IgA and subclasses IgA1 and IgA2 (Nordic Immunological Laboratories and Becton Dickinson Monoclonal Center), eight (53.3%) had deposits of IgA1 alone, and seven (46.7%) had IgA1 and IgA2 deposits in the glomerular mesangium. The IgA2 deposits were of weaker intensity. These conflicting results from a number of different countries may relate to both geographic or racial differences, as well as to methodology. It is also probable that both subclasses IgA1 and IgA2 may be present in IgA nephropathy.

Recent work has shown that polymeric IgA has an equal distribution between the IgA1 and IgA2 subclasses [62] and heterogeneity in the intestine, with predominance of IgA1 in the oropharynx or upper respiratory tract and IgA2 in the small intestine [64]. It is possible that antigenic stimulation of a mucosa will cause local S-IgA2 secretion in the mucosa, but preferentially IgA1 synthesis in the associated lymphoid tissue [34]. It is possible that the deposition of predominantly macromolecular IgA1 in patients with IgA nephropathy is due to an increase of plasma cells producing IgA dimers or polymers in the mucosal system or in the bone marrow, or to impaired elimination. The exact reasons for IgA1 predominance over IgA2 in the glomerular mesangium are unknown. More than one factor or agent may be responsible for IgA deposition nephropathy because the synthesis of IgA1 and IgA2 seems to be regulated to different and unidentified factors [64].

J piece was observed rarely, and only with IgM rather than IgA by some workers [57, 61, 65], causing the authors to conclude that mesangial deposits in IgA nephropathy are composed of monomeric IgA1. However, others reported J piece in all or nearly all biopsies [34, 55, 66–68]. Previous failure to demonstrate J chain may be due to no acid urea pretreatment or pretreatment of too long duration. It is unlikely that deposited glomerular IgA is a consequence of immune complexes with IgA as an antigen, since a substantial number of patients showed IgA deposits as the only immunoglobulin [19, 23, 39, 43, 49, 69], and no antibody activity against IgA was found in the circulation [49]. The granular pattern of the glomerular IgA depositions, occasional deposits in the skin [70, 71], and recurrence in renal allografts [72] suggested an immune complex disease, which was later demonstrated by López-Trascasa and colleagues [73]. Immune complexes formed in vivo or in vitro with monomeric IgA failed to induce glomerulonephritis [74], whereas polymeric IgA was found in IgA nephropathy [68]. As the disease often follows upper respiratory infections, it seems probable that the source of the infection is there. The IgA is involved as an antibody against an antigen(s), either at the mucus membrane, in the circulation, or within the mesangium.

Light microscopy

Initial reports by Berger [1, 2] and others [11, 12, 35] described a predominantly focal and segmental type of lesion, with minor changes in the majority of glomeruli, in IgA nephropathy. Later observations reported variable glomerular morphology [4, 18–20, 22, 24, 50, 75]. Many of the differences were due to the initial small number of cases, and also possibly to differences in the criteria used for the classification of the changes in IgA nephropathy. Several publications have attempted to classify these glomerular lesions into types, grades, groups, or classes, based on the severity of the glomerular pathology [16, 19, 20, 42, 43, 76–80].

Glomerular lesions

To enable comparative studies to be made on renal diseases, it would be useful to agree on criteria for diagnosis. The uniform system for Classification of Glomerular Diseases, proposed by the World Health Organization Committee [81], has been used in the classification of the light-microscopic lesions of IgA nephropathy [80]. Five major classes of glomerular lesions can be seen in Berger's disease:

I. Minimal lesions, appearing "normal" on light microscopy.
II. Minor change, with widening of the mesangium with increased cellularity of groups of up to three cells per area in the periphery of glomeruli.
III. Focal and segmental glomerulonephritis, with less than 50% of the glomeruli showing localized or segmental sclerosis, mesangial cell proliferation, or infrequently necrosis; the remaining glomeruli showing minor changes.
IV. Diffuse mesangial cell proliferation, with varying degrees of hypercellularity, and irregular in distribution. This group subdivided into mild, moderate, and marked mesangial cell hyperplasia. Class IV lesions were categorized into: IVa, where there are no superimposed glomerular lesions; and IVb, where there are additional lesions of capsular adhesions, glomerular sclerosis, and crescents.
V. Diffuse sclerosing glomerulonephritis, with involvement of >80% of glomeruli.

Table 6-2. Patterns of glomerular lesions in IgA nephropathy

		Types of glomerular lesions (%)				
Reference	No. of cases	Minimal/ minor changes	Focal prolifera- tive GN	Diffuse prolifera- tive GN	Diffuse proliferation with crescents	Diffuse sclerosing GN
Levy et al. 1973 [20]	36	33.3	47.2		19.4	
McCoy et al. 1974 [22]	20	10	50	25	15	
Zimmerman and Burkholder 1975 [35]	18	33.6	66.7			
Ueda et al. 1977 [39]	85	21.2	22.4	38.8	17.6	
Yokoska et al. 1978 [40]	67	10		71.6	1.5	7.5
Sakai et al. 1979 [17]	130	19.2	19.2	44.6	16.9	
Sinniah et al. 1981 [19]	239	35.6	28.1	22.2	13.4	0.3
Hogg and Silva 1984 [76]	83	30.1	36.1	33.7		
Mihatsch et al. 1984 [77]	48	28.0	54.0		12.0	6.0

Table 6-2 shows the distribution of glomerular lesions on light microscopy in IgA nephropathy, from several centers, demonstrating the variable glomerular pathology in Berger's type nephritis.

From a large series of 268 cases with IgA nephropathy, the glomerular lesions at initial biopsy were grouped into five classes (table 6-3): class I minimal lesion accounting for 3.7%; class II minor changes (figure 6-3) with a few lobular tufts showing increased cellularity of up to three nuclei per mesangial area in approximately 30% of the cases; class III focal and segmental glomerulonephritis in approximately 30% of cases, with 14 (17.7%) of the 79 patients showing segmental proliferation (figure 6-4a), and the remaining 65 (82.3%) with segmental sclerosis (figure 6-4b), adhesions, necrosis or crescents (figure 6-4c); class IVa diffuse mesangial cell proliferation (figure 6-5) in 4.9% (13) of cases, and class IVb diffuse mesangial proliferation with superimposed lesions of sclerosis, adhesions, necrosis, and crescents in 31.3% (84) of patients; and class V lesions of diffuse sclerosing glomerulonephritis, an infrequent finding at initial biopsy.

Superimposed glomerular lesions of focal and segmental lobular tuft necrosis were seen in focal proliferative and diffuse mesangial proliferative lesions [22]. Occasional glomerular capillary aneurysms (figure 6-6) were found. Crescents were frequently associated with lobular tuft necrosis indicative of a possible causal relationship. There was significantly increased glomerular sclerosis and crescents formation in diffuse mesangial cell proliferation than in focal glomerulonephritis ($p < 0.01$), indicating that the severity of diffuse mesangial cell hyperplasia is the most important factor in IgA nephropathy. Mesangial interposition along some glomerular capillaries was seen in cases with diffuse mesangial cell proliferation, but no definite mesangiocapillary glomerulonephritis was seen [19, 28]. Circumferential crescents were rare

Table 6-3. IgA nephropathy: correlation of glomerular lesions with tubulointerstitial and vascular changes

		Superimposed glomerular lesions					Tubulointerstitial lesion grades			
Glomerular lesion class	No. of cases	Segmental prolif.	Sclerosis	Adhesions	Necrosis	Crescents	1	2	3	Vascular Lesions
I. Minimal change	10 (3.7%)									
II. Minor change	80 (29.9%)						2			
III. Focal GN	79 (29.5%)	14 (17.7%)	58[a] (73.4%)	18 (22.5%)	4 (5.1%)	24[a] (30.4%)	9	8 (21.5%)	0	2 (2.5%)
(i) Segmental proliferation	14	14	2		3	10	2	8		2
(ii) Segmental sclerosis, etc.	65		56	18	1	14	7	8		2
IVa. Diffuse mes. proliferation	13 (4.9%)									
b. Diffuse mes. proliferation with superimposed lesions	84 (31.3%)		78[a] (92.9%)	20 (23.8%)	5 (6%)	46[a] (54.8%)	20 (40.5%)	14		10 (11.9%)
(i) Mild	48		42	9	1	18	3	2		
(ii) Moderate	30		30	5	3	22	10	13		
(iii) Severe	6		6	6	1	6			6	3
V. Diffuse sclerosing GN	2(0.7%)								2	2
Total	268									

[a]Statistically significant differences between FGN and DMP ($p < 0.01$).
The distributions are not statistically significant except for: (1) sclerosis: FGN 73.4% vs 92.9% diff. prolif., $\chi^2 = 9.77$, *df* (degree of freedom) = 1; $p < 0.01$; and (2) crescent FGN 30.4% vs 54.8% diff. prolif., $\chi^2 = 8.9$, $df = 1$, $p < 0.01$.

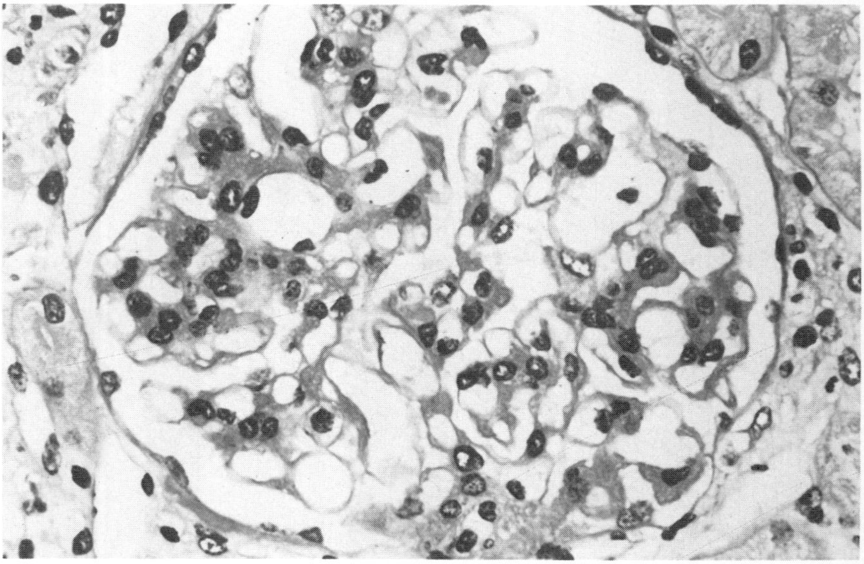

Figure 6-3. Minor change, with segmental increase in mesangial cell nuclei up to three per mesangial area. PAS, ×640.

[17, 28, 39]. In all classes of lesions, there were varying degrees of mesangial enlargement, and spread from a segmental to a global pattern. IgA nephropathy is characterized by diffuse mesangial widening, positive for argyrophilic deposits (figure 6-7a), with the involvement of focal lesions or diffuse proliferations. Mesangial deposits as discrete droplets (figure 6-7b) were detected in up to 30% of cases, with PAS, Martius scarlet blue (MSB), and Masson's trichrome stains, as discrete droplets (figure 6-7b).

Tubulointerstitial lesions

The severity of tubulointerstitial lesions correlated well with the severity of glomerular changes. Focal interstitial edema and lymphocytic cell infiltrates were found in 36% of cases [80]. Tubulointerstitial damage was graded 1 to 3, based on the degree of tubular necrosis, atrophy, and interstitial fibrosis, with inflammatory cell infiltration, predominantly lymphocytes. The frequency and severity of tubulointerstitial damage (figure 6-8) were more marked in the more severe glomerular lesions. These observations have been well documented [16, 20, 28, 35, 76, 82, 83]. In cases with class I and II glomerular lesions, interstitial mononuclear cellular infiltrates were absent or minimal. Class III and IV glomerular lesions showed increasing degrees of tubular destruction and interstitial fibrosis, with the most severe pathology seen in patients with class IVb glomerular lesions.

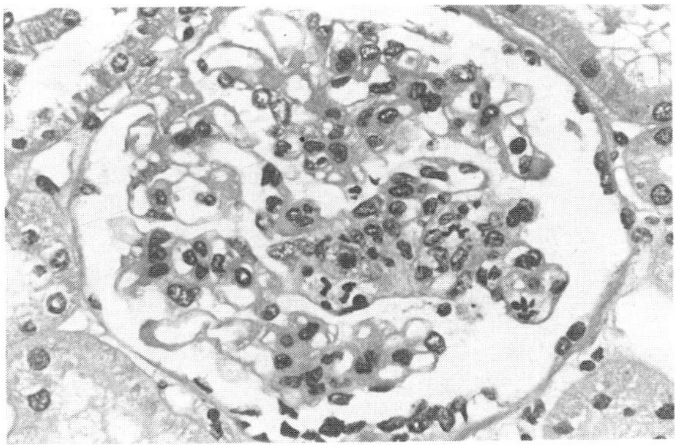

A

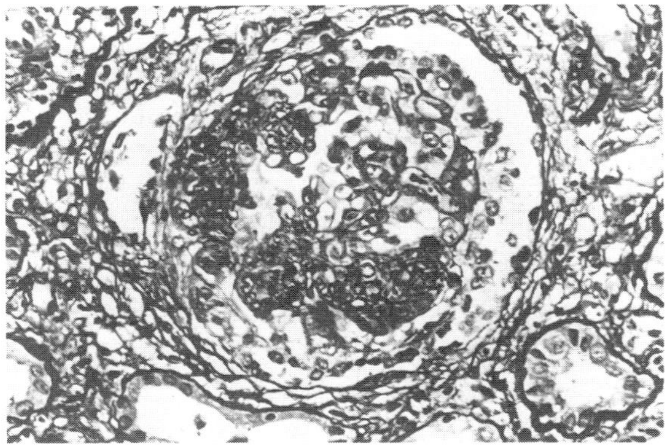

B

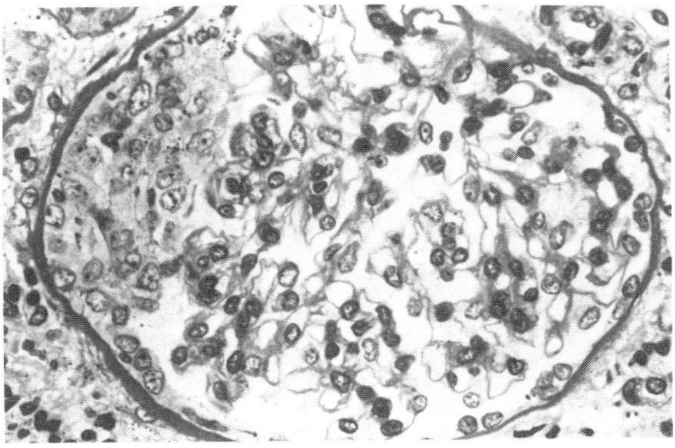

C

Figure 6-4. (**a**) Focal segmental glomerulonephritis; segmental lobular tuft proliferation of predominantly mesangial cells. H & E, ×640. (**b**) Focal segmental glomerulonephritis; segmental glomerular sclerosis with crown of hypertrophied podocytes. PAS–silver, ×400. (**c**) Focal and segmental crescent compressing peripheral glomerular capillaries. PAS, ×640.

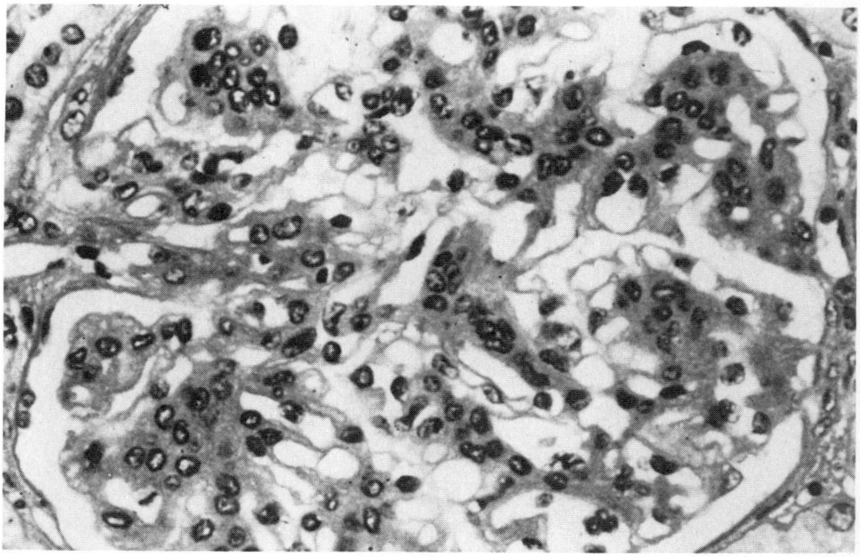

Figure 6-5. Diffuse mesangial proliferative glomerulonephritis, showing widening of the mesangium by mesangial cell hyperplasia and deposition of matrix. H & E, ×640.

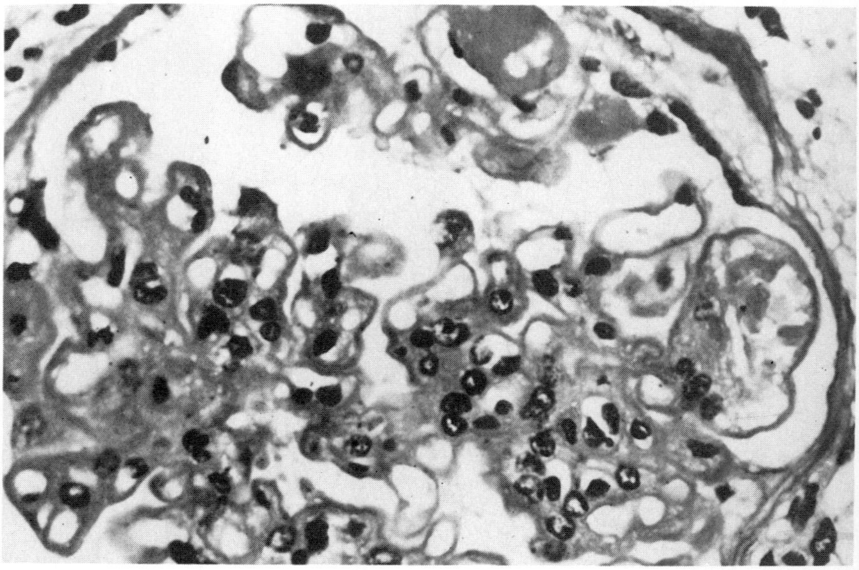

Figure 6-6. Glomerular capillary aneurysms in a case of IgA nephropathy. PAS, ×640.

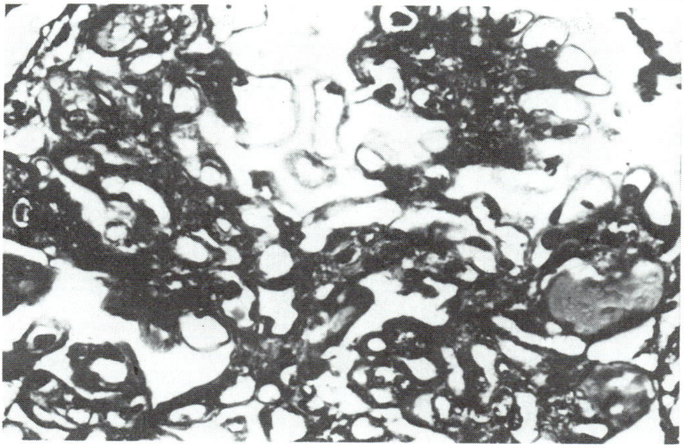

A

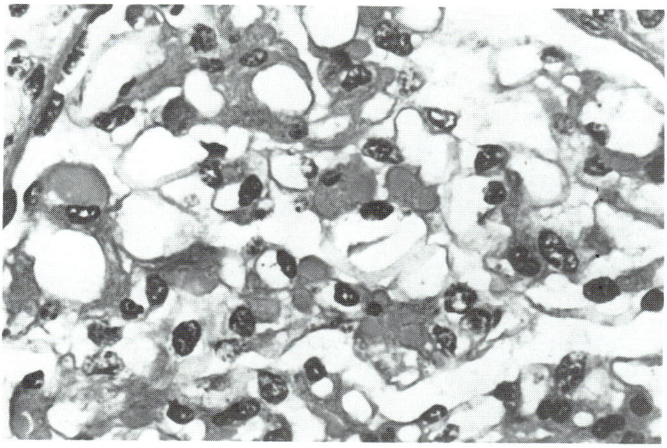

B

Figure 6-7. (**a**) Glomerulus showing marked widening of the centrilobular mesangial stalks by argyrophilic deposits, in a case of IgA nephropathy. PAS–silver, ×640. (**b**) Discrete droplets in the mesangium in a case of IgA nephropathy. Masson's trichrome, ×900.

Vascular lesions of arteriolosclerosis with hyalinosis and arteriosclerosis (figure 6-9) were seen in the more severe types of glomerulonephritis and correlated with the extent of the glomerular sclerotic lesions [16, 19, 28]. The strong correlation between vascular sclerosis and glomerulosclerosis indicates a causal relationship whose precise manner is uncertain. It has been suggested that arteriosclerosis may lead to glomerular ischemia, collapse, and sclerosis [4, 84, 85]. The vascular sclerosis with medial hypertrophy and hyalinization with increased disease formed clustered vessels, which may be due to a combination of parenchymal loss with relative increase in vessel mass, or to vascular hypertrophy with tortuosity of the blood vessels. The exact relation-

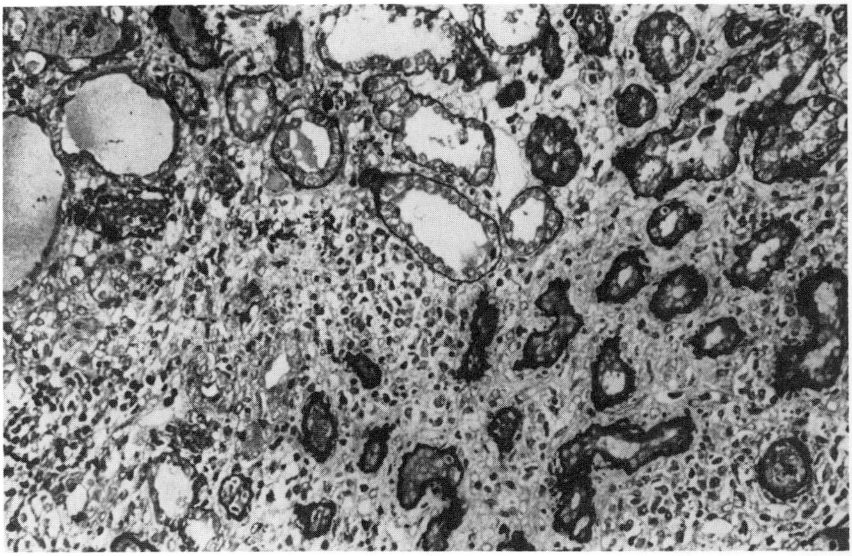

Figure 6-8. Tubulointerstitial lesions in IgA nephropathy. There is tubular necrosis and atrophy, with interstitial fibrosis and lymphocytic cells infiltrates. PAS–silver, ×250.

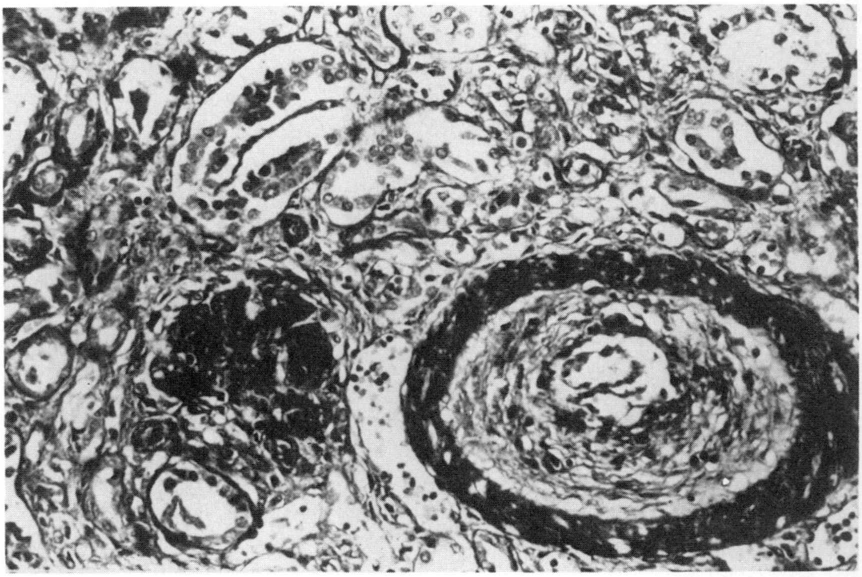

Figure 6-9. Vascular lesion of medial hypertrophy and luminal narrowing in an advanced case of IgA nephropathy. Masson's trichrome, ×350.

ship between vascular sclerosis and glomerulosclerosis is uncertain, and it has been suggested that it may be hemodynamically mediated [85].

Electron microscopy

Sites of deposits

In IgA nephropathy, the constant findings are massive electron-dense deposits in the mesangium intermingled with the mesangial matrix (figure 6-10). The quantity of dense deposits varies from region to region within a glomerulus and among glomeruli. Electron-dense deposits have been known to extend into the peripheral subendothelium of the capillary loops in some cases (figure 6-11) [4, 19, 28, 35, 48, 86]. A number of authors have stated that subendothelial and subepithelial humps were rare or absent in the peripheral capillary loops of their cases [16, 20, 22, 78, 87], but others have seen peripheral deposits in the subendothelial and subepithelial positions [19, 24, 88, 89]. Detailed study of 78 cases of IgA nephropathy by electron microscopy (table 6-4) showed peripheral subendothelial deposits in 61.6% of cases (16.7% with subepithelial deposits as well), and mesangial with subepithelial deposits (figure 6-12) in 3.8% (3) of patients.

Mesangial changes

The mesangium is enlarged by cytoplasm and matrix. Many of these mesangial changes have been well documented in a number of studies [16, 19, 20, 22, 28, 79, 87, 90, 91]. In the acute and active stages of the disease, the mesangial cells show abundant cytoplasm with numerous mitochondria and prominent endoplasmic reticulum. Collagen fibers may be found in the mesangial matrix in biopsies with mesangial sclerosis. The thickened and serpigineous matrix appears to encroach on the mesangial cells and capillary loops (figure 6-13), leading to glomerular obsolescence. These mesangial changes appear to be preceded by mesangiolysis probably caused by the deposits of immunoproteins within the matrix (figure 6-14).

Peripheral glomerular capillary wall abnormalities have been seen in 40% [88] to over 50% (table 6-5) of cases. Peripheral capillary wall thinning, splitting, lamination, membranolysis, disruption of lamina densa, aneurysmal dilatation, and irregular thickening of the glomerular basement membrane have been documented (4, 19, 24, 35, 79, 87, 92]. There is subendothelial widening with electron-lucent substance admixed with granules (figure 6-15) in the peripheral glomerular capillary loops. The changes are similar to hemolytic-uremic syndrome, malignant hypertension, and toxemia found during pregnancy [93]. All these conditions are known to include hypertension or intravascular coagulation, which was not the case in our patients. Irregular thickening of the glomerular basement membrane is seen in over 50% of the cases, due to the presence of basement membrane-like material, irregular layers of electron-lucent and medium electron-dense material with

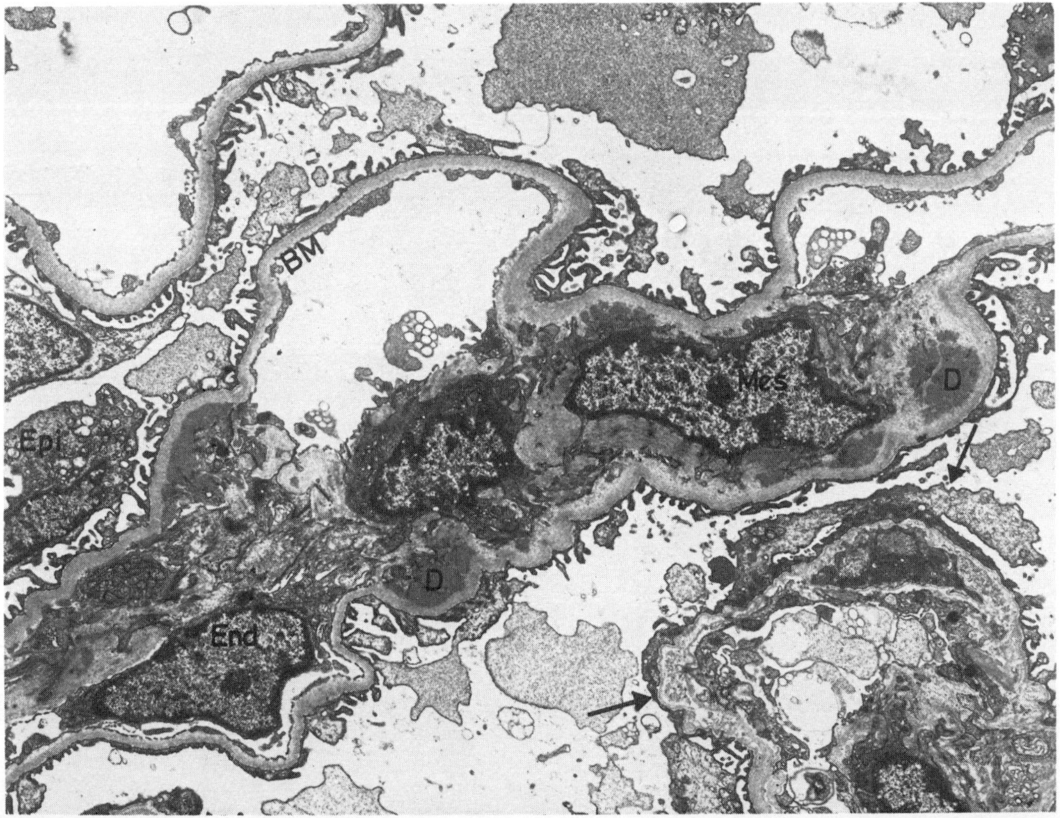

Figure 6-10. Electron micrograph of part of a glomerulus shows electron-dense deposits in the mesangium. Part of a capillary loop (*arrows*) shows damage to the glomerular basement membrane. *End*, endothelial cell; *Mes*, mesangial cell; *BM*, basement membrane; *Epi*, epithelial cell; and *D* dense deposits. ×6300.

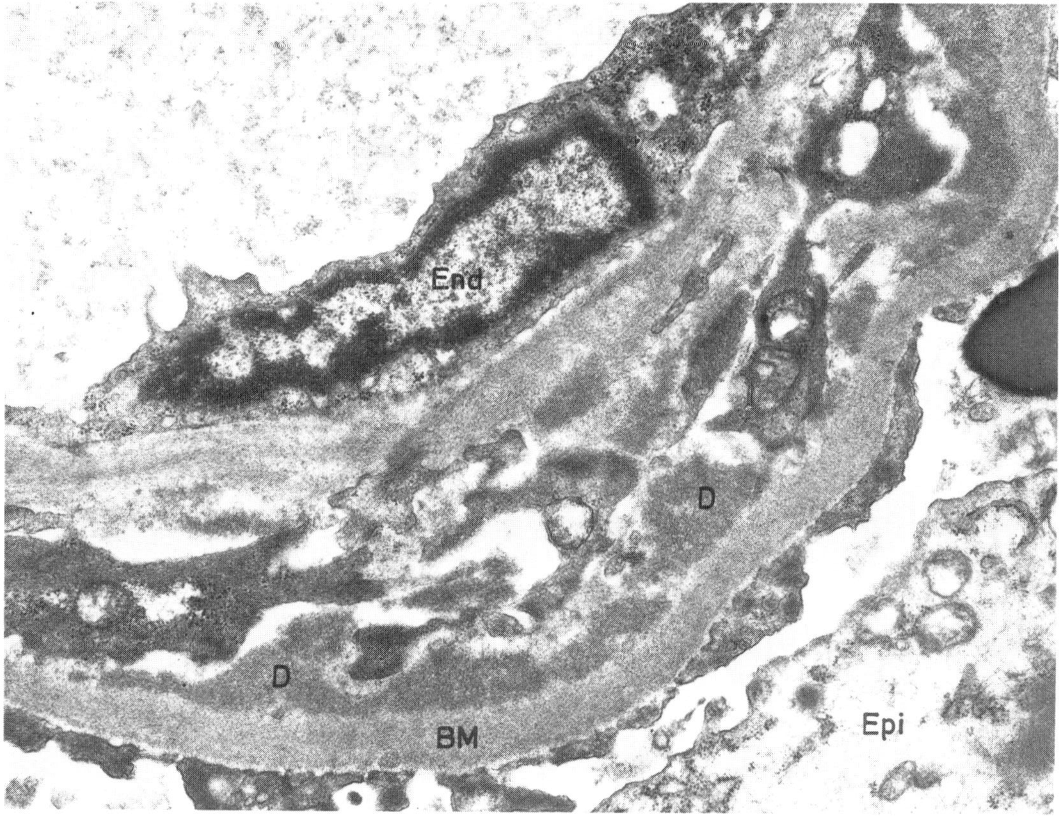

Figure 6-11. Segment of a peripheral glomerular capillary loop shows mesangial interposition along the subendothelium, with reduplication of basement membrane, and electron-dense deposits in the subendothelium. *End*, endothelial cell; *D*, dense deposits; *BM*, basement membrane; and *Epi*, epithelial cell. ×29,250.

Table 6-4. Electron microscopy of IgA nephropathy: sites of deposits and mesangial changes

		Sites of electron-dense deposits				Mesangial changes			
Light-microscopy class	No. of cases	Mesangium	Subendo-thelium	Subendo-thelium/ subepi-thelium	Subepi-thelium	Increased matrix	Increased cells	Lysis	Collagen fibers
I. Minimal change	3	3	2			3		1	
II. Minor change	25	25	8	4		23	10	1	
III. (i) Focal segmental proliferation, crescents	8	8	5			7	6	1	1
(ii) Focal segmental sclerosis	13	13	10			13	9	3	
IVa. Diffuse mesangial proliferation	8	8	1	1	1	8	8		
b. (i) Diffuse mesangial proliferation with sclerosis	7	7	4			7	7	4	1
(ii) Diffuse mesangial proliferation, sclerosis and crescents	14	14	5	8	1	14	14	4	
Total	78	78	35 (44.9%)	13 (16.7%)	3 (3.8%)			14	

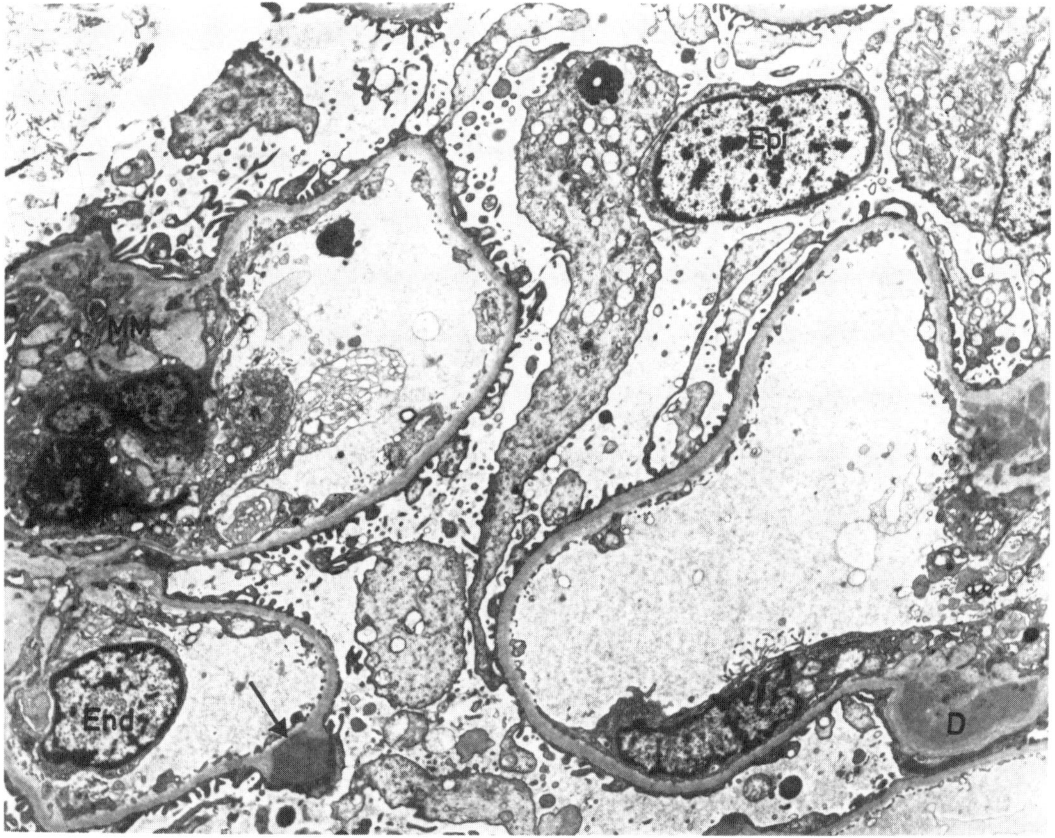

Figure 6-12. Electron micrograph of part of a glomerulus shows electron-dense deposits in the mesangium and in the subepithelium of a peripheral capillary (*arrow*). The podocytes show microvilli. *MM*, mesangial matrix; *End*, endothelial cell; *Epi*, epithelial cell; and *BM*, basement membrane. ×6300.

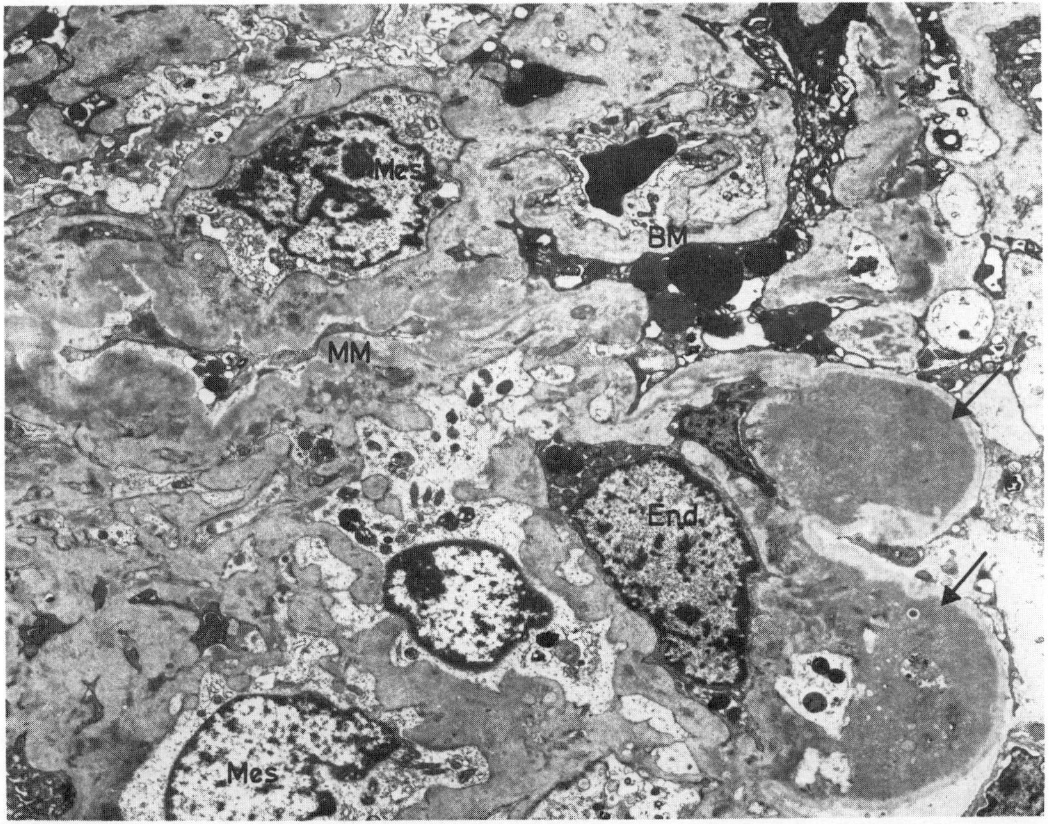

Figure 6-13. Electron micrograph of part of a glomerulus shows marked increase in mesangial matrix, containing scattered electron-dense deposits. There is encroachment of the mesangial sclerotic nodule into the glomerular capillary lumen, which also shows hyalinosis (*arrows*). *MM*, mesangial matrix; *Mes*, mesangial cell; *End*, endothelial cell; and BM, *basement membrane*. ×*6300*.

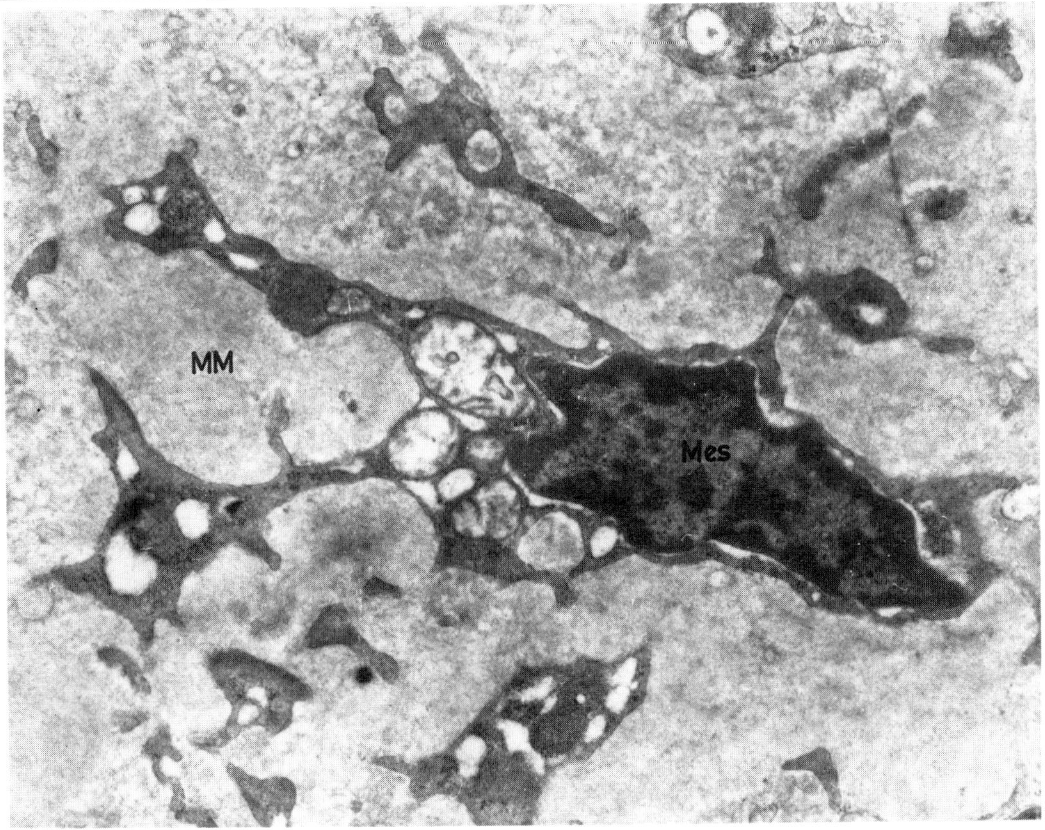

Figure 6-14. Electron micrograph of the mesangium shows dissolution or mesangiolysis of the matrix; related to the dense deposits. *MM*, mesangial matrix; and *Mes*, mesangial cell. ×33,000.

Table 6-5. Electron microscopy of IgA nephropathy: peripheral capillaries' changes

Light-microscopy class	No. of cases	Subendothelium fluffy, granules lamination	Lysis of GBM	Aneurysm	Thickening of GBM	Dense deposits	Reduplication of GBM	Dense deposits	Thinning of GBM	Podocyte necrosis	Podocyte effacement	Polymorphs in lumen	Tubuloreticular particles
I. Minimal change	3	2			1	1				1	1		
II. Minor change	25	7	3		12	4	6	3	8	1	11	4	1
III. (i) Focal segmental proliferation, crescents	8	3	3	1	3		3	3		1	2·	3	
(ii) Focal segmental sclerosis	13	5			9	3	8	3	5	1	6	5	
IVa. Diffuse mesangial proliferation	8	3	1		5	1	5	1	1	1	1	2	2
b. (i) Diffuse mesangial proliferation, sclerosis	7	2	4	3	4	2	5	1	1	2	1	1	1
(ii) Diffuse mesangial proliferation, sclerosis, crescents	14	4	5	2	7	6	6	3		4	5	4	3
Total	78	26 (33.3%)	16 (20.5%)	6 (7.7%)	41 (52.3%)	17	33 (42.3%)	14	15 (19.2%)	11 (14.1%)	27 (34.6%)	19 (24.4%)	7 (9%)

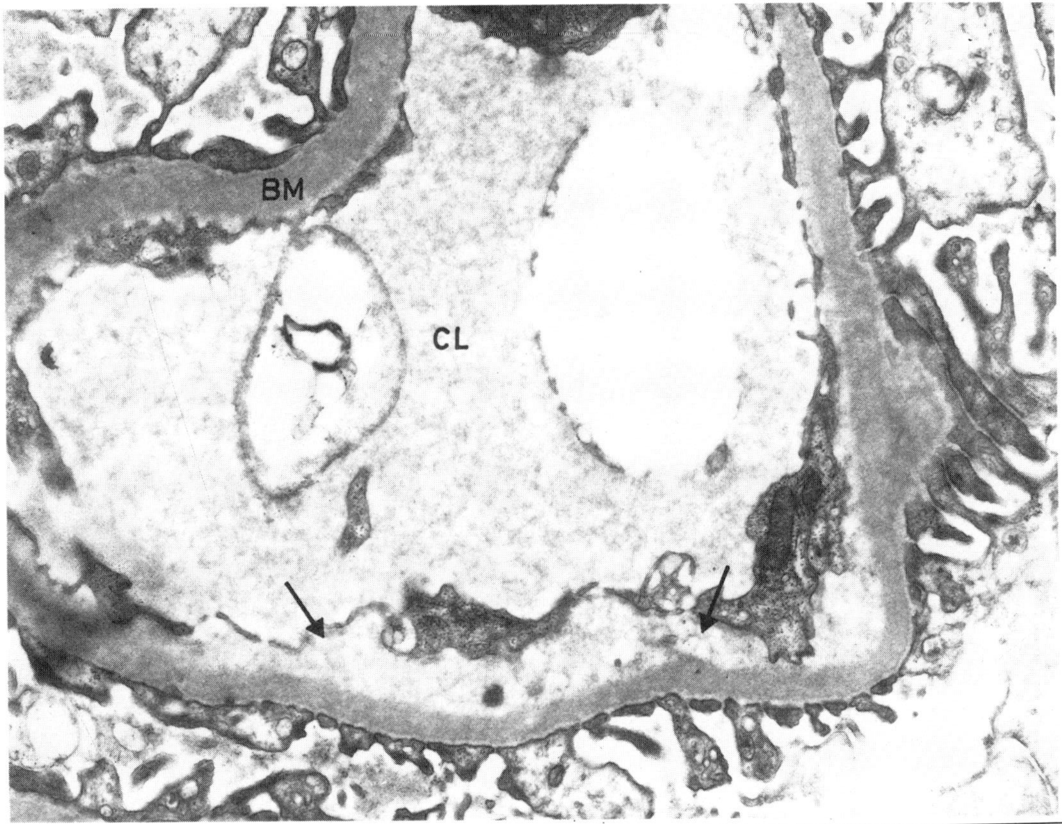

Figure 6-15. Segment of glomerular capillary loop shows widening of the lamina rara interna with lucent granular materials (*arrows*). *CL*, capillary lumen; and *BM*, basement membrane. ×18,000.

foci of entrapped vesicular and cytoplasmic structures, probably of both mesangial and endothelial cell origin. Mesangial interposition in capillary loops with focal and segmental reduplication is also a frequent finding. There are also foci of membranolysis, with aneurysmal dilatation of segmental peripheral capillary loops (figure 6-16). These aneurysms show disruption and loss of the lamina densa and the presence of granular and fibrillar materials within a lucent substance with features similar to plasma insudates.

Focal and segmental thinning of the glomerular basement membrane is seen in approximately 20% of cases. There is thinning of the lamina densa with, in some cases, detachment and necrosis of the overlying podocytes and foot processes (figure 6-17). The other frequent changes are focal widening or effacement of foot processes, with epithelial hypertrophy and microvilli formation. Mesangial and visceral epithelial cells contain dense vesicles, which are phagolysosomes [19, 20, 24, 87]. Tubuloreticular particles are seen infrequently (9%) in the endothelial cytoplasm (figure 6-18) in the cases with IgA nephropathy in contrast to lupus nephritis, which is found in over 90% of patients [3].

Pathogenesis of glomerular damage

The large amount of glomerular deposits located in the mesangium and peripheral capillary walls could lead to glomerular mesangial and endothelial damage. The mesangial deposits appear to stimulate increased production of mesangial matrix, which may be preceded by mesangiolysis. There is deposition of collagen within the matrix, and the sclerotic mesangium encroaches on the mesangial cells with subsequent loss of these cells. The glomerular basement membrane changes are most likely a result of damage to the peripheral capillary wall by the immune deposits, which activate complement, and possibly the release of lysosomes by the attracted polymorphonuclear neutrophils and monocytes may have a role to play. Thinning of the peripheral glomerular basement membrane and aneurysm formation may represent acute lesions. These may lead to disruption of the basement membrane and subsequent escape of intraluminal material into the Bowman's space, and eventually result in the formation of crescents and adhesions [28, 87, 88]. Thickening and reduplication of the glomerular basement membrane may represent later stages of the disease and the encroachment of the chronic mesangial changes of increased matrix formation into the lumen of the peripheral glomerular capillaries.

The IgA complexes have been demonstrated to be small (7–13 s) or intermediate (13–17 s) in size [94]. Also, IgA nephropathy patients at different periods of time show some changes in IgA complex size [95]. This may explain the localization of the deposits in the mesangium and at various sites in the peripheral glomerular capillary loops. There is no significant difference in the histologic type of glomerular lesions between patients with

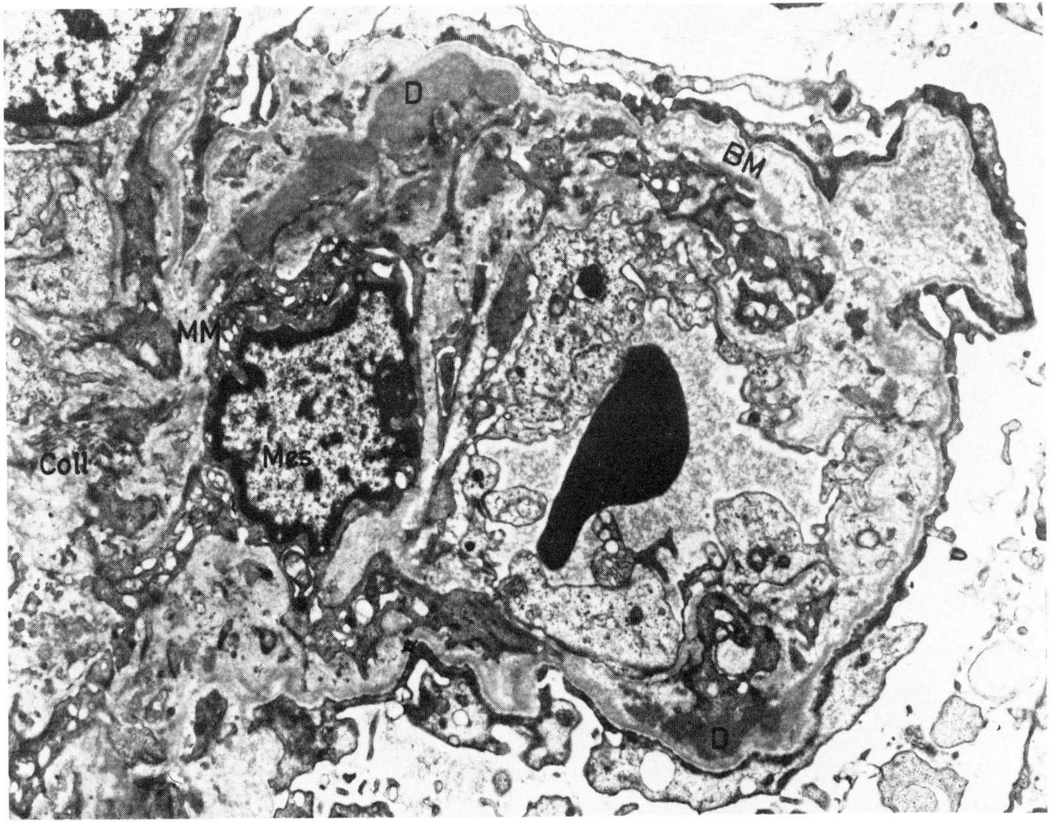

Figure 6-16. Electron micrograph of part of a glomerulus in IgA nephropathy. There is increased mesangial matrix containing collagen fibers. There are electron-dense deposits in the mesangium–paramesangium and peripheral subendothelium. There is segmental mesangial interposition with reduplication of the basement membrane. There is severe membranolysis with glomerular capillary aneurysms. The podocytes show obliteration of foot processes. *MM*, mesangial matrix; *Mes*, mesangial cell; *BM*, basement membrane; *Coll*, collagen fibers; and *D*, dense deposits. ×12,600.

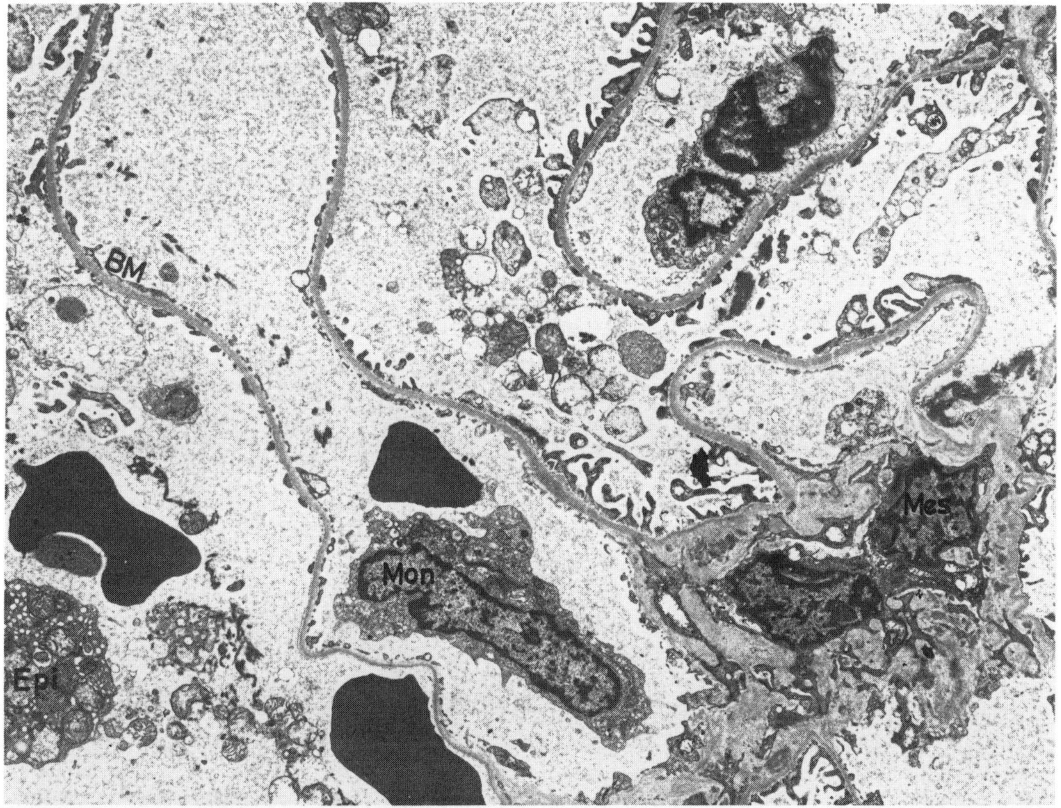

Figure 6-17. Electron micrograph of part of a glomerulus shows thinning of the basement membrane; necrosis and detachment of the podocytes in a case of IgA nephropathy. *Mes*, mesangial cell; *Mon*, monocyte; *BM* basement membrane; and *Epi*, epithelial cell. ×6300.

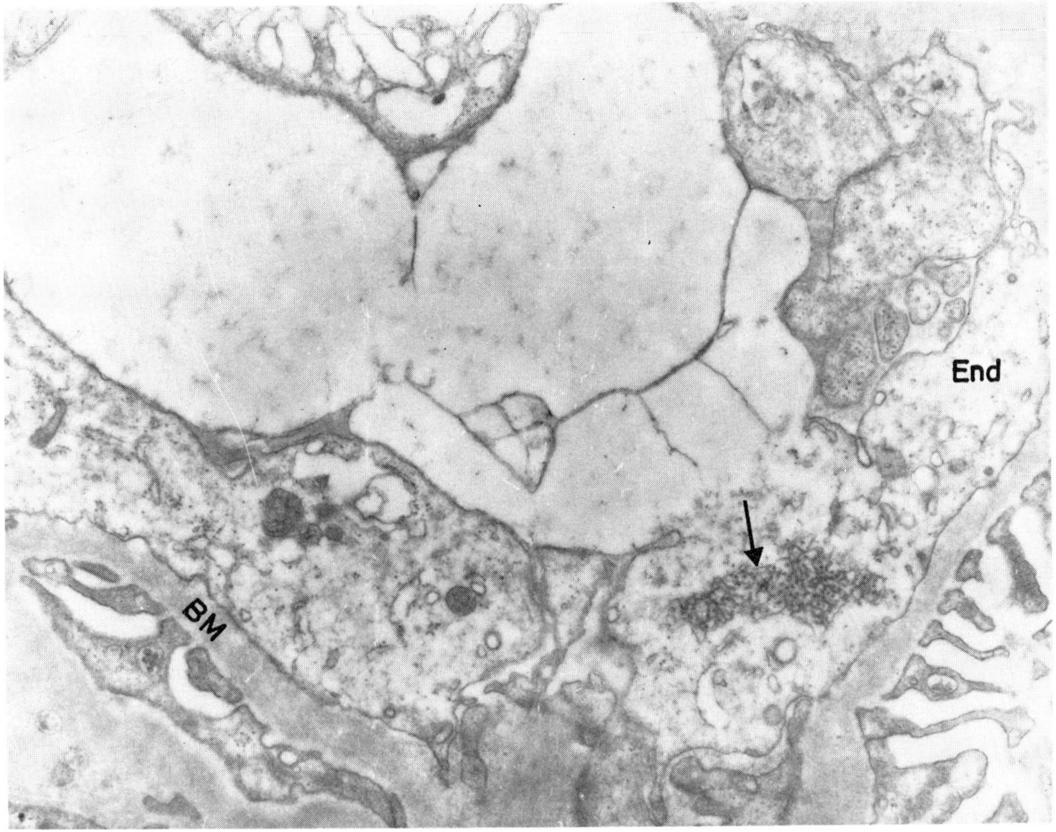

Figure 6-18. Electron micrograph of part of a glomerulus shows tubuloreticular particles (*arrows*) in the endothelial cytoplasm. *End*, endothelium; and *BM*, basement membrane. ×33,000.

peripheral capillary wall lesions and those without. In patients with the most severe proliferative and sclerotic glomerular damage observed by light microscopy, there is greater mesangial sclerosis with collagen fibers, with increased mesangial cells and matrix [48, 79, 90]. Electron-microscopic studies have shown clearly that the combination of damage to the mesangium and the peripheral glomerular capillaries manifests in a varied clinical presentation of the disease. The mesangial and capillary wall damage leads to eventual glomerular obsolescence and a diffuse sclerosing glomerulonephritis with tubulointerstitial damage and vascular lesions. The combined renal parenchymal loss and vascular sclerosis lead to end-stage renal disease that can be treated only by dialysis and/or renal transplantation. Therefore the understanding of the basic pathology of this widespread kidney disease is of utmost importance to nephrologists.

REFERENCES

1. Berger J, Hinglais N: Les dépôts intercapillaires d'IgA-IgG. J Urol (Paris) 74:694–695, 1968.
2. Berger J: IgA glomerular deposits in renal disease. Transplant Proc 1:934–944, 1969.
3. Sinniah R, Feng PH: Lupus nephritis: correlation between light, electron microscopic and immunofluorescent findings and renal function. Clin Nephrol 6:340–351, 1976.
4. Clarkson AR, Seymour AE, Thompson AJ, Haynes WDG, Chan YL, Jackson B: IgA nephropathy: a syndrome of uniform morphology, diverse clinical features, and uncertain prognosis. Clin Nephrol 8:459–471, 1977.
5. Sinniah R, Feng PH, Chen BTM: Henoch-Schönlein syndrome: a clinical and morphological study of renal biopsies. Clin Nephrol 9:219–228, 1978.
6. Callard P, Feldmann G, Prandi P, Belair MF, Maudet C, Weiss Y, Druet P, Benhamou JP, Bariety J: Immune complex type glomerulonephritis in cirrhosis of the liver. Am J Pathol 80:329–337, 1975.
7. Berger J, Yaneva H, Nabarra B: Glomerular changes in patients with cirrhosis of the liver. In: Hamburger J, Crosnier J, Maxwell H (eds) Advances in nephrology. Chicago: Year Book Medical, 1978, pp. 3–14.
8. Sinniah R: Heterogeneous IgA glomerulonephropathy in liver cirrhosis. Histopathology 8:947–962, 1984.
9. Sinniah R: Mucin secreting cancer with mesangial IgA deposits. Pathology 14:303–308, 1982.
10. Mustonen J, Pasternack A, Helin H: IgA mesangial nephropathy in neoplastic diseases. In: D'Amico G, Minetti L, Ponticelli C (eds) IgA mesangial nephropathy. Basel: Karger, 1984, pp 283–291.
11. Morel-Maroger L, Leathem A, Richet G: Glomerular abnormalities in non-systemic diseases: relationship between findings by light microscopy and immunofluorescence in 433 renal biopsy specimens. Am J Med 53:170–184, 1972.
12. Droz D: Natural history of primary glomerulonephritis with mesangial deposits of IgA. Contrib Nephrol 2:150–157, 1976.
13. Di Belgiojoso GB, Tarantino A, Civati G, Limido D, Minetti L: Glomerulonefrite A depositi intercapillari di IgA-IgG: studio clinico E. morfologico di 63 casi. Rincera Clin Lab 3:30–62, 1973.
14. Colasanti G, Banfi G, Di Belgiojoso B, Bertoli S, Fogazzi G, Rangni A, Ponticelli C, Minetti L, D'Amico G: Idiopathic IgA mesangial nephropathy: clinical features. Contrib Nephrol 18:147–156, 1984.
15. D'Amico G: Natural history and treatment of idiopathic IgA nephropathy. In: Robinson RR, et al. [eds] Nephrology, vol 1: proceedings of the 9th international congress of nephrology. New York: Springer-Verlag, 1984, pp 686–701.
16. Shirai T, Tomino Y, Sato M, Yoshiki T, Itoh T: IgA nephropathy: clinicopathology and immunopathology. Contrib Nephrol 9:88–100, 1978.

17. Sakai O, Kitajima T, Kawamma K, Ueda Y: Clinicopathological studies on IgA glomerulonephritis: In: Yoshitoshi Y, Ueda Y (eds) Glomerulonephritis: proceedings of the international symposium on glomerulonephritis, Tokyo 1977. Tokyo: University of Tokyo Press, 1979, pp 167–180.
18. Sinniah R, Pwee HS, Lim CH: Renal glomerular lesions in patients with asymptomatic microscopic haematuria–proteinuria discovered on a routine medical examination. Ann Acad Med [suppl] 4:11–16, 1975.
19. Sinniah R, Javier AR, Ku G: The pathology of mesangial IgA nephritis with clinical correlation. Histopathology 5:469–490, 1981.
20. Levy M, Beaufils H, Gubler MC, Habib R: Idiopathic recurrent macroscopic haematuria and mesangial IgA-IgG deposits in children (Berger's disease). Clin Nephrol 1:63–69, 1973.
21. Hyman LR, Wagnild JP, Beirne GJ, Burkholder PM: Immunoglobulin-A distribution in glomerular disease: analysis of immunofluorescence localization and pathogenetic significance. Kidney Int 3:397–408, 1973.
22. McCoy RC, Abramowsky CR, Tisher CC: IgA nephropathy. Am J Pathol 76:123–144, 1974.
23. Sissons JGP, Woodrow DF, Curtis JR, Evans DJ, Gower PE, Sloper JC, Peters DK: Isolated glomerulonephritis with mesangial IgA deposits. Br Med J 3:611–614, 1975.
24. Sinniah R, Pwee HS, Lim CH: Glomerular lesions in asymptomatic microscopic haematuria discovered on routine medical examination. Clin Nephrol 5:216–228, 1976.
25. Bariety J, Druet PH: Résultats de l'immunohistochimie de 589 biopsies rénales (transplantés exclus). Ann Med Int 122:63–69, 1971.
26. Woodroffe AJ, Thompson NM, Meadows R, Lawrence JR: IgA-associated glomerulonephritis. Aust NZ J Med 5:97–100, 1975.
27. Alexander F, Barabas AZ, Jack RGJ: IgA nephropathy. Hum Pathol 8:173–185, 1977.
28. D'Amico G: Idiopathic mesangial IgA nephropathy. In: Bertani T, Remuzzi G (eds) Glomerular Injury 300 years after Morgagni. Milan: Wichtig Editore, 1983, pp 205–228.
29. Druet P, Bariety J, Bernard D, Lagrue G: Les glomérulopathies primitives à dépôts mésangiaux d'IgA et d'IgG: étude clinique et morphologique de 52 cas. Presse Med 78:583–587, 1970.
30. Davies DR, Tighe JR, Jones NF, Brown GW: Recurrent haematuria and mesangial IgA deposition. J Clin Pathol 26:672–677, 1973.
31. Covarsi A, Flores R, Barcelo P, Santaularia JM, Ballarin J, Del Rio G: Glomerulonephritis por depositos mesangiales de IgA (enfermedad de Berger) Parametros evolutivos. Nefrologia 1:1–12, 1981.
32. Mandreoli M, Pasquali S, Donini V, Casanova S, Cagnoli L: Correlazioni anotomo-cliniche in corso di malattia di Berger. Nefrol Dial 1:9–16, 1981.
33. Vangelista A, Frasca GM, Mardini S, Bonomini V: Idiopathic IgA mesangial nephropathy: immunohistological features. Contrib Nephrol 40:167–173, 1984.
34. Waldherr R, Rambausek M, Rauterberg W, Andrassy K, Ritz E: Immunohistochemical features of mesangial IgA glomerulonephritis. Contrib Nephrol 40:99–106, 1984.
35. Zimmerman SW, Burkholder PM: Immunoglobulin A nephropathy. Arch Intern Med 135:1217–1223, 1975.
36. Katz A, Underdown BJ, Minta JO, Lepow IH: Glomerulonephritis with mesangial deposits of IgA unassociated with systemic disease. CMA J 114:209–216, 1976.
37. Burkholder PM, Zimmermann SW, Moorthy AV: A clinicopathologic study of the natural history of mesangial IgA nephropathy. In: Yoshitoshi Y, Ueda Y (eds) Glomerulonephritis: progression and regression. Baltimore: University Park Press, 1979, pp 143–166.
38. Woodroffe AJ, Gormly AA, McKenzie PE, Wootton AM, Thompson AJ, Seymour AE, Clarkson AR: Immunologic studies in IgA nephropathy. Kidney Int 18:366–372, 1980.
39. Ueda Y, Sakai O, Yamagata M, Kitajima T, Kawamura K: IgA glomerulonephritis in Japan. Contrib Nephrol 4:36–47, 1977.
40. Yokoska H, Nagase M, Maeda T, Koide K: Mesangial IgA glomerulonephritis: clinicopathological study of 85 cases. Contrib Nephrol 9:101–110, 1978.
41. Nakamoto Y, Asano Y, Dohi K, Fujioka M, Iida H, Kida H, Kibe Y, Hattori N, Takeuchi J: Primary IgA glomerulonephritis and Schönlein-Henoch purpura nephritis: clinicopathological and immunohistological characteristics. Q J Med 47:495–516, 1978.
42. Ng WL, Chan CW, Yeung CK, Hua SP: The pathology of primary IgA glomerulonephritis: a renal biopsy study. Pathology 13:137–143, 1981.

43. Sinniah R, Ku G: Clinicopathologic correlations in IgA nephropathy. In: Robinson RR, et al. (ed) Nephrology, vol 1, New York: Springer-Verlag, 1984, pp 665–685.
44. Juncos L, Schlein E, Teague P, Waldman R, Cade R: Immunoglobulin A glomerulonephritis: a clinicopathologic study. Lab Invest 32:140–148, 1975.
45. Götze O, Müller-Eberhard HJ: The C3-activator system an alternate pathway of complement activation. J Exp Med 134:90–108, 1971.
46. Evans DJ, Williams GD, Peters DK, Sissons JGP, Boulton-Jones JM, Ogg CS, Cameron JS, Hoffbrand B: Glomerular deposition of properdin in Henoch-Schönlein syndrome and idiopathic focal nephritis. Br Med J 3:326–328, 1973.
47. Southwest Pediatric Nephrology Study Group: A multicentric study of IgA nephropathy in children. Kidney Int 22:643–652, 1982.
48. Hara M, Endo Y, Nihei H, Hara S, Fukushima O, Mimura N: IgA glomerulonephritis with subendothelial deposits. Virchows Arch [Pathol Anat] 386:249–263, 1980.
49. Lowance DC, Mullins JD, McPhaul JJ: Immunoglobulin A (IgA) associated glomerulonephritis. Kidney Int 3:167–176, 1973.
50. Dobrin RS, Knudson FE, Michael AF: The secretory immune system and renal disease. Clin Exp Immunol 21:318–328, 1975.
51. Tsuchida H, Shishido H, Koyama A, Hirose K, Narita M, Tojo S, Ito H, Iwama H, Sanada T, Mitsuhashi S, Okada M: Chance hematuria and/or proteinuria: immunopathologic studies on Japanese patients with special reference to mesangial IgA nephropathy [abstr 359]. In: 4th international congress of nephrology, Florence, 1975.
52. Tourville DR, Adler RH, Bienenstock J, Tomasi TB: The human secretory immunoglobulin system: immunohistological localization of gamma A, secretory "piece" and lactoferrin in normal human tissues. J Exp Med 129:411–429, 1969.
53. Lomax-Smith JD, Zabrowarny LA, Howarth GS, Seymour AE, Woodroffe AJ: The immunochemical characterization of mesangial IgA deposits. Am J Pathol 113:359–364, 1983.
54. André C, Berthoux FC, André F, Gillon J, Genin C, Sabatier J-C: Prevalence of IgA2 deposits in IgA nephropathies: a clue to their pathogenesis. N Engl J Med 303:1343–1346, 1980.
55. Bene MC, Faure G, Levy M, Duheille J: Identification de la sous-classe IgA1 et/ou IgA2 des dépôts mésangiaux d'IgA. Nouv Presse Med 11:2639–2640, 1982.
56. Conley ME, Cooper MD, Michael AF: Selective deposition of immunoglobulin A1 in immunoglobulin A nephropathy, anaphylactoid purpura nephritis, and systemic lupus erythematosus. J Clin Invest 66:1432–1436, 1980.
57. Tomino Y, Endoh M, Nomoto Y, Sakai H: Immunoglobulin A1 in IgA Nephropathy. N Engl J Med 305:1159–1160, 1981.
58. Tomino Y, Sakai M, Miura M, Endoh M, Nomoto Y: Detection of polymeric IgA in glomeruli from patients with IgA nephropathy. Clin Exp Immunol 49:419–425, 1982.
59. Hall RP, Stachura I, Cason J, Whiteside TL, Lawley TL: IgA-containing circulating immune complexes in patients with IgA nephropathy. Am J Med 74:56–63, 1983.
60. Valentijn RM, Radl J, Haaiman JJ, Daha MR, Van Es LA: Circulating macromolecular IgA-1 and mesangial secretory component-binding IgA-1 in primary IgA nephropathy [abstr] Kidney Int 24:408, 1983.
61. Katz A, Newkirk MH, Klein MH: Circulating and mesangial IgA in IgA nephropathy. In: D'Amico G, Minetti L, Ponticelli C (eds) IgA mesangial nephropathy. Contrib Nephrol 40:74–79, 1984.
62. Delacroix DL, Liroux E, Vaerman JP: High proportion of polymeric IgA in young infants' sera and independence between IgA-size and IgA subclass distributions. J Clin Immunol 3:53–58, 1983.
63. Crago SS, Kutteh WH, Prince SJ, Radl J, Haajman JJ, Mestecky J: Distribution of IgA1 and IgA2 subclasses in human tissue: correlation with the presence of J-chain. Ann NY Acad Sci 409:803–805, 1983.
64. Conley ME, Koopman WJ: Serum IgA1 and IgA2 in normal adults and patients with systemic lupus erythematosus and hepatic disease. Clin Immunol Immunopathol 26:390–397, 1983.
65. Murakami T, Furuse A, Hattori S, Kobayashi K, Matsuda I: Glomerular IgA1 and IgA2 deposits in IgA nephropathies. Nephron 35:120–123, 1983.

66. Bene MC, Faure G, Duheille J: IgA-nephropathy: characterization of the polymeric nature of mesangial deposits by in vitro binding of free secretory component. Clin Exp Immunol 47:527–534, 1982.
67. Komatsu N, Nagura H, Watanabe K, Nomoto Y, Kobayashi K: Mesangial deposition of J chain-linked polymeric IgA in IgA Nephropathy. Nephron 33:61–64, 1983.
68. Egido J, Sancho J, Mampaso F, Lopez-Trascasa M, Sanchez-Crespo M, Blasco R, Hernando L: A possible common pathogenesis of the mesangial IgA glomerulonephritis in patients with Berger's disease and Schönlein-Henoch syndrome. Proc Eur Dial Transplant Assoc 17:660-666, 1980.
69. De Werra P, Morel-Maroger L, Leroux-Robert C, Richet G: Glomérulites à dépôts d'IgA diffus dans le mèsangium: étude de 96 cas chez l'adulte. Schweiz Med Wochenschr 103:761–768 and 797–803, 1973.
70. Baart de la Faille-Kuyper EH, Kater L, Kuigten RH, Kooiker CJ, Wagenaar SS, Van der Zuuwen P, Dorhout Mees EJ: Occurrence of vascular IgA deposits in clinical normal skin of patients with renal disease. Kidney Int 9:424–429, 1976.
71. Ku G, Sinniah R, Seah PP, Loke GKF, Lau YK, Chan HL, Tay L, Khoo OT: Simultaneous analysis of renal biopsy, immunochemistry and immunofluorescent studies of clinically normal skin in glomerulonephritis. J Med Assoc Thai [Suppl 1] 61:3–9, 1978.
72. Berger J, Yaneva H, Nabarra B, Barbanel C: Recurrence of mesangial deposition of IgA after renal transplantation. Kidney Int 7:232–241, 1975.
73. López-Trascasa M, Egido J, Sancho J, Hernando L: IgA glomerulonephritis (Berger's disease): evidence of higher serum levels of polymeric IgA. Clin Exp Immunol 42:247–254, 1980.
74. Rifai A, Small PA Jr, Teague PO, Ayoub EM: Experimental IgA nephropathy. J Exp Med 150:1161–1173, 1979.
75. Kurt Lee SM, Rao VM, Franklin WA, Schiffer MS, Aronson AJ, Spargo BH, Katz AI: IgA nephropathy: morphologic predictors of progressive renal disease. Hum Pathol 13:314–322, 1982.
76. Hogg RJ, Silva FG: IgA nephropathy: natural history and prognostic indices in children. Contrib Nephrol 40:214–221, 1984.
77. Mihatsch MJ, Imbasciati E, Fogazzi G, Giani M, Chio L, Gaboardi F: Ultrastructural lesions of Henoch-Schönlein syndrome and IgA nephropathy: similarities and differences. Contrib Nephrol 40:255–263, 1984.
78. Kupor LR, Mullins JD, McPhaul JJ Jr: Immunopathologic findings in idiopathic renal hematuria. Arch Intern Med 135:1204–1211, 1975.
79. Finlayson G, Alexander R, Juncos L, Schlein E, Teague P, Waldman R, Cade R: Immunoglobulin A glomerulonephritis: a clinicopathologic study. Lab Invest 32:140–148, 1975.
80. Sinniah R: IgA mesangial nephropathy: Berger's disease. [editorial review]. Am J Nephrol 5:73–83, 1985.
81. Churg J, in collaboration with LH Sobin and pathologists and nephrologists in 14 countries: Renal disease: classification and atlas of glomerular diseases. Tokyo: Igaku-Shoin, 1982.
82. Droz D, Kramar A, Nawar T, Noel LH: Primary IgA nephropathy: prognostic factors. Contrib Nephrol 40:202–207, 1984.
83. D'Amico G, Di Belgiojoso B, Imbasciati E, Fogazzi G, Radaelli L, Ferrario F, Fellin G, Ponticelli C, Minetti L: Idiopathic IgA mesangial nephropathy: natural history. Contrib Nephrol 40:208–213, 1984.
84. Clarkson AR, Seymour AE, Woodroffe AJ: Primary renal hematuria: IgA nephropathy. In: Massry SG, Glassock RJ (eds) Text book of nephrology, vol 1. Baltimore: Williams and Wilkins, 1983, pp 6.56–6.61.
85. Feiner HD, Galvin S, Neelakantappa K, Baldwin D, Gallo GR: Vessel sclerosis and progression in IgA nephropathy. Contrib Nephrol 40:222–227, 1984.
86. Navas-Palacios JJ, Gutierrez-Millet LV, Usera-Sárraga G, Garzón-Martin A: IgA nephropathy: an ultrastructural study. Ultrastruct Pathol 2:151–161, 1981.
87. Okada M, Tsuchida H, Yamamoto S: Familial mesangial IgA Nephropathy. In: Yoshitoshi Y, Ueda Y (eds) Glomerulonephritis progression and regression. Baltimore: University Park Press, 1978, pp 201–223.
88. Ng WL, Chan KW, Yeung CK, Kwan S: Peripheral glomerular capillary wall lesions in IgA nephropathy and their implications. Pathology 16:324–330, 1984.

89. Singer DB, Hill LL, Rosenberg HS, Marshall J, Swenson R: Recurrent hematuria in childhood. N Engl J Med 279:7–12, 1968.
90. Sinniah R, Churg J: Effect of IgA deposits on the glomerular mesangium in Berger's disease. Ultrastruct Pathol 4:9–22, 1983.
91. Vernier RL, Resnick JS, Mauer SM: Recurrent hematuria and focal glomerulonephritis. Kidney Int 7:224–231, 1975.
92. Shigematsu H, Kobayashi Y, Tateno S, Hiki Y, Kuwao S: Ultrastructural glomerular loop abnormalities in IgA nephropathy. Nephron 30:1–7, 1982.
93. Sinclair RA, Antonovych TT, Mostofi FK: Renal proliferative arteriopathies and associated glomerular changes: a light and electron microscopic study. Hum Pathol 7:565–588, 1976.
94. Valentijn RM, Kauffmann RH, Brutel de La Rivière G, Daha MR, Van Es LA: Presence of circulating macromolecular IgA in patients with hematuria due to primary IgA nephropathy. Am J Med 74:375–381, 1983.
95. Egido J, Sancho J, Rivera F, Hernando L: The role of IgA and IgG immune complexes in IgA nephropathy. Nephron 36:59–66, 1984.

7. IgA NEPHROPATHY: CLINICOPATHOLOGIC CORRELATIONS

DOMINIQUE DROZ

IgA nephropathy is now accepted as a clinicopathologic entity characterized by diffuse glomerular mesangial deposition of IgA as the predominant immunoglobulin [1, 2]. As pointed out by Berger in his first description, clinical presentation and symptoms as well as glomerular aspects by light microscopy vary from patient to patient. Some present with recurrent macroscopic hematuria while in the others the disease is discovered by "chance" finding of proteinuria. Although the mode of presentation of IgA nephropathy may be influenced by renal biopsy policy, obvious differences are observed between pediatric and adult reports, on the one hand, and among different countries, on the other. For instance, in France, gross hematuria is the presenting symptom in 40% of adults and 80% of children [3, 4] while, in Japan, gross hematuria is the initial symptom in only 14% of adults and children [5]. In the majority of patients, the evolution is chronic during several years with persistent urinary abnormalities. Episodes of macroscopic hematuria are more frequent during the first years of the course and then tend to disappear [3, 4, 6, 7]. Long-standing clinical remission may occur in a few patients, especially in children [7]. However, 15–25% of all patients develop progressive renal failure [6, 8]. A few of them follow a direct, rapid course to terminal renal failure and are thus referred to as having "malignant" IgA nephropathy [9]. Hypertension develops during the course in a significant number of cases [6, 8, 10, 11] preceding or not the appearance of renal insufficiency.

A wide spectrum of glomerular lesions are observed by light microscopy, leading to various terminology and classifications (see chapter 6). Mesangial involvement with increase in mesangial matrix, presence of fibrinoid deposits, and some focal degree of hypercellularity characterize the "mesangiopathic" aspect or minor changes [12]. In the majority of the cases, superimposed focal and segmental glomerular lesions are present [2, 3, 7]. It is widely accepted that all the different types of these focal and segmental lesions represent the various evolutive stages of a continuum, although the nature of the pathogenic process remains unknown: segmental thrombosis, then necrosis with consecutive epithelial crescents progressing to fibrous cellular adhesion, and finally ending with permanent segmental or global glomerular fibrosis or hyalinosis. Focal glomerular tuft necrosis and extracapillary proliferation may reflect active stages of the disease. On the other hand, the estimation of the number of glomeruli affected by segmental lesions is important in assessing the severity of the disease and its prognosis [8]. A small number of patients have diffuse glomerular lesions characterized by diffuse endocapillary proliferation with segmental epithelial crescents (endo-extraproliferative glomerulonephritis) [3, 7]. It has been established by several groups that the tubular interstitial lesions parallel the intensity and diffusion of the glomerular lesions [6, 8, 13, 14] (table 7-1).

Bearing these preliminary remarks in mind, we will now discuss the clinicopathologic correlations in IgA nephropathy.

SEX, AGE AT ONSET, DURATION OF THE DISEASE PRIOR TO BIOPSY

Female sex appears to be associated with minor glomerular lesions, as compared with those in males, either in adults or in children [8, 15], which would account for the better prognosis observed in females [6, 8, 11] (table 7-1). Late age at onset is related to more extensive global glomerular sclerosis, interstitial fibrosis, and vascular damage [6, 16]. A prebiopsy follow-up of long duration is also associated with more severe lesions on biopsy, especially sclerotic lesions ("inactive" type) [12, 13, 17, 18]. Minor changes or mesangiopathic lesions are more frequently observed in biopsies made within one year of the clinical onset as compared with those taken at later stages [12]. In our experience (table 7-1) the number of glomeruli with segmental lesions increases with the duration of prebiopsy follow-up. However, there is no statistically significant difference in prebiopsy duration of the disease between patients with minor changes, or those with focal glomerulonephritis or those with diffuse endo-extraproliferative glomerulonephritis. Therefore, the glomerular lesions are likely to develop and to progress variably in each case, suggesting that the course of the disease is particular to each patient.

PROTEINURIA, NEPHROTIC SYNDROME

Persistent proteinuria exceeding 0.5 g/day is rarely observed less than five years from the documented onset of symptoms, which suggests that pro-

Table 7-1. Clinicopathologic correlations (232 patients)

						At the time of biopsy					Evolution	
	Glom	I nb pts	V nb pts	♂/♀ nb pts	Median age at onset (years)	Median prebiopsy interval (months)	RGH nb pts	Median Pu g/day	HT nb pts	RI nb pts	HT nb pts	RI nb pts
Minor	45	1	4	30/15	27	38	29 (65%)	0.3	3 (7%)	0	10 (23%)	1 (2%)
FSG_1	119	14	13	77/42	28	28	42 (35%)	0.6	19 (16%)	3 (25%)	46 (39%)	13 (10%)
FSG_2	43	33	17	39/4	33	41	15 (35%)	1.4*	15 (35%)	13 (30%)	24 (55%)	26 (60%)
FSG_3	16	16	11	14/2	32	54	3 (20%)	2.8**	12 (75%)	14 (87%)	14 (87%)	16 (100%)
EE	9	9	5	8/1	25	41	4 (45%)	2.2***	2 (22%)	4 (45%)	5 (55%)	7 (78%)

Glom, glomerular lesions; I, severe tubulointerstitial fibrosis; V, severe vascular lesions; nb pts, number of patients; minor, increase in mesangial matrix ± deposits ± segmental mesangial hypercellularity; FSG_1, minor + 0–30% glomeruli with segmental lesions; FSG_2, minor + 30–60% glomeruli with segmental lesions; FSG_3, minor + >60% glomeruli with segmental lesions; EE, diffuse endo-extracapillary proliferative glomerulonephritis; RGH, recurrent gross hematuria prior to biopsy; Pu, proteinuria (*nephrotic range Pu (>3 g/24 h) (* 5pts, ** 7 pts, and *** 2 pts); HT, hypertension; and RI, renal insufficiency.

teinuria is a late manifestation in IgA nephropathy [19]. This is emphasized by the observation of transplanted patients with IgA recurrent disease, indicating that the presence of IgA mesangial deposits antedates the appearance of proteinuria by several months [20].

It is widely recognized that, in both children and adults, the level of proteinuria is well correlated to the severity and extent of the glomerular lesions, whatever the mode of histologic grading used [6, 14–17, 21, 22]. In adults, proteinuria level is higher at diagnosis in older patients, and in those with a long duration of the disease, which is correlated to the extent of focal glomerular sclerosis and of interstitial fibrosis [6, 10, 16, 17]. In our experience, patients who have only minor changes have proteinuria <0.5 g/day at the time of biopsy. The level of proteinuria increases with the number of glomeruli involved by segmental lesions. In the patients with diffuse endocapillary proliferative glomerulonephritis with focal crescents, proteinuria is over 2 g/day (table 7-1).

In a few patients, proteinuria may reach the nephrotic range and then is associated with impaired renal function [24]. In these cases, the renal biopsy consistently shows severe glomerular lesions characterized by diffuse mesangial cell proliferation with numerous focal epithelial crescents or focal sclerosis. Extensive tubulointerstitial lesions are always present [3, 7, 14, 23, 24] (table 7-1). Disappearance of the podocyte foot processes can be noted by electron microscopy [24] and IgA deposits are frequently observed in both mesangial and parietal topography [7, 25].

These patients, with severe glomerular lesions, nephrotic syndrome, and poor prognosis, must be distinguished from the few patients recently described who have steroid-responsive nephrotic syndrome and associated mesangial IgA deposits [26–28]. Such patients, either children or adults, have a fully-developed nephrotic syndrome with dramatic response to steroids but with frequent relapses. Renal biopsy, which was indicated in some patients

Table 7-2. Long-standing clinical remission in IgA nephropathy

	Age at onset	RGH	Glom. lesions	Delay onset → remission	Follow-up
1 ♂	32	+	FSG_1	7	13*
2 ♂	38	+	minor	17	0
3 ♂	26	0	FSG_1	13	0
4 ♂	10	+	FSG_1	11	3*
5 ♂	24	+**	minor	7	3
6 ♀	15	+	FSG_1	10	4*
7 ♂	19	0	FSG_1	2	9

*Second biopsy: patient one, minor changes; patient 4, FSG_1 lesions; and patient six, minor changes.
**Daily gross hematuria during 3½ years.

because of gross hematuria, showed minimal glomerular lesions or mild mesangial lesions [26–28]. In one case, however, the presence of segmental and focal glomerular lesions has been reported [28]. Immunofluorescence discloses IgA mesangial deposits. To date, none of these patients has developed renal insufficiency. Such observations may at the present time represent the coincidental occurrence of nephrosis and IgA nephropathy.

GROSS HEMATURIA

Many reports have dealt with the correlation between macroscopic hematuria and pathologic findings, but they have led to differing conclusions. Some authors found more severe glomerular changes in patients who had a history of gross hematuria [15, 29] while, on the contrary, others found minor lesions in these patients, compared with those without a history of macroscopic hematuria [6, 14, 22]; others found no correlation between the severity of glomerular lesions and previous gross hematuria [8, 10, 30]. As underlined above, several factors such as patient age and duration of prebiopsy follow-up could explain these discrepancies.

The significance of gross hematuria in terms of the underlying glomerular lesion has been studied by Bennett and Kincaid-Smith [29]. In all adults in whom renal biopsy was carried out during an episode of macroscopic hematuria, they found the presence of epithelial crescents. Moreover, 91% of biopsies done within 30 days of an episode of macroscopic hematuria showed crescents. Similarly, the presence of crescents on the biopsy was related to high urinary erythrocyte counts, being observed in 79% of biopsies when over 10^6 RBC/ml and only in 4% of biopsies when below 10^6 RBC/ml [29]. In eight (61%) of 13 of our patients with more than 10^6 RBC/min at the time of biopsy (four having gross hematuria), the presence of segmental epithelial crescents and/or areas of tuft necrosis was observed in variable numbers ($<$10% in two, 10–19% in two, and 20–50% in four). However, in two of these patients who had more than ten gross hematuria episodes prior to biopsy all the glomeruli looked entirely normal and in the three remaining cases only fibrous segmental lesions were present in less than 10% of the glomeruli. On the other hand, 21 (32%) of 68 patients with less than 10^5 RBC/min at the time of biopsy had epithelial crescents by light microscopy ($<$10% of the glomeruli in nine, 10–19% in six, and 20–50% in seven cases) and 17 of them had no episode of gross hematuria during the year preceding the biopsy. Therefore at least in adult patients, gross hematuria seems to be associated with focal glomerular necrosis and crescents and thus reflects an "active" lesional process; however, there is no good correlation between the number of glomeruli with crescents and the level of urinary red blood cell counts.

It would be expected that more extensive segmental or global scarring glomerular lesions should be found in patients who had a history of recurrent macroscopic hematuria prior to biopsy. However, such a relationship could not be established in several large studies [6, 8]. Moreover, in the study by Levy et al., 28 (45%) of 64 children with gross hematuria episodes prior to biopsy were found to have only minor glomerular abnormalities without any global sclerosis or segmental lesions [7]. It has recently been reported, on the basis of repeat biopsies performed in children with Henoch-Schönlein purpura nephritis, that, surprisingly, epithelial crescents may apparently resolve without leaving any glomerular scar [31]. One can speculate that a similar phenomenon may spontaneously occur in IgA nephropathy, at least in young patients, and would explain why, beyond the problem of sampling, numerous macroscopic hematuria episodes may apparently result in few glomerular changes. In the study by Levy et al., 26 of 31 children with recurrent macroscopic hematuria had, at the end of follow-up, normal urinalysis and normal renal function [7]. Similarly, five of seven of our patients with long-standing spontaneous clinical remission had macroscopic hematuria episodes during the course (daily episodes during three years in one patient) (table 7-2). Therefore, the presence of macroscopic hematuria episodes does not have a worse prognostic significance.

ACUTE NEPHRITIS EPISODES (ACUTE RENAL FAILURE EPISODES)

Acute nephritis episodes may occur during the course of some patients [7, 10, 11, 32, 33]. They present with macroscopic hematuria, acute deterioration in renal function, and sometimes hypertension, edema, and loin pain. They resolve spontaneously within a few weeks or months [7, 11, 32, 33] or in coincidence with treatment [10]. In such cases, the renal failure is not related to the extent of glomerular crescents, which are occasional, but to the presence of acute tubular necrosis [7] or in some cases to the presence of erythrocytic casts occluding the tubular lumens [32, 34] (figure 7-1). In one patient with biopsy-proven chronic IgA nephropathy, we observed a resolutive episode of acute renal failure following streptococcal tonsillitis infection. The renal biopsy performed at that time surprisingly showed a pattern of postinfectious acute glomerular nephritis with the presence of numerous polymorphs in the capillary loops. Parietal granular C3 deposits were present while IgA mesangial deposits were markedly diminished as compared with the initial biopsy. This observation suggests that acute renal failure in IgA nephropathy can also be related to superimposed glomerulonephritis of other types [35].

HYPERTENSION

Hypertension occurs in a large number of adult patients [6, 8, 10, 11], but its incidence in children remains low (5%). In our experience, 6.8% of patients had hypertension at the first examination and 41% were hypertensive at the end of follow-up [8] (table 7-1). The occurrence of hypertension was similar

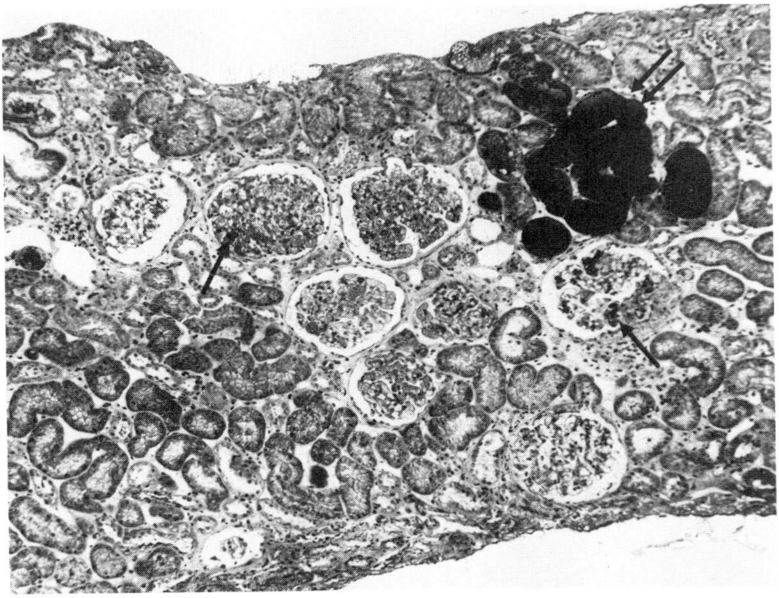

Figure 7-1. Renal biopsy. Masson trichrome with light green, ×160. Patient presenting with acute renal failure, gross hematuria, and proteinuria. Acute renal failure spontaneously resolves. Note the presence of glomerular tuft necrosis and epithelial crescents (↑) and the numerous erythrocytic tubular casts (↑ ↑).

in both sexes in patients under 35 years at the time of onset (35%), but was more frequently observed in patients whose disease began after the age of 35 years (64%) [8]. We observed the same incidence of hypertension in patients with membranoproliferative glomerulonephritis (45% of 188 patients) (unpublished results) while the incidence of hypertension in patients with membranous glomerulonephritis was lower (25% of 116 patients) [36]. The presence of vascular lesions on biopsy (arteriosclerosis and fibrous endarteritis) is noted in nearly half of adult patients with IgA nephropathy [6, 8, 10] whether the patients were hypertensive or not at the time of biopsy. All the patients who were hypertensive at the time of biopsy had vascular lesions, but, conversely, similar lesions were also found in normotensive patients [8]. The severity of vascular lesions parallels the extent of glomerular damage [6, 8] (table 7-1). In addition, a good correlation is found among the patients' age, hypertension, vascular sclerosis, and glomerular sclerosis [6, 10, 12].

A key point is whether vascular lesions are secondary to glomerular damage or play a role in progressive glomerular damage through ischemia. By analyzing the morphologic pattern of glomerular sclerosis (global tuft collapse or disorganization of glomerular structure), Feiner suggested that glomerular sclerosis may be mediated, not solely by a continued immunologic injury, but also by vascular sclerosis or alteration of intrarenal hemodynamics [37]. Another alternative would be an immunologic mechanism affecting both glomeruli and vessels. IgA deposits were found within normal cutaneous blood vessels in patients with IgA nephropathy [38]. It has thus been suggested that similar IgA deposits could be present in renal arterioles. However, although IgA deposits may be abundant in the lacis areas at the vascular pole, none could be demonstrated in the renal interstitial arterioles [7, 8, 12] (Berger, personal communication).

Another point relies upon the relationship between hypertension and vascular damage. Vascular lesions could cause hypertension by inducing ischemia and increased renin release. In IgA nephropathy, however, the presence of vascular damage is not accompanied by high plasma renin activity (PRA) values either in normotensive or hypertensive patients. Moreover, high PRA levels are present in normotensive patients without vascular lesions or glomerular sclerosis, which would suggest that mesangial lesions could per se lead to renin release [39].

PROGRESSION TO RENAL FAILURE

Progressive evolution to renal failure

As one might expect, there is a consensus that severe histologic damage correlates well with a progression to renal insufficiency [3, 6–8, 10, 13, 14, 17, 40]. The estimation of severity and especially the extent of glomerular lesions on the first biopsy appears to be, in many studies, a good indicator of prognosis [6–8, 41, 42]. In Levy's study, none of 70 children who had either minimal glomerular abnormalities or focal and segmental glomerulonephritis affecting less than 30% of the glomeruli progressed toward renal failure during the follow-up while eight of 21 of those who had diffuse proliferative glomerulonephritis with segmental crescents did. In our experience, the relative risk of evolution toward renal insufficiency is ten times lower in patients with minor abnormalities than in those with more than 30% of affected glomeruli [8]. Even when adjusted on glomerular lesions, the proteinuria level maintains a statistical prognostic significance, which indicates that the degree of proteinuria is a better indicator of prognosis than is the extent of glomerular lesions [8]. On the other hand, when adjusted on glomerular lesions, the degree of interstitial fibrosis and of vascular changes loses its statistical prognostic significance [8]. However, four of 14 of our patients with severe tubular interstitial lesions and apparently mild glomerular changes developed renal insufficiency, suggesting that in some cases the tubular interstitial lesion is a better reflection of the renal damage as compared with glomerular involvement (personal observation). The amounts of IgA mesangial deposits are not related to the severity of histologic lesions or to outcome [7, 11, 21, 43].

Rapid progression to renal failure

In several reports, a few patients, mainly males, reach terminal renal failure in a short period of time and belong to the group termed *malignant* IgA nephropathy [9]. Presence of numerous epithelial crescents, affecting more than 50% of glomeruli, is characteristic in these patients [7, 9, 23]. In one 14-year-old boy with recurrent macroscopic hematuria of four-year duration, normal renal function, and 0.7 g/day proteinuria, the first renal biopsy showed the presence of segmental crescents in two of 35 and segmental fibrosis in seven of 35; 18 months later, a second biopsy was performed because of persistent hematuria, proteinuria of 6 g/day, and renal failure and showed a diffuse endo-extracapillary proliferative glomerulonephritis [44]. In this case, the sudden deterioration of the renal function corresponded to the transformation of focal to diffuse glomerulonephritis with diffuse crescents. Similar histologic transformations have been reported in adult patients with sudden deterioration of renal function, but remain rare [6].

CLINICAL REMISSION

Long-standing spontaneous clinical remission (i.e., absence of urinary abnormalities and normal renal function) occurs in nearly 10% of the children [7, 45] and 5% of the adults [1] (personal observation and table 7-2). Such clinical remissions occur only in patients with mild glomerular lesions on the first biopsy [7, 11] (personal cases). Some serial biopsies have been performed in adults with clinical remission (five in the series of Nicholls [11] and three personal cases): the persistance of IgA mesangial deposits has always been observed despite a follow-up as long as 13 years [11] (table 7-2).

ACKNOWLEDGMENTS

The author would like to thank Mr. A. Kramar (Institut de Statistiques, Villejuif, France) for statistical analysis, Dr. L.-H. Noel and Dr. J.-P. Grunfeld for helpful critical review and advice, Ms. M. Kadouche for photographs, and Ms. D. Broneer for efficient secretarial assistance and review of the English text.

REFERENCES

1. Berger J, Hinglais N: Les dépôts intercapillaires d'IgA-IgG. J Urol Néphrol 74:694–695, 1968.
2. Berger J: IgA glomerular deposits in renal disease. Transplant Proc 1:939–944, 1969.
3. Droz D: Natural history of primary glomerulonephritis with mesangial deposits of IgA. Contrib Nephrol 2:150–157, 1976.
4. Levy M, Beaufils H, Gubler MC, Habib R: Idiopathic recurrent hematuria and mesangial IgA-IgG deposits in children (Berger's disease). Clin Nephrol 1:63–69, 1973.
5. Kitajima T, Murakami M, Sakai O: Clinicopathological features in the Japanese patients with IgA nephropathy. Jpn J Med 22:219–222, 1983.
6. D'Amico G, Imbasciati E, Barbiano di Belgioioso G, Bertoli S, Fogazzi G, Ferrario F, Fellin G, Ragni A, Colasanti G, Minetti L, Ponticelli C: Idiopathic IgA mesangial nephropathy: clinical and histological study of 374 patients. Medicine 64:49–60, 1985.

7. Levy M, Gonzales S, Domergues JP, Foulard M, Sorez JP, Broyer M, Habib R: Berger's disease in children: natural history and outcome. Medicine 64:157–180, 1985.
8. Droz D, Kramar A, Nawar T, Noel LH: Primary IgA nephropathy: prognostic factors. Contrib Nephrol 40:202–207, 1984.
9. Nicholls K, Walker RG, Dowling JP, Kincaid-Smith P: "Malignant" IgA nephropathy. Am J Kidney Dis 5:42–46, 1985.
10. Clarkson AR, Seymour AE, Thompson AJ, Haynes WDG, Chan YL, Jackson B: IgA nephropathy: a syndrome of uniform morphology, diverse clinical features and uncertain prognosis. Clin Nephrol 8:459–471, 1977.
11. Nicholls KM, Fairley KF, Dowling JP, Kincaid-Smith P: The clinical course of mesangial IgA associated nephropathy in adults. Q J Med 53:227–250, 1984.
12. Sinniah R, Javier AR, Ku G: The pathology of mesangial IgA nephritis with clinical correlation. Histopathology 5:469–490, 1981.
13. De Werra P, Morel Maroger L, Leroux-Robert C, Richet G: Glomerulites à dépôts d'IgA diffus dans le mésangium: étude de 96 cas chez l'adulte. Schweiz Med Wochenschr 103:761–768, 1973.
14. Shirai T, Tomino Y, Sato M, Yoshiki T, Itoh T: IgA nephropathy: clinicopathology and immunopathology. Contrib Nephrol 9:88–100, 1978.
15. Hogg RJ, Silva F, Walker P, Weinberg AG et al.: A multicenter study of IgA nephropathy in children: a report of the Southwest Pediatric Nephrology Study Group. Kidney Int 22:643–652, 1982.
16. Croker BP, Dawson DV, Sanfilippo F: IgA nephropathy: correlation of clinical and histologic features. Lab Invest 48:19–35, 1983.
17. Van der Peet J, Brentjens DRH, Marrink J, Hoedemaeker Ph J: The clinical course of IgA nephropathy in adults. Clin Nephrol 8:335–340, 1977.
18. Schmekel B, Sualander C, Bucht H, Westberg NG: Mesangial IgA glomerulonephritis in adults: clinical and histopathological observations. Acta Med Scand 210:363–372, 1981.
19. Kincaid-Smith P, Nicholls K: Mesangial IgA nephropathy. Am J Kidney Dis 3: 90–102, 1983.
20. Berger J, Yaneva H, Nabarra B, Barbanel C: Recurrence of mesangial deposition of IgA after renal transplantation. Kidney Int 7:232–241, 1975.
21. Roy PL, Fish AJ, Vernier RL, Michael AF: Recurrent macroscopic hematuria, focal nephritis, and mesangial deposition of immunoglobulin and complement. J Pediatr 82:767–772, 1973.
22. Gartner HV, Honlein F, Traub U, Bohle A: IgA-nephropathy (IgA-IgG-nephropathy/IgA-nephritis): a disease entity? Virchows Arch [Pathol Anat] 385:1–27, 1979.
23. Katz A, Walker JF, Landy PJ: IgA nephritis with nephrotic range proteinuria. Clin Nephrol 20:67–71, 1983.
24. Abuelo JG, Esparza AR, Matarese RA, Endreny RG, Carvalho JS, Allegra SR: Crescentic IgA nephropathy. Medicine 63:396–406, 1984.
25. Hara M, Endo Y, Nihei H, Hara S, Fukushima O, Mimura N: IgA nephropathy with subendothelial deposits. Virchows Arch [Pathol Anat] 386:249–263, 1980.
26. Mustonen J, Pasternack A, Rantala I: The nephrotic syndrome in IgA glomerulonephritis: response to corticosteroid therapy. Clin Nephrol 20:172–176, 1983.
27. Herve JP, Cledes J, Leroy JP, Simon P, Ramee MP, Legall E: Syndromes néphrotiques cortico-sensibles avec dépôts mésangiaux d'IgA: 4 observations. Néphrologie 5:46, 1984.
28. Hogg RJ (a report of the Southwest Pediatric Nephrology Study Group): Association of IgA nephropathy with steroid-responsive nephrotic syndrome. Am J Kidney Dis 5:157–164, 1985.
29. Bennett WM, Kincaid-Smith P: Macroscopic hematuria in mesangial IgA nephropathy: correlation with glomerular crescents and renal dysfunction. Kidney Int 23:393–400, 1983.
30. Sissons JGP, Woodrow DF, Curtis JR, Evans DJ, Gower PE, Sloper JC, Peters DK: Isolated glomerulonephritis with mesangial IgA deposits. Br Med J 3:611–614, 1975.
31. Niaudet P, Levy M, Broyer M, Habib R: Clinicopathologic correlations in severe forms of Henoch-Schönlein purpura nephritis based on repeat biopsies. Contrib Nephrol 40:250–254, 1984.
32. Praga M, Millet VG, Navas J, Morales JM, Ruilope LM, Alcazar JM, Rodicio JL: Acute worsening of renal function during episodes of macroscopic hematuria [abstr 119A]. In: 9th international congress on nephrology, Los Angeles, 1984.

33. Talwalkar YB, Price WH, Musgrave JE: Recurrent resolving renal failure in IgA nephropathy. J Pediatr 92:596–597, 1978.
34. Kincaid-Smith P, Bennett WM, Dowling JP, Ryan BG: Acute renal failure and tubular necrosis associated with hematuria due to glomerulonephritis. Clin Nephrol 19:206–210, 1983.
35. Simon P, Ramee MP, Grunfeld JP, Droz D, Grateau G, Cam G, Ang KS: Disparition des dépôts d'IgA au cours d'une glomerulonéphrite aigue post-infectieuse chez deux patients atteints d'une néphropathie à IgA. Néphrologie 6:213, 1985.
36. Noel LH, Zanetti M, Droz D, Barbanel C: Long-term prognosis of idiopathic membranous glomerulonephritis (study of 116 untreated patients). Am J Med 66:82–90, 1979.
37. Feiner HD, Cabili S, Baldwin DS, Schacht RG, Gallo GR: Intrarenal vascular sclerosis in IgA nephroapthy. Clin Nephrol 18:183–192, 1982.
38. Baart de la Faille-Kuyper EH, Kater L, Kuijten RH, Kooiker CJ, Wagenaar SS, Van der Zouwen P, Dorhout Mees EJ: Occurrence of vascular IgA deposits in clinically normal skin of patients with renal disease. Kidney Int 9:424–429, 1976.
39. Degli Esposti E, Zuchelli P, Chiarini C, Santoro A, Sturani A, Zuccala A, Cagnoli L, Donini U, Mandreoli M, Pasquali S: Berger's nephropathy: relationship between histological pattern, blood pressure and renin. Proc Eur Dial Transplant Assoc 19:696–700, 1982.
40. Hood SA, Velosa JA, Holley KE, Donadio JV: IgA-IgG nephropathy: predictive indices of progressive disease. Clin Nephrol 16:55–62, 1981.
41. D'Amico G, Ferrario F, Colosanti G, Ragni A, Bestetti Bosisio M: IgA-mesangial nephropathy (Berger's disease) with rapid decline in renal function. Clin Nephrol 16:251–257, 1981.
42. Lee SMK, Rao MV, Franklin WA, Schiffer MS, Aronson AJ, Spargo BH, Katz AI: IgA nephropathy: morphologic predictors of progressive renal disease. Hum Pathol 13:314–322, 1982.
43. Kher KK, Makker SP, Moorthy B: IgA nephropathy (Berger's disease): a clinicopathologic study in children. Int J Pediatr Nephrol 4:11–18, 1983.
44. Martini A, Magrini U, Scelsi M, Capelli V, Barberis L: Chronic mesangioproliferative IgA glomerulonephritis complicated by a rapidly progressive course in a 14-year-old boy. Nephron 29:164–166, 1981.
45. McCoy RC, Abramowsky CR, Tisher CC: IgA nephropathy. Am J Pathol 76:123–140, 1974.

8. NATURAL HISTORY AND PROGNOSIS

GIUSEPPE D'AMICO

NATURAL HISTORY AND OUTCOME

Our knowledge of the natural history of idiopathic IgA mesangial nephropathy is still incomplete for two major reasons: (a) the disease has been characterized and recognized as a distinct clinical and pathologic entity only in these last 15 years, with the worldwide application of immunofluorescence microscopy to renal biopsies, and therefore clinical data from long-term observations of large series of patients are still scarce; and (b) for the subgroup of patients whose disease is discovered by chance because of asymptomatic urinary abnormalities, it is impossible to identify the time of onset.

Recent long-term follow-up studies in sufficiently large cohorts of patients have not confirmed the initial prevailing belief that this nephropathy is benign [1–37]. There is accumulating evidence that it relentlessly progresses into chronic renal failure in a number of patients and, in many countries throughout the world, IgA mesangial nephropathy is now recognized as one the most frequent single causes of end-stage chronic renal failure requiring dialysis. The Australian and New Zealand Dialysis and Transplant Registry data [30], the data for France reported by Berger [16] and our data for Italy [3, 14, 28, 29, 35] show that this disease was the underlying cause in approximately 10% of patients given dialysis treatment for end-stage chronic renal failure.

The rapidity of this progression appears to vary greatly. Some patients arrive at renal death quite soon after the apparent onset of the disease, even when this coincides with the first episode of macroscopic hematuria, which probably marks the true onset of the disease [35]. Others have normal renal function for more than 30 years after the first episode of gross hematuria or the first chance discovery of urinary abnormalities. We and many other investigators have seen complete clinical resolution of the disease, with disappearance of all the urinary abnormalities even for some years [23, 31, 33, 38]. In the 140 patients studied in Spain by Rodicio [31] for periods of from four months to four years, it occurred in 15% of cases. Kitajama et al. [23] reported clinical remission in 20% of 481 children after a mean follow-up of 29 months and in 6.5% of 1349 adults after 39 months. Of the 217 patients studied in Australia by Nicholls et al. [33], 15 also had complete disappearance of all clinical signs of the disease. Some of these patients were rebiopsied and these subsequent specimens showed persisting mesangial proliferative glomerulonephritis and mesangial deposition of IgA [33]. To our knowledge, spontaneous disappearance of the mesangial deposits of IgA, which are characteristic of the disease and probably responsible for the glomerular damage, has never been described. We agree with the recent statement of Kincaid-Smith [36] that, probably, once the condition has reached a stage at which it can be diagnosed, the histologic lesions persist indefinitely.

There is still considerable debate about the overall incidence of renal insufficiency and the average rate of its progression to end-stage. Table 8-1 summarizes some of the reported data on this incidence at the end of sufficiently long follow-up observations. The extreme variability of this incidence could be due to differences in the numbers of patients studied and in the criteria used to select patients for biopsy. In the different surveys listed in the table, the percentages of patients diagnosed and enrolled in the follow-up study because of the routine screening of urine of a healthy population or because of the discovery of urinary abnormalities vary considerably, as estimated from the incidence of patients without history of macroscopic hematuria.

Data on actuarial renal survival from different geographic areas, summarized in table 8-2, are probably better indices of the average rate of progression of the disease to end-stage. They are more concordant. They indicate that only 15–20% of patients developed end-stage renal failure within ten years after apparent onset. Since the true onset can considerably antedate the apparent onset from which survival was calculated, at least in the subgroup of patients who did not have gross hematuria to mark the start of the disease, we can estimate that renal survival in idiopathic IgA mesangial nephropathy is greater than 90% at ten years and 75% at 20 years.

According to Legrain et al. [42], the only ones who have compared renal survival in their populations of patients with different types of primary glomerulonephritis, survival with IgA neprhopathy was similar to that with

Table 8-1. Incidence of renal failure and arterial hypertension after variable periods of follow-up, in different series of patients with IgA nephropathy

Reference				Duration of follow-up						
No.	Authors	No. of patients	% with macroscopic hematuria	Total duration of the disease (years) Mean	(Min.–Max.)	Duration of postbiopsy follow-up (years) Mean	(Min.–Max.)	% of patients with reduced GFR at the end of follow-up[a]		% of patients with high blood pressure at the end of follow-up
[39]	De Werra et al. 1973	96	46	6.5	(0.5–36)	—	—	9		11
[1]	Droz 1976	179	44		(1–32)	—	—	23.6	(18)	40
[2]	Clarkson et al. 1977	50	34		(1–18)		(0.2–3.0)	70	—	62
[4]	Van der Peet et al. 1977	25	37	6.3	(0.5–18)	3.9	(0.2–8.7)	40	(20)	—
[11]	Burkholder et al. 1979	34	22	6.3	(1.8–19)	2.9	(0.2–7.0)	13	—	—
[9]	Sakai et al. 1979	101	15	—	—	—	(1.5–10.0)	34	(4)	24
[18]	Gutierrez-Millet et al. 1982	40	80	5.0	(0.5–29)	—	—	22.5	(7.5)	22.5
[15]	Hood et al. 1981	37	78	5.5	(1.2–21)	2.8	(0.7–6.7)	24.3	(13.5)	—
[20]	Southwest Pediatric Nephrology study group 1982	39	87	—	(0.1–75)	2		15	(3)	5
[40]	Abe et al. 1983	177	—	6.4	(2–19)	—	—	—	(11)	—
[26]	Rambausek et al. 1983	50	68	5.7	(0.5–15.5)	—	—	34	(6)	44
[32]	Droz et al. 1984	244	—	—	—	—	—	25.8	(10.6)	41
[41]	Simon et al. 1984	58	45	6.0	(1.5–22)	—	—	36	(8.5)	—
[31]	Rodicio 1984	140	76	—	(2–15)	—	—	—	(8)	29
[33]	Nicholls et al. 1984	217	59	5.0	(1–21)	—	—	43	(9)	53
[35]	D'Amico et al. 1985	267	56	6.5	(1–45)	3.5	(1–13)	37.8	(14.6)	54

[a]In parentheses, % of patients with renal death.

Table 8-2. Actuarial renal survival at 10 years and at 20 years for patients with idiopathic IgA nephropathy, according to different investigators

No.	Reference	No. of patients	Renal survival at 10 years	Renal survival at 20 years
[42]	Legrain et al. 1978	75	85%	—
[12]	Egido et al. 1981	80	78%	—
[43]	Droz and Noel 1983	260	85%	75%
[44]	Beukhof et al. 1983	75	80%	72%
[31]	Rodicio 1984	140	87%	80%
[29]	D'Amico 1984	365	84.7%	66.2%

membranous glomerulonephritis, but definitely better than that with focal glomerulosclerosis or membranoproliferative glomerulonephritis.

In the course of the disease, there are usually very few clinical signs. For years, microscopic hematuria and a proteinuria that is usually mild and without casts may be the only signs in both patients whose disease started with an episode of macroscopic hematuria and those who never experienced such episodes. Recurrent episodes of gross hematuria may occur in the former group of patients after periods of time varying from a few weeks to many years. In the latter group of patients, whose disease was discovered by chance during a routine urinalysis or because of signs such as nephrotic syndrome, chronic renal insufficiency, or arterial hypertension, an episode of gross hematuria during the subsequent follow-up examinations is an exceptional phenomenon in our experience, which make us think that the first episode of macroscopic hematuria usually coincides with the true onset of disease.

In patients with recurrent macroscopic hematuria, the number of recurrences ranges from only a few to more than 20; the interval between episodes tends to become longer with time [35]. In those patients who reported infection at the time of the first episode, the recurrence is often closely associated with a recurrence of the same type of infection. The interval between the precipitating infectious event and the appearance of gross hematuria is characteristically very short (24–48 h) as it was in the first episode. The same occasional infectious diseases that precipitate the new episodes of gross hematuria in the subgroup of patients with recurrent macroscopic hematuria may cause a transitory increase in the number of urinary red cells and/or in the amount of proteinuria in the subgroup of patients without any history of macroscopic hematuria. Such a transitory increase may take place sometimes without any recognizable cause and in some patients represents the first sign of a progressive course. The increase in the amount of proteinuria may be so massive as to cause a humoral or clinically evident nephrotic syndrome. This complication during the course of the disease has been described in some reports from different countries in percentages of patients as high as 24% [24], but is very uncommon in our experience [35] as in that of many other investigators [1, 6, 9, 11, 18, 39, 45].

When arterial hypertension is not already present at the time of diagnosis, it tends to appear during the follow-up examinations, often before the serum creatinine increases to pathologic levels (table 8-1). We demonstrated [46] that the incidence of high blood pressure at different degrees of renal insufficiency is no higher in this glomerulonephritis than in other types of primary glomerulonephritis, such as membanous or membranoproliferative glomerulonephritis, and that it is lower than it is in focal glomerulosclerosis.

The incidence of malignant hypertension appears to vary in the different reports. It is very low in our experience, but was 7% in the study of Clarkson et al. [2] and 10% in that of Rambausek et al. [26]. A very rapid decline in renal function, with the clinical syndrome of acute renal failure, may develop during the course of the disease even without the previous or concomitant appearance of malignant hypertension. We observed two such patients in whom serum creatinine reached 7.5 and 13 mg/dl [35]. The first one showed this abrupt deterioration after more than one year of a clinical course characterized by two episodes of macroscopic hematuria and normal renal function. In the second, the acute syndrome developed after only two months of a history of gross hematuria and mild edema. No precipitating events could be detected for either patient. Renal biopsy examination at that time revealed cellular circumferential crescents in 50% and 67% of glomeruli, respectively. Similar patients with crescents in the majority of glomeruli have been described by others [2, 20, 47, 48].

Serum IgA concentrations do not change much during follow-up. Patients with initially high concentrations usually continue at high concentrations, and those with initially normal levels show no tendency to develop an abnormal elevation. After repeated long-term monitoring (1–8 years) of serum IgA concentrations in 66 patients, in the latest determination we observed abnormal increases in only three of 35 patients with initially normal concentrations (<350 mg/dl), and decreases to normal in only six of 31 with initially high concentrations (>350 mg/dl). Pregnancy is usually well tolerated by patients and does not result in deterioration of renal function or a rise in blood pressure [1, 39, 49]. IgA mesangial nephropathy recurs very frequently after transplantations, within 1–4 years [1, 50, 51]. So far, the clinical course of the recurrent disease appears to be mild, with light proteinuria and microscopic hematuria usually the only clinical manifestations. In contrast, transplantation of donor kidneys with mesangial IgA deposits into patients with previous non-IgA-related disease results in disappearance of the deposits [52–54].

CLINICAL AND HISTOLOGIC PROGNOSTIC INDICATORS

The variable rate of progression of IgA mesangial nephropathy justifies an attempt to identify clear prognostic indicators to apply when an individual patient is first evaluated. Early identification of those patients who are likely to progress would allow us to select a group for whom therapeutic intervention is justifiable and a controlled trial would give reliable results.

Some recent studies have demonstrated that certain clinical signs and histologic features can be of assistance for prediction of the clinical course of the disease, even though, with a few exceptions, too few patients have been studied to allow firm conclusions to be drawn.

Clinical indicators of unfavorable prognosis

The following clinical features have been correlated with more frequent and faster deterioration of renal function:

Older age at the onset. The majority of investigators agree that renal function of older patients deteriorates more frequently [12, 22, 25, 29, 32, 35]. Since the disease is discovered in nearly half of patients during routine medical examinations, and hence the time of onset of the disease cannot be defined, it is possible that older patients are those in whom the disease did not start later but was discovered later. However, even in the subgroup of our patients in whom an episode of macroscopic hematuria probably heralded the true onset of the disease, those with an older age at onset had less favorable prognoses (G. D'Amico, unpublished observations).

Male sex. Some investigators reported more severe renal lesions and/or a less favorable prognosis for male patients [10, 17, 20, 22, 32, 33]. We could not confirm any prognostic role of sex in a large population of 374 patients studied in Milan [35].

No history of macroscopic hematuria. Many investigators [2, 10, 12, 22, 32, 35, 55], including ourselves, have reported the unexpected phenomenon that patients with recurrent episodes of macroscopic hematuria have a more favorable prognosis than those who never experienced such episodes. In our experience, those patients that had a single episode of macroscopic hematuria had an actuarial renal survival that was intermediate between that of patients with recurrent episodes and those without episodes [29]. This could be due to earlier detection of the disease in patients with macroscopic hematuria, so that their progression appears longer. However, in the two subgroups of our patients with recurrent episodes or with an isolated episode of macroscopic hematuria, in whom the true onset of the disease could be established with comparable accuracy, the probability of developing renal failure appeared to be inversely proportional to the number of episodes of macroscopic hematuria, the opposite of what one would expect [29]. To explain it, we suggest that there is a discontinuous effect of the injurious mechanism, limited to the clinical exacerbations, in patients with recurrent macroscopic hematuria, as opposed to a continuous effect in patients without episodes of macroscopic hematuria. Beukhof et al. [56] have recently reported that these two subgroups of patients have different genetic markers and probably represent two different subentities of IgA mesangial nephropathy. Patients with recurrent macroscopic hematuria are in general younger than those without it, and Droz et al. [32] believe that their different prognosis is age related. However, we demonstrated that, even in the same age group, renal survival of patients with recurrent macroscopic hematuria is better than that of patients without macroscopic hematuria [29]. Kincaid-Smith et al. [33, 36] have a completely different opinion about the role of hematuria as prognostic factor. According to this Australian group, when patients are closely age and sex matched, macroscopic hematuria is associated with a worse prognosis. In the absence of macroscopic hematuria, continuing heavy microscopic hematuria (over 100,000 erythrocytes/ml) was associated with greater risk of deterioration of renal function [33].

Decreased glomerular filtration rate at the time of biopsy. As would be expected, stable impairment of renal function at the time of biopsy is associated with an increased risk of subsequent fast deterioration [4, 11, 17, 25, 33, 35, 44].

Arterial hypertension at the time of biopsy. The majority of investigators agree on its bad prognostic significance [4, 7, 11, 12, 15, 17, 18, 22, 25, 29, 33, 35, 43].

Heavy proteinuria at the time of biopsy. According to all investigators, patients who during the course of the disease and/or at the time of biopsy have severe proteinuria (>1 g/day) or a nephrotic syndrome have a less favorable outcome [2, 12, 15, 18, 20, 22, 24, 25, 27, 29, 32–35].

Another clinical feature that has been widely analyzed for its possible prognostic value is an abnormally high titer of serum IgA. All investigators have concluded that the prognosis for patients with high serum IgA is no worse than for those with normal serum IgA [2, 7, 12, 15, 18, 32, 33, 57].

Histologic indicators of unfavorable prognosis

There is good agreement among the different investigators that prognosis correlates well with the overall severity of the proliferative and sclerotic lesions, as scored histologically on the basis of increasing severity and extension of mesangial proliferation and of glomerular sclerosis, as proposed by Sinniah et al. [13], Hood et al. [15], and Lee et al. [17].

When the prognostic roles of the different histologic lesions were analyzed separately, the following results were obtained:

Glomerular sclerosis. All studies indicate that it is a strong indicator of an unfavorable prognosis [2, 7, 11, 12, 15, 18, 22, 25, 29, 33, 35, 36]. This is not unexpected, since glomerular segmental sclerosis and glomerular obsolescence increase with time, as repeat biopsies show [33, 35], probably because of the progressive mesangial damage consequent to the chronic stimulation and overload due to the continuous deposition of IgA immune complexes.

Interstitial sclerosis. This feature is also a recognized indicator for an unfavorable prognosis [11, 18, 22, 35, 40]. Univariate and multivariate renal survival analysis of our patients indicate that it remains a significant predictor even when data are adjusted for the concomitant glomerular sclerosis (D'Amico et al., unpublished observation), and is therefore an independent prognostic marker.

Intracapillary proliferation. Patients with diffuse and severe proliferation have a significantly worse prognosis than those with focal and segmental proliferation or with minimal lesions by light microscopy [11, 18, 29, 35]. We demonstrated that the extent and diffusion of the intracapillary proliferative lesions are not progressive [35]. In our opinion, some patients tend to develop more severe and widespread histologic lesions from the onset of the disease, and these patients progress more frequently and faster to renal failure.

Extracapillary proliferation. A distinction must be made between widespread circumferential crescents, which are found infrequently in this disease, and the small noncircumferential areas of extracapillary proliferation that are rather often present in IgA nephropathy. While the former are usually associated with rapid progressive disease and/or with episodes of acute renal failure, the prognostic value of the latter is still controversial. Many investigators, including ourselves, believe that the presence of even small noncircumferential crescents in a large percentage of glomeruli is an indicator for an unfavorable prognosis [17, 18, 29, 33].

Segmental thickening of glomerular basement membrane. This lesion is rather infrequent in IgA nephropathy. Investigators agree that, when present, it is a sign of more severe disease [34, 58, 59]. Renal survival analysis shows that it is a statistically significant negative prognostic indicator [29].

Extension of immunofluorescent deposits to the peripheral capillary walls. In a variable percentage of cases, the deposition of IgA at immunofluorescence is not exclusively restricted to the mesangial areas, but shows some parietal extension. We [29, 35] and Kobayashi et al. [25] have recently demonstrated that this immunohistologic feature is also a prognosticator of more rapid deterioration of renal function. We suggest that this feature and the presence of the lesions of the GBM described above indicate a more marked engulfment of the mesangial cells by IgA immune complexes, which overflow the mesangial areas and produce lesions of the peripheral capillary walls, therefore favoring a more rapid progression of the disease.

Other immunohistologic features that have been considered predictors of faster progression of the disease include a more massive deposition of C3 [7, 18] or the codeposition of IgG and/or IgM [2, 60, 61]. In our experience, none of these features is prognostic [29, 35].

In conclusion, we are beginning to individuate some clinical, histologic, and immunohistologic factors that seem to be correlated with prognosis. In our experience, however, a prognosis based on such findings for an individual patient is often imprecise, and no numerical score based on their quantitative or semiquantitative evaluation accurately predicts the rate of progression to end-stage renal failure. This is understandable since in IgA nephropathy the immunologically mediated mechanism that seems to be responsible for the disease probably continues to operate up to the latest stages, perhaps with intermittent phases of remission and flare-up, which from time to time modify the rate of progression and of deterioration of renal function.

ACKNOWLEDGMENTS

The work was partly supported by Consiglio Nazionale delle Ricerche (Roma, Italy) grant 84.1985.04. We thank Mrs. Mascia Marchesini and Mrs. Marisa Zanini for typing the manuscript.

REFERENCES

1. Droz D: Natural history of primary glomerulonephritis with mesangial deposits of IgA. Contrib Nephrol 2:150–156, 1976.
2. Clarkson AR, Seymour AE, Thompson AJ, Haynes WDG, Chan YL, Jackson B: IgA nephropathy: a syndrome of uniform morphology, diverse clinical features and uncertain prognosis. Clin Nephrol 8:459–471, 1977.
3. Imbasciati E, Colasanti G, Barbiano di Belgioioso, Banfi G, Durante A, Ragni A, Ponticelli C, Minetti L, D'Amico G: Long-term follow-up of IgA mesangial deposits glomerulonephritis. Proc Eur Dial Transplant Assoc 14:472–475, 1977.
4. Van der Peet J, Arisz L, Brentjens JRH, Marrink J, Hoedemaeker PJ: The clinical course of IgA nephropathy in adults. Clin Nephrol 8:335–340, 1977.
5. Ueda Y, Sakai O, Yamagata M, Kitajima T, Kawamura K: IgA glomerulonephritis in Japan. Contrib Nephrol 4:36–47, 1977.
6. Yokoska H, Nagase M, Maeda K: Mesangial IgA glomerulonephritis: clinicopathological study of 85 cases. Contrib Nephrol 9:101–110, 1978.
7. Shirai T, Tomino Y, Yoshiki T, Itoh T: IgA nephropathy: clinicopathology and immunopathology. Contrib Nephrol 9:88–100, 1978.
8. Nakamoto Y, Asano Y, Dohi K, Fujioka M, Iida H, Kibe Y, Hattori N, Takeuchi J: Primary IgA glomerulonephritis and Schönlein-Henoch purpura nephritis: clinicopathological and immunohistological characteristics. Q J Med 47:495–516, 1978.
9. Sakai O, Kitajima T, Kawamura K, Ueda Y: Clinicopathological studies on IgA glomerulonephritis. In: Yoshitoshi Y, Ueda Y (eds) Glomerulonephritis. Baltimore: University Park Press 1979, p 167.
10. Gärtner HV, Honlein F, Traub U, Bohle A: IgA-nephropathy (IgA-IgG nephropathy, IgA-nephritis): a disease entity? Virchows Arch [Pathol Anat] 385:1–27, 1979.
11. Burkholder PM, Zimmerman SW, Moorthy AV: A clinicopathological study of the natural history of mesangial IgA nephropathy. In: Yoshitoshi Y, Ueda Y (eds) Glomerulonephritis. Baltimore: University Park Press, 1979, p 143.
12. Egido J, Riviera Hernandez F, Sancho J, Moreno M, Kreisler M, Hernando L: Estudio del sistema HLA yy factores de riesgo para la insuficiencia renal en la glomerulonephritis mesangial IgA. Nefrologia 1:21–27, 1981.
13. Sinniah R, Javier AR, Ku G: The pathology of mesangial IgA nephritis with clinical correlation. Histopathology 5:469–490, 1981.
14. D'Amico G, Ferrario F, Colasanti G, Ragni A, Bestetti M: IgA mesangial nephropathy (Berger'S disease) with rapid decline in renal function. Clin Nephrol 16:251–257, 1981.
15. Hood SA, Velosa JA, Holley KE, Donadio JV: IgA-IgG-nephropathy: predictive indices of progressive disease. Clin Nephrol 16:55–62, 1981.
16. Berger J, Yaneva H, Crosnier J: La glomérulonephrite à dépôts mésangiaux d'IgA: une cause fréquente d'insuffisance rénale terminale. Nouv Presse Med 9:219–221, 1980.
17. Lee SMK, Rao MV, Franklin WA, Schiffer MS, Aronson AJ, Spargo BK, KAtz AI: IgA

negphropathy: morphologic predictors of progressive renal disease. Hum Pathol 13:314–322, 1982.
18. Gutierrez-Millet V, Navas Palacios JJ, Prieto C, Ruilope LM, Usera G, Barrientos A, Alcazar JM, Perez AJ, Jarillo MD, Rodicio JL: Glomerulonephritis mesangial IgA idiopatica: estudio clinico e immunopathologico de 40 casos y revision de la literatura. Nefrologia 2:21–34, 1982.
19. Feiner HD, Cabili S, Baldwin DS, Schacht RG, Gallo GR: Intrarenal vascular sclerosis in IgA nephropathy. Clin Nephrol 18:183–192, 1982.
20. Southwest Pediatric Nephrology Study Group: A multicentric study of IgA nephropathy in children. Kidney Int 22:643–652, 1982.
21. Coppo R, Basolo B, Martina G, Rollino C, De Marchi M, Giacchino F, Mazzucco G, Messina M, Piccoli G: Circulating immune complexes containing IgA and IgM in patients with primary IgA nephropathy and with Henoch-Schönlein nephritis: correlation with clinical and histologic signs of activity. Clin Nephrol 18:230–239, 1982.
22. Rambausek WL, Seeling HP, Andrassy K, Waldherr R, Kehry I, Lenhard V, Ritz E: Mesangial IgA-Glomerulonephritis: neue Aspekte zur Diagnose, Klinik und Prognose. Dtsch Med Wochenschr 108:125–130, 1983.
23. Kitajima T, Murakami M, Sakai O: Clinicopathological features in the Japanese patients with IgA nephropathy. Jpn J Med 22:219–222, 1983.
24. Croker BP, Dawson DV, Sanfilippo F: IgA nephropathy: correlation of clinical and histologic features. Lab Invest 48:19–24, 1983.
25. Kobayashi Y, Tateno S, Hiki Y, Shigematsu H: IgA nephropathy: prognostic significance of proteinuria and histological alteration. Nephron 34:146–153, 1983.
26. Rambausek M, Seeling HP, Andrassy K, Waldherr R, Lenhard V, Ritz E: Clinical and serological features of mesangial IgA glomerulonephritis. Proc Eur Dial Transplant Assoc 19:663–668, 1983.
27. Katz A, Walker JF, Landy PJ: IgA nephritis with nephrotic range proteinuria. Clin Nephrol 20:67–71, 1983.
28. D'Amico G, Barbiano di Belgioioso G, Imbasciati E, Fogazzi G, Radaelli L, Ferrario F, Fellin G, Ponticelli C, Minetti L: Idiopathic IgA mesangial nephropathy: natural history. Contrib Nephrol 40:208–213, 1984.
29. D'Amico G: Natural history and treatment of idiopathic IgA nephropathy. In: Robinson RR (ed) Nephrology. New York: Springer, 1984, p 686.
30. Clarkson AR, Woodroffe AJ, Bannister KM, Lomax-Smith JD, Aarons I: The syndrome of IgA nephropathy. Clin Nephrol 21:7–14, 1984.
31. Rodicio JL: Idiopathic IgA nephropathy. Kidney Int 25:717–729, 1984.
32. Droz D, Kramar A, Nawar T, Noel LH: Primary IgA nephropathy: prognostic factors. Contrib Nephrol 40:202–207, 1984.
33. Nicholls KM, Fairley KF, Dowling JP, Kincaid-Smith P: The clinical course of mesangial IgA-associated nephropathy in adults. Q J Med 210:227–250, 1984.
34. Beukhof JR, Ockhuizen Th, Halie LM, Westra J, Beelen JM, Donker AJ M, Hoedemaeker Ph J, Van der Hem GK: Subentities within adult primary IgA-nephropathy. Clin Nephrol 22:195–199, 1984.
35. D'Amico G, Imbasciati E, Barbiano di Belgioioso G, Bertoli S, Fogazzi G, Ferrario F, Fellin G, Ragni A, Colasanti G, Minetti L, Ponticelli C: Idiopathic IgA mesangial nephropathy: clinical and histological study of 374 patients. Medicine 64:49–60, 1985.
36. Kincaid-Smith PS: Mesangial IgA nephropathy. Br Med J: 96–97, 1985.
37. Sinniah R: IgA mesangial nephropathy: Berger's disease. Am J Nephrol 5:73–83, 1985.
38. Glassock RJ, Kurotawa KV: IgA nephropathy in Japan. Am J Nephrol 5:127–137, 1985.
39. De Werra P, Morel-Maroger L, Leroux-Robert C, Richet G: Glomérulites à dépôts d'IgA diffus dans le mésangium: étude de 96 cas chez l'adulte. Schweiz Med Wochenschr 103:761–803, 1973.
40. Abe T, Kida H, Yokoyama H, Hattori N: Significance of extracapillary lesions (ECL) for IgA nephropathy [abstr] In: Proceedings of the second Asian Pacific congress of nephrology, Melbourne, 1983, p 17.
41. Simon P, Ang KS, Bavay P, Cloup C, Miguard JP, Ramee MP: Glomérulonéprite à immunoglobulines A: epidémiologie dans une population de 250,000 habitants. Nouv Presse Med 13:257–260, 1984.

42. Legrain M, Salah H, Beaufils H, Flores Esteves L, Guedon J: Le prognostic de glomérulonéphrites chroniques primitives de l'adulte. Nouv Presse Med 7:533–538, 1978.
43. Droz D, Noel LH: Ré-evaluation du prognostic des glomerulonéphrites à dépôts intracapillaires d'IgA. Semin Nephrol Pediatr 26–31, 1983.
44. Beukhof JR, Anema J, Halic LM, Fleuren GJ, Van der Hem GK: Prognosis of adult primary IgA nephropathy [abstr]. Kidney Int 24:408, 1983.
45. Mustonen J, Pasternak A, Helin H, Rilva A, Penttinen K, Wager O, Harmoinen A: Circulating immune complexes, the concentration of serum IgA and the distribution of HLA antigens in IgA nephropathy. Nephron 29:170–175, 1981.
46. Vendemia F, Fornasieri A, Velis O, Baroni M, Scarduelli B, D'Amico G: Different prevalence rates of hypertension in various renoparenchimal diseases. In: Blaufox MD, Bianchi C (eds) Secondary forms of hypertension. New York: Grune and Stratton, 1980, p 89.
47. Martini A, Magrini U, Scelsi M, Capelli V, Barberis L: Chronic membranoproliferative IgA glomerulonephritis comlicated by a rapidly progressive course in a 14 years old boy. Nephron 29:164–166, 1981.
48. Abuelo JG, Esparza AR, Matarese RA, Endreny RG, Carvalho JS, Allegra SR: Crescentic IgA nephropathy. Medicine 63:396–406, 1984.
49. Surian M, Imbasciati E, Cosci P, Barbiano di Belgioioso G, Brancaccio D, Minetti L, Ponticelli C: Glomerular disease and pregnancy: a study of 123 pregnancies in patients with primary and secondary glomerular diseases. Nephron 36:101–105, 1984.
50. Berger J, Yaneva H, Nabarra B, Barbanel C: Recurrences of mesangial deposition of IgA after renal transplantation. Kidney Int 7:232–241, 1975.
51. Cameron JS, Turner DR: Recurrent glomerulonephritis in allografted kidneys. Clin Nephrol 7:47–54, 1977.
52. Limas C, Spector D, Wright JR: Histologic changes in preserved cadaveric renal transplants. Am J Pathol 88:403–428 1977.
53. Sanfilippo F, Croker BP, Bollinger RR: Fate of four cadaveric donor renal allografts with mesangial IgA deposits. Transplantation 33:370–376, 1982.
54. Silva FG, Chander P, Pirani CL: Disappearance of glomerular mesangial IgA deposits after renal allograft transplantation. Transplantation 33:214–216, 1982.
55. Sissons JGP, Woodrow DF, Curtis JR, Evans DJ, Gover PE, Sloper JC, Peters DK: Isolated glomerulonephritis with mesangial IgA deposits. Br Med J 3:611–614, 1985.
56. Beukhof JR, Kardaun O, Schaafsma W: Individual prognosis of patients with IgA-nephropathy on basis of the proportional hazard model, (in press).
57. Schmeckel B, Svalander C, Bucht H, Westberg NG: Mesangial IgA glomerulonephritis in adults. Acta Med Scand 363–372, 1981.
58. Shigematsu H, Kobayashi Y, Tateno S, Hiki Y, Kuwao S: Ultrastructural glomerular loop abnormalities in IgA nephritis. Nephron 30:1–7, 1982.
59. Ng WL, Chan CW, Yeung CK, Hua SP: The pathology of primary IgA glomerulonephritis: a renal biopsy study. Pathology 13:137–143, 1981.
60. McCoy RC, Abramowsky CR, Tisher CC: IgA nephropathy. Am J Pathol 76:123–144, 1974.
61. Sinniah R, Pwee HS, Lim CH: Glomerular lesions in asymptomatic microscopic hematuria discovered on routine medical examination. Clin Nephrol 5:216–228, 1976.

9. THE GLOMERULAR MESANGIUM

ANTHONY R. CLARKSON

GLOMERULAR MESANGIUM

The brunt of immune complex deposition in IgA nephropathy is borne by the glomerular mesangium. Glomerular capillary wall deposits of varying extent and severity do occur, however, and these may account for symptoms such as hematuria and morphologic lesions such as acute glomerular necrosis, inflammation, and crescent formation. These seem unlikely, on the other hand, to account for the progressive decline in renal function, development of hypertension, increasing mesangial expansion, and glomerular sclerosis that typify the patient with progressive disease. These features are most likely to be a result of persisting mesangial deposition. Several glomerular diseases leading to chronic renal failure are characterized by similar changes although, in IgA nephropathy, the mesangial pathology clearly is related to deposition of immune material. Others include diabetic glomerulosclerosis, focal glomerulosclerosis, and hereditary glomerulonephritis. It seems, therefore, that alteration in mesangial function as well as structure plays an important role in progressive reduction in glomerular filtration rate in several diseases. In this chapter, their relevance to IgA nephropathy is discussed.

MESANGIAL STRUCTURE (figure 9-1)

Classic electron-microscopic studies have defined the features of the glomerular mesangium and its relationship to surrounding structures.

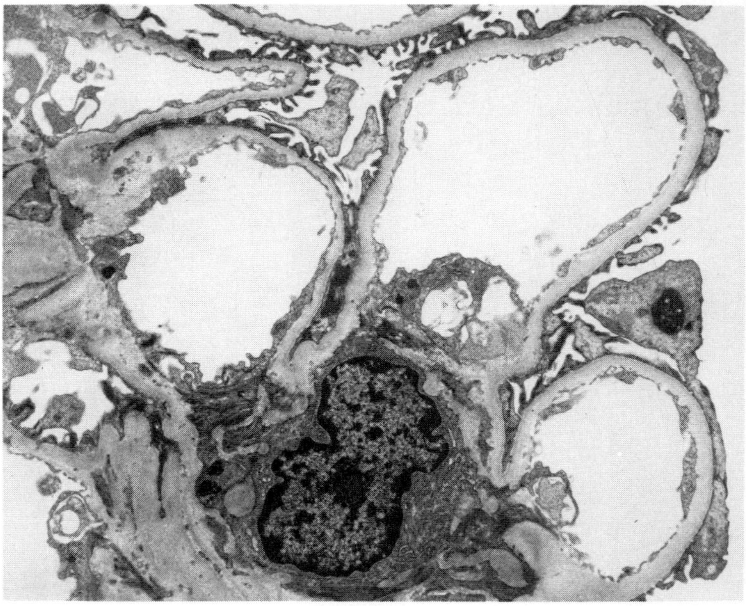

Figure 9-1. Electron micrograph of normal glomerulus. The mesangium occupies the lower portion of the micrograph and consists predominantly of mesangial cell cytoplasm surrounding the indented nucleus. Mesangial matrix is seen between digitations of mesangial cell cytoplasm and is similar in appearance to the glomerular capillary basement membrane. The basement membrane is a continuous structure surrounding glomerular capillaries, save for the area of the capillary adjacent to the mesangium, and is reflected round the mesangium to the next capillary. The mesangium is separated from capillary lumens by the fenestrated endothelial cell cytoplasm.

Mesangial cells (stalk cells, intercapillary cells) and matrix together form the mesangium which forms a support structure upon which the glomerular capillaries are hung or attached. Glomerular capillaries are separated from the mesangium by fenestrated endothelial cells and the glomerular capillary basement membrane (GBM) is in direct continuity with the basement membrane surrounding the mesangium. Through the matrix run channels that are thought to connect the capillary lumen with the region of the juxtaglomerular apparatus (JGA). The mesangium is a continuous structure extending from the region of the JGA, where it is relatively wider at the infundibulum of the glomerulus, to the periphery of the stalk, where it is comparatively narrow. Mesangial cells contain numerous microfilaments both in the perinuclear cytoplasm and extended cell processes. In addition to ribosomes and other cellular microtubules, these microfilaments are thought to contain actomyosin [1–3]. There is a well-developed Golgi apparatus, but few lysosomes. On occasions, cellular processes or pseudopodia may extend to the capillary lumen. The mesangial cell nuclei are slightly notched, a feature thought to indicate activation. In the rat, there normally exists a subpopulation of mesangial cells bearing Ia determinants, resembling mononuclear phagocytes [4]. These cells grown in culture take up antigen and stimulate lymphocytes, both syngeneic and allogeneic.

Mesangial matrix fills the rest of the mesangial area. It is an amorphous substance similar in density to the basement membrane and is in continuity with the lamina rara interna of the basement membrane. Collagen is usually absent and, if present in any quantity, indicates disease. Recently, analysis of mesangial matrix using immunohistochemical and monclonal antibody probes has provided further knowledge of its structure. Collagen types IV and V, fibronectin, and laminin are found in matrix and lamina rara interna [5], but the roles of these components in health and disease have not, as yet, been determined. Information from several laboratories also indicates that the mesangial matrix contains charge sites of heparan and chondroitin sulfates. On the basis of cell culture studies, it is thought that matrix is produced by the mesangial cells [3].

Of considerable importance to the understanding of mesangial function is the close anatomic relationship of the mesangium in the hilum of the glomerulus to the lacis cells of the JGA which, in turn, merge with the epithelioid granular cells of the afferent arteriole and macula densa. This close anatomic juxtaposition indicates a close functional integration and in particular a dependence of glomerular filtration rate on mesangial function.

FUNCTION

Like the trunk of a tree, the mesangium is more than a support structure for its peripheral foliage, the glomerular capillaries. Studies using different macromolecular probes have confirmed the mesangium as a zone of plasmatic flow and transit. Inorganic suspensions, polysaccharides [34], proteins, aggregated proteins, and immune complexes have been administered intravenously to animals and their transit determined using immunohistochemical, electron-microscopic, and immune electron-microscopic techniques, and by kinetic studies [6]. Macromolecular tracers gain access to the mesangium via endothelial fenestrae although entry into the lamina rara interna at the periphery and migration into the mesangium may occur.

Transit through the mesangium occurs via the intercellular channels to the region of the lacis cells, their fate thereafter being a matter of debate. They may enter lymphatics and venules or be excreted via renal tubules. Evidence in support of the latter is found after ureteric ligation in rats in which the kinetics of administered aggregated human immunoglobulin are markedly altered [7]. In addition, exit via the overlying epithelium into the urinary space may occur, thereby contributing to glomerular filtration. This route of exit may explain why large concentrations of tracers (and immune proteins) are found beneath the basement membrane in paramesangial areas [8]. Kinetic studies have reinforced the ultrastructural and immunohistochemical analyses suggesting that passage of inorganic suspensions differs from that of polysaccharides and proteins. Accumulation of aggregated proteins and immune complexes within the mesangium occurs within 4 h of administration and they subsequently disappear over 24–72 h. Their accumulation is dependent on the concentration achieved within the circulation and therefore on the disappearance rate from the blood [9]. Activity of the systemic mononuclear phagocytic system is the predominant determinant of blood clearance. Molecular size [10], type, charge, and the biologic properties of the macromolecules [11] also determine rate of accumulation and clearance. Considerable controversy exists as to the part played by phagocytosis in the clearance of macromolecules by resident mesangial cells. While clearly this occurs with some tracers and immune complexes [12, 13], its contribution to total clearance is probably small. Movement into and out of the mesangium may arbitrarily be separated into afferent and efferent limbs [6]. Its study and the factors that influence such movement are of important relevance to IgA nephropathy and its progression.

Factors affecting mesangial uptake (afferent limb) mentioned above include blood levels, which are related to the state of the reticuloendothelial system, size, type, and digestibility of the molecules, glomerular capillary characteristics such as permeability, and hemodynamic factors. In addition, corticosteroid administration [14], endotoxin [15], and systemic infections [16] may lead to increased uptake in experimental animals. Factors affecting the efferent limb or egress from the mesangium include phagocytosis, transport via intercellular channels to the stalk, regurgitation into glomerular capillaries, passage into the urinary space, and the pressure and flow relationships induced by glomerular and arteriolar hemodynamic changes. Lastly, ureteric obstruction is followed by increased mesangial accumulation of macromolecules [7].

HEMODYNAMIC FACTORS

Mesangial cells have characteristics similar to smooth muscle cells and their surface contains receptors that bind a variety of vasoactive substances, particularly angiotension II [17]. Contraction of the glomerular mesangium alters the size of mesangial channels, thereby influencing movement of plasma and macromolecules. Mesangial contraction may also change glomerular filtration by altering glomerular capillary surface area. As well as angiotensin II, vasopressin and thromboxane A_2 cause mesangial contraction while prostaglandin E_2, prostacyclin, and α-1-adrenergic antagonists cause mesangial relaxation [18]. These authors have demonstrated that angiotensin II increases the mesangial uptake and delays mesangial clearance of infused

IgG in rats and postulate that angiotension II may trigger release of other vasoactive substances capable of influencing movement of macromolecules through the mesangium [19]. Renal vasodilators such as diazoxide also increase mesangial uptake of macromolecules while causing systemic blood pressure to fall. This action may be explained by virtue of angiotension II stimulation. Infusion of angiotension II into man increases urinary PGE_2 excretion and PGE release [20, 21] from the kidney. Studies using angiotensin blockade with saralasin and angiotensin-converting enzyme (ACE) inhibitor drugs suggest that prostaglandin release by the kidney is mediated directly by angiotensin II [22]. There is no evidence that saralasin and ACE inhibitors work in a manner similar to indomethacin, which inhibits prostaglandin synthesis directly. Mesangial cells in culture produce PGE_2 and prostacyclin [23].

MESANGIAL CELL ANTIGENS

The glomerular mesangium contains at least two and possibly more cell subpopulations. The predominant mesangial cell is of renal origin and resembles smooth muscle [33], is contractile, and bears angiotensin II receptors. It is probably nonphagocytic. Bone-marrow-derived monocytes may also enter the mesangium and 50–60% of these cells bear the Ia antigen [4, 24]. The role of these cells in cellular immune reactions within the glomerulus is unclear although striking T-cell accumulation and subsequent macrophage-induced injury may occur in experimental anti-GBM glomerulonephritis in rats [25]. These phagocytes also bear Fc receptors.

The theta or Thy-1.1 antigen recently has been localized to mesangial cells in the rat [2] where it is also present on thymocytes, nucleated bone marrow cells including the pluripotential stem cell, and some of its lymphoid (both T and B) and nonlymphoid descendants. Relatively large amounts of Thy-1 are also present in dog and human kidneys [26–28]. In the rat, the majority of mesangial cells, including the native contractile cell, possess the Thy-1.1 antigen, but any role in antigen processing and initiation of cellular responses is as yet unclear. Evidence is available, however, that mouse mesangial cells (bearing microfilaments) produce a factor that stimulates lymphocyte proliferation with macrophages acting as intermediaries [29]. This factor may be interleukin 1, which is known to be produced by mesangial cells [30], although prostaglandins and free oxygen radicals may also be immunoregulatory. The interaction between monocytes/phagocytes and mesangial cells is, however, probably bidirectional. Mononuclear cell products exert an effect on mesangial cell proliferation, on the one hand, while the mesangial cells in turn regulate the function of the infiltrating monocytes. Thus the Ia-bearing cells act to present antigen while the contractile cell provides an amplification signal for further monocyte accumulation. These observations may be of considerable importance in the development of mesangial proliferation due to immunologic stimuli.

THE MESANGIUM AND DISEASE

The glomerular mesangium seems to be directly or indirectly involved with the evolution of several renal diseases, both immunologic and nonimmunologic. Of the latter, perhaps diabetes mellitus, focal glomerulosclerosis, and hereditary glomerulonephritis are prime examples. Mesangiocapillary glomerulonephritis, lupus nephritis, and IgA nephropathy are examples of immunologically mediated diseases while, in preeclampsia, the nature of the mesangial injury is unknown.

Abnormal mesangial function and structure is widely recognized in experimental animals with diabetes and in puromycin-induced nephrosis which is similar to focal glomerulosclerosis in man [19]. In mice with nephritis induced by lymphocytic choriomeningitis virus infection [16] and in rats where nephritis was produced by intraperitoneal administration of ferritin [31], mesangial localization of immune complexes is associated with abnormal mesangial function. In the ferritin-treated animals, decrease occurred in glomerular filtration rate (GFR), single nephron GFR, single nephron plasma flow, and glomerular capillary pressure. It was concluded that the functional alterations induced by immunologically induced mesangial injury resulted from increased afferent and efferent arteriolar resistance.

In human IgA nephropathy, immune proteins appear to gain access to the mesangium from the capillary lumen via endothelial fenestrae or channels between endothelial cells. The contractility of the mesangial cells may account for movement of deposits to the hilus for possible removal. Partial dissolution of deposits occurs within mesangial matrix, but little evidence exists for any significant intracellular phagocytosis or digestion. The mesangial deposits appear directly or indirectly to stimulate cellular hypertrophy and hyperplasia and increased deposition of mesangial matrix. This is accompanied by formation of collagen fibrils within the thickened matrix, atrophy of mesangial cells, and sclerosis of glomeruli [32].

IgA nephropathy shares with the diseases mentioned above the potential for disease progression, development of hypertension and renal impairment associated with increasing mesangial expansion, focal glomerular sclerosis, global sclerosis, vascular changes of hypertension, and tubulointerstitial scarring.

Evidence is accumulating rapidly pointing to chronic mesangial injury as the common denominator of this pathophysiologic sequence.

REFERENCES

1. Becker CG: Demonstration of actomyosin in mesangial cells of the renal glomerulus. Am J Pathol 66:97–110, 1972.

2. Paul LC, Rennke HG, Milford EL, Carpenter CB: Thy-1.1 in glomeruli of rat kidneys. Kidney Int 25:771–777, 1984.
3. Schienman JI, Fish AJ, Brown DM, Michael AF: Human glomerular smooth muscle (mesangial) cells in culture. Lab Invest 34:150–158, 1976.
4. Schreiner GF, Kiely J-M. Cotran RS, Unanue EG: Characterization of resident glomerular cells in the rat expressing Ia determinants and manifesting genetically restricted interactions with lymphocytes. J Clin Invest 68:920–931, 1981.
5. Michael, AF: The glomerular mesangium. Contrib Nephrol 40:7–16, 1984.
6. Michael AF, Keane WF, Raij L, Vernier RL, Mauer SM: The glomerular mesangium. Kidney Int 17:141–154, 1980.
7. Raij L, Keane WF, Osswald H, Michael AF: Mesangial function in ureteral obstruction in the rat: blockade of the efferent limb. J Clin Invest 64:1204–1212, 1979.
8. Latta H, Fligiel S: Mesangial fenestrations, sieving, filtration and flow. Lab Invest 52:591–598, 1985.
9. Michael AF, Fish AJ, Good RA: Glomerular localization and transport of aggregated protein in mice. Lab Invest 17:14–29, 1967.
10. Mauer SM, Fish AJ, Blau EB, Michael AF: The glomerular mesangium. I. Kinetic studies of macromolecular uptake in normal and nephrotic rats. J Clin Invest 51:1092–1101, 1972.
11. Batsford SR, Weghaupt R, Takamiya H, Vogt A: Studies on the mesangial handling of protein antigens: infuence of size, charge and biologic activity. Nephron 41:146–151, 1985.
12. Cattell V, Gaskin de Urdaneta A, Arlidge S, Collar JE, Roberts A, Smith J: Uptake and clearance of ferritin by the glomerular mesangium I: phagocytosis by mesangial cells and blood monocytes. Lab Invest 47:296–303, 1982.
13. Seiler MW, Hoyer JR, Sterzl RB: Role of macrophages in the glomerular mesangial uptake of polyvinyl alcohol in rats. Lab Invest 49:26–33, 1983.
14. Haakenstad AO, Case, JB, Mannik M: Effect of cortisone on the disappearance kinetics and tissue localization of soluble immune complexes. J Immunol 114:1153–1160, 1975.
15. Shvil Y, Michael AF, Mauer SM: Uptake of aggregated immunoglobulin by the mouse kidney. 1. Effect of endotoxin. Br J Exp Pathol 61:22–29, 1980.
16. Hoffstein PE, Swerdlin A, Bartell M, Hill CL, Venverloh J, Brotherson K, Klahr S: Reticulo-endothelial and mesangial function in murine immune complex glomerulonephritis. Kidney Int 15:144–151, 1979.
17. Sraer JD, Sraer J, Ardaillou R, Mimoune D: Evidence of renal glomerular receptors for angiotensin II. Kidney Int 6:241–246, 1974.
18. Raij L, Keane WF: Glomerular mesangium: its function and relationship to angiotensin II. Am J Med 79:24–30, 1985.
19. Keane WF, Raij L: Angiotensin II modulates afferent and efferent limb [abstr]. Kidney Int 23:184H, 1983.
20. Danon A, Chang LCT, Sweetman BJ, Nies AS, Oates JA: Synthesis of prostaglandin by the rat papilla in vitro: mechanisms of stimulation by angiotensin II. Biochem Biophys Acta 388:71–75, 1975.
21. Frolich JC, Wilson TW, Sweetman BJ, Smigel M, Nies AS, Carr K, Watson JT, Oates JA: Urinary prostaglandins: identification and origin. J Clin Invest. 55:763–770, 1975.
22. Lee JB: Prostaglandins and the renin–angiotensin axis. Clin Nephrol 14:159–163, 1980.
23. Kreisberg JI, Karnovsky MJ, Levine L: Prostaglandin production by homogeneous cultures of rat glomerular epithelial and mesangial cells. Kidney Int 22:355–359, 1982.
24. Striker GE, Mannik M, Tung MY: Role of marrow-derived monocytes and mesangial cells in removal of immune complexes from renal glomeruli. J Exp Med 149:127–136, 1979.
25. Tipping PG, Neale TJ, Holdsworth SR: T-lymphocyte participation in antibody-induced experimental glomerulonephritis. Kidney Int 27:530–537, 1985.
26. Dalchau R, Fabre JW: Identification and unusual tissue distribution of the canine and human homologues of Thy-1 (θ). J Exp Med 149:576–591, 1979.
27. McKenzie JL, Fabre JW: Studies with a monoclonal antibody on the distribution of Thy-1 in the lymphoid and extracellular connective tissues of the dog. Transplantation 31:275–282, 1981.
28. McKenzie JL, Fabre JW: Human Thy-1: unusual localization and possible functional significance in lymphoid tissues. J Immunol 126:843–850, 1981.

29. MacCarthy EP, Hsu A, Ooi YM, Ooi BS: Evidence for a mouse mesangial cell-derived factor that stimulates lymphocyte proliferation. J Clin Invest 76:426–430, 1985.
30. Lovett DH, Ryan JL, Sterzl RB: A thymocyte-activity factor derived from glomerular mesangial cells. J Immunol 130:1796–1808, 1983.
31. Michels LD, Davidman M, Keane WF: The effects of chronic mesangial immune injury on glomerular function. J Lab Clin Med 96:396–407, 1980.
32. Sinniah R, Churg J: Effects of IgA deposits on the glomerular mesangium in Berger's disease. Ultrastructur Pathol 4:9–22, 1983.
33. Pease DC: Myoid features of renal corpuscles and tubules. J Ultrastruct Res 23:304–320, 1968.
34. Sterzl, RB, Eisenbach GM, Seiler MW, Hoyer JR: Uptake of polyvinyl alcohol by macrophages in the glomerular mesangium of rats. Am J Pathol 111:247–255, 1983.

10. THE BIOLOGY OF IgA MUCOSAL IMMUNITY

RANDALL A. ALLARDYCE

The body of clinical and experimental evidence relating to the pathogenesis and course of IgA nephropathy is consistent with the development of a mucosally derived IgA immune complex-mediated disease process. Of course, to obtain conclusive evidence for immune complex pathogenesis, it is necessary to demonstrate that the same antigen and antibody present in the serum are also present in glomerular mesangial deposits. Although this proof does not currently exist for antigen, the evidence strongly supports the view that the immunoglobulins deposited in the glomeruli are the same as those in circulating complexes. It is of value to note that, although a number of experimental animal models of IgA nephropathy can be attributed to the continued mucosal administration of antigen, no such direct evidence exists in man. However, the frequent observation of recurrent infections of the upper respiratory tract, often preceding renal involvement, suggests a possible etiopathologic pattern for IgA nephropathy. Such a sweeping view is not without obvious pitfalls and the occurrence of mesangial polymeric IgA deposits secondary to impaired hepatic function highlights this. Indeed, Clarkson and his colleagues regard IgA nephropathy as a syndrome rather than an immunopathologic entity [17].

Nevertheless, one has attempted to describe the role and functions of mucosally derived IgA as it might be viewed in the context of current thinking on IgA nephropathy. This has involved descriptions of the mechanism controlling IgA generation and production, regulation and transport. Finally, a few areas of speculation have been raised. On the debit side of the ledger: this is not a review of mucosal immunity per se. Such an approach has inevitably led to omissions of subjects such as IgE, breast feeding, and neonatal mucosal development, atopy, genetic susceptibility to infection, the influences of MHC gene products, and cell-mediated mucosal immunity.

IgA NEPHROPATHY AND THE MUCOSAL IMMUNE SYSTEM

It is the spectrum of pathologic features of IgA nephropathy and its various animal models that focus attention on IgA in general, and polymeric IgA and the mucosal immune system in particular. The experimental findings using a variety of animal models have recently been summarized by Woodroffe and Lomax-Smith [1]. In the murine model, it was found that mesangial deposition of IgA followed the intravenous administration of aggregated polymeric IgA [2, 3] or IgA and hapten carrier protein (dinitrophenyl-bovine serum albumin) immune complexes [4]. It was of particular note that the feature critical to mesangial deposition was the polymeric nature of the IgA aggregate or immune complex. Further experiments in which mice were actively immunized showed that oral doses of ovalbumin, bovine gamma globulin, and horse spleen ferritin resulted in the formation of IgA immune complexes that were deposited in the mesangium [5, 6]. In addition, it was found that the parenteral administration of dextran (known to block the uptake of polymeric IgA and IgA immune complexes by the reticuloendothelial system) had similar effect [7, 8]. Other situations in which liver function may be impaired by parasitic infection (as in the case of hepatasplenic schistosomiasis [9] or partial ligation of the portal vein or bile duct [9, 10]) have also resulted in mesangial IgA deposits. Further observations on carbon tetrachloride-treated cirrhotic rats indicated that the degree of mesangial deposition of IgA, C3 and, to a minor extent, IgG, and IgM, increased with the duration of the experiment [1]. These pathologic changes in the mesangium secondary to presumed impairment of liver function are also seen in Aleutian disease of mink in which raised serum levels of IgA, glomerular AD viral antigens, and associated antiviral antibodies have been described [11].

In the clinical setting, IgA-containing circulating immune complexes have been extensively described [12, 13] as has the mesangial deposition of polymeric IgA immune complexes in patients with IgA nephropathy [14–16]. As discussed later, there exists some uncertainty concerning the subclass of IgA antibody involved in the renal deposits observed by a number of workers [13, 17, 18]. However, experimental and clinical studies have indicated that mesangial IgA can be deposited in either antibody or antigen excess and the actual amounts of antibody and antigens in the circulation appear to be more important than the ratio of the two. Analogies drawn between the experimental models cited and human IgA nephropathy are consistent with the concept of mucosally derived antigen and subsequent immune responses leading to the production of polymeric IgA immune complexes.

Overlying the broad considerations of IgA immune reactivity to a spectrum of mucosae-associated antigens are the features of IgA nephropathy that are secondarily related to experimental manipulations or disease processes known to alter IgA concentration, clearance, catabolism, or circulation pattern. It is well recognized that polymeric IgA immune complexes are cleared by secretory component (SC) present on the hepatocytes of some rodents [19–22]. Additional clearance of both monomeric and polymeric IgA complexes is mediated by IgA heavy-chain membrane receptors (Fcα) on both hepatocytes and Kupffer cells [23]. Processing of soluble IgA immune complexes by the liver is impaired in human [24] as well as murine [13] cirrhosis.

Another feature of high levels of circulating polymeric IgA or IgA immune complexes includes the suppression of chemotaxis and phagocytosis of polymorphonuclear leukocytes (PMN) [25]. Additional studies have shown that peripheral blood PMN from IgA nephropathy patients do not adhere to glomeruli in frozen sections of specimens from patients with IgA nephropathy in as great numbers as to those from healthy subjects [26]. Linking this observation with previous studies, indicating depressed neutrophil phagocytic activity and intracytoplasmic inclusions containing IgA, and Wilton's observation that aggregated IgA depresses PMN phagocytosis in vitro [27], Sato and his colleagues [26] have drawn attention to the generally depressed nature of PMN function in IgA nephropathy. Of further possible significance is the isolation of antiidiotype antibody to antibovine serum albumin (mostly of the IgA class) in the sera of two patients with IgA nephropathy [13]. This observation could suggest that in some patients the idiotype–antiidiotype network of antibodies may participate in immune complex formation in vivo. Although the significance of this observation cannot be evaluated at this time, it is important to note that idiotype–anti-idiotype mesangial complexes have been found in an experimental nephritis [28].

A number of the characteristic pathogenetic features of IgA nephropathy do not fit easily into a generalized scheme of systemic autoimmune or immunecomplex-mediated diseases such as hemolytic anemia, systemic lupus erythematosis, or myasethenia gravis [29]. For example, serum concentrations of polymeric IgA and IgA-containing immune complexes are associated with the deposition of J-chain-containing oligomeric IgA complexes in the renal mesangium [15, 30, 31]. Also the intermittent or chronic nature of these immune complexes is suggestive of continuing antigenic stimulation of mucosal associated lymphoid tissues (MALT) [30] and not systemic immune reactivity. This link is further strengthened by an increased association of IgA nephropathy with inflammatory conditions and infections of mucosal surfaces [32]. The additional lack of marked or prolonged systemic IgG or IgM involvement in the development of IgA nephropathy gives further cause for consideration of the mucosal immune system and mucosally derived IgA in the generation and maintenance of the disease.

THE CONCEPTUAL BASIS FOR THE MUCOSAL IMMUNE SYSTEM

In many respiratory and intestinal infections, the presence of specific antibodies in mucosal secretions is better correlated with resistance than with those in serum. This is also the situation for the surface of the nose, salivary, lacrimal, and mammary glands and the female reproductive tract where, like the gut and upper respiratory tract, IgA is the predominant immunoglobulin isotype. It is the site-specific defense and regulatory roles of IgA, together with its local synthesis, transport, and secretion, that set mucosal apart from systemic immunity [33–35]. It is fair to comment that, since the cause-and-effect relationship between IgA and host resistance has not been conclusively proven, additional factors such as cellular mechanisms and nonspecific humoral factors in secretions may all contribute significantly to host protection.

Quite apart from playing a front-line role in the defense against pathogens, mucosal surfaces form the interfaces through which most of the essential transactions between the individual and its environment are undertaken. Thus the mucosal immune system may serve to generate vehicles to transport and direct nutrients, microorganism metabolites, and environmental toxins for effective catabolism or excretion as well as to regulate subsequent mucosal and systemic immune reactivity. For example, the specific binding of mucosally derived IgA may mask the active sites of absorbed toxins while directing these and other absorbed molecules to the liver without stimulating additional clones of reactive and memory lymphocytes or generating a network of antiidiotypic antibodies that might compromise subsequent protective immunity. In addition, the binding of mucosally derived immunoglobulins to absorbed antigens has been shown to regulate a wide spectrum of mucosal and systemic cell types [36–38].

As will be discussed later, the selective patterns of lymphocyte migration and localization between mucosal tissues suggest that it may be possible to immunize mucosal tissues distant from the site to which antigen is originally presented. The factors that regulate this localization depend on many mechanisms, including the presence of antigen [39, 40]. For example, in the mouse, mesenteric lymph node (MLN) bone-marrow-derived (B) lymphoblasts selectively localize, under hormonal control, to the breast and cervix where they predominantly produce IgA [41]. Moreover, after feeding ferritin, IgA antibody-containing cells of presumed MLN origin are found in the gut, lung, mammary, and parotid glands of mice [42, 43]. Although the mucosal immune system appears to be effectively compartmentalized, it is not exclusive. For once inflammation is induced in a mucosal tissue, the patterns of cellular traffic and localization change and a response characteristic of systemic immunity may supervene at that site [36, 39]. This general concept of a common mucosal immunologic system or network may not only apply to cellular traffic, but also extends to the selective mucosal and hepatic localization of intravascular dimeric IgA2 synthesized at distant sites [35, 44, 45].

THE ROLES OF IgA

Two major roles have been attributed to IgA [37]. The first involves host defense against invasion and infection by microorganisms. The second relates to the clearance of dietary and environmental materials that may gain access across the various mucosal surfaces and the regulation of immune reactions to them. Closely related to these roles of IgA is the maintenance of immunologic and physiologic homeostasis at mucosal surfaces.

Antigens gaining access through mucosal membranes may meet IgG, IgA, or IgM antibodies. Both IgG and IgM immune complexes may fix complement components also present in the mucosa and induce the full cascade of inflammatory mediators locally. The presence of IgA of local or remote origin may moderate these inflammatory mechanisms either by blocking polymorph involvement [25–27] or inhibiting the complement-mediated effects of corresponding IgG and IgM antibodies [46, 47]. The balance may be a fine one. Too much IgA might predispose toward an increased susceptibility to disseminated disease through the lack of serum bactericidal activity [48]. Too much IgM and IgG might alternatively lead to the large-scale production of complement activation products leading to severe local inflammatory changes and enhanced mucosal penetrability [49]. These elements, acting to maintain mucosal homeostasis, form only a part of the complex palimpsest of effectors and regulators such as the various thymus-dependent (T) cell subsets, mucus-secreting cells, and other nonimmune defense molecules present in mucosal secretions. The importance of these becomes apparent since many children with X-linked hypogammaglobulinemia and adults with common variable immunodeficiencies show no clinical, function, or structural abnormalities of the gut [51]. It is also true that, because of the interrelated activities of specific and nonspecific systemic and mucosally derived effectors and regulators, it is not possible at this time to attribute exact in vivo protective or homeostatic roles exclusively to secretory IgA.

Despite the obvious complexities, it is, however, possible to envisage two levels of immune activity in response to mucosal antigens, each with distinctly different local and systemic consequences. Relatively minor disturbances in immunologic homeostasis can occur when secretory IgA and IgM confront antigens or noxious substances. Their effects are counterbalanced with the resolution of minor changes that might temporarily compromise mucosal stability.

On the other hand, should the initial secretory response fail to cope with a persistent or overwhelming antigen or toxin load, there is accompanying proliferation of IgG- and IgE-producing lymphocytes. In attempting to limit the dissemination of the noxious factors, the release and activation of these products induce severe changes locally and encourage the recruitment of systemic inflammatory elements that further destabilize the mucosal surface [36, 39]. With normal local mucosal homeostasis and function altered, the perpetuation of inflammatory reactions may serve as part of the mechanism leading to the development of chronic mucosal inflammatory diseases such as coeliac disease, ulcerative colitis, and Crohn's disease.

Mucosally derived IgA

The composition of IgA in mucosal tissues differs from the circulating form produced in the systemic and peripheral lymphoid tissues or bone marrow. Dimeric IgA2 associated with a relatively short joining or "J" polypeptide chain, is produced by plasma cells in the mucosal lamina propria and transported onto the mucosal surface by two means that will be described in greater detail later in this chapter. Briefly however, locally diffusing IgA2 is transported in vesicles across mucosal columnar epithelial cells and secreted by exocytosis into the intestinal lumen after complexing with membrane-associated secretory component (SC) displayed on the surface of epithelial cells [52, 53]. Alternatively, dimeric IgA2 may enter the intestinal lumen indirectly via the bile. In many animals, hepatic parenchymal cells display surface SC or Fcα receptors and transport IgA2 and IgA2-containing immune complexes into their biliary systems [23, 44]. Monomeric IgA and IgA2 SC are not transported into the bile by SC-bearing hepatocytes. The extent of IgA2 transport by hepatic mechanisms in man is not yet certain.

Although the fluids associated with mucosal surfaces contain secretory IgA, the local tissues may differ in their expression of surface SC or the presence of IgA-producing plasma cells. Gut and bronchus, for example, contain both, whereas sweat glands, kidney, urinary bladder, hepatic parenchymal cells, amnion, fallopian tubes, ulterine mucosa, and the thymus express SC, but do not produce or have IgA plasma cells (the liver as a whole appears to contain considerable numbers of immunoglobulin-producing cells [44, 54]). The ureter, esophagus, vagina, gingiva, and buccal squamous epithelia appear to have neither surface SC nor resident IgA plasma cells.

Secretory IgA is highly resistant to the activities of most proteolytic enzymes and is therefore well adapted to function in a hostile environment. For example, much of the secretory IgA in breast milk can be found intact in baby's stools. However, several bacterial pathogens (e.g., *Streptococcus sanguis*, Neisseria gonorrhoeae, N. mengitidis, *Streptococcus pneumoniae*, and *Hemophilus influenzae*) secrete enzymes that specifically degrade only the IgA1 class [55–57]. This IgA protease is associated with pathogenicity in several *Neisseria* and *Streptococcus* strains [55, 56]. There is also data showing that the resulting molecule generated by the action of IgA protease has defective antibody function [58]. The observation that *Klebsiella pneumoniae* and group-

A streptococci are protease negative [59] indicates, however, that other factors are also involved in pathogenicity.

Epithelial surfaces do not constitute complete barriers to the environment. Dietary antigens, viruses, bacteria, starch (25 μ), and even asbestos particles (90 μ) may be found in free or complexed form in the circulation following ingestion [60]. Moreover, the infectivity of many bacterial pathogens is related to their adherence to mucosal surfaces. Secretory IgA present as a result of any of the mechanisms discussed, or passively transferred in milk, can effectively block both bacterial adherence and antigen association with enterocyte membranes, thereby reducing or eliminating mucosal penetration [35].

Viral infections

The attention of those concerned with IgA nephropathy has been focused upon the potential role of viruses because they are common inhabitants of the upper respiratory tract [6], are associated with the mesangium in Aleutian mink disease [11], and because "viral-like" inclusions have been identified in renal tissues of patients with IgA nephropathy [62]. The situation concerning the protective role of IgA in mucosal virus infection is not altogether clear. Although external transfer of IgA is increased during infection, in the acute phase, secretory antibody may have little specific protective value. In this early phase, IgA lacks high-affinity specific antibody activity. This may relate to the broad spectrum of low-affinity antibody specificities exhibited by secretory IgA as opposed to serum IgG following vaccination [63, 64]. Viruses such as rotavirus, parainfluenza, rhinovirus, adenovirus, and respiratory syncytial virus colonize mucosal surfaces producing disease locally with little or no systemic spread. Secretory IgA antibody levels correlate more closely with protection in these cases, possibly due to viral neutralization, than do serum antiviral antibody titers and appear to prevent the mucosal carrier state of viruses such as polio [34].

Bacterial infections

A full review of this area is well beyond the scope of this chapter; however, there exists a close relationship between the site of bacterial colonization and the local secretion of specific IgA at mucosal surfaces. There is also a clear demonstration of the dissociation between the local antibody responses to bacteria and that detected in serum. Likewise, IgA antibody-secreting cells and specific IgA antibodies in breast milk reflect specificities for bacterial antigenic stimuli originating in the gastrointestinal tract that are absent from the serum [65–67].

Intestinal secretory IgA antibodies are protective in experimental cholera in that they inhibit the adherence of *Vibrio cholerae* to enterocytes [68]. Antibodies to enterotoxins have also been demonstrated in the milk of women from developing countries, and in rats it has been shown that intestinal antibodies inhibit the binding of enterotoxin to intestinal microvillus membranes [69]. Additional support for the protective role of secretory IgA in the gut is demonstrated when colostral and intestinal IgA antibodies obtained from immune adult mice transfer protection against infections with *Taenia taenioformis* to neonatal mice [70]. Moreover, the demonstration of specific IgA directed against all areas of the surface of *Giardia lamblia* trophozoites suggests several mechanisms by which the clearance of parasites as well as bacterial pathogens might be facilitated by this antibody. These include interference with adherence to the enterocytes, agglutination, binding to flagella, and hindering motility and participating in antibody-dependent cell-mediated cytotoxicity [71].

IgG and especially IgA secretory antibodies against *Escherichia coli* O and K antigens of patients with acute urinary tract infections can prevent *E. coli* adherence to uroepithelial cells [72, 73]. It may be of significance, therefore, that bacteria with the ability to adhere are found in the urine of patients with asymptomatic bacteriuria demonstrate greatly reduced adherence. Furthermore, effective local immunity to urinary tract infections has been generated in experimental animal models [74].

In the human respiratory tract, locally formed secretory antibodies have been demonstrated against pneumococcal, meningococcal, staphylococcal, and mycoplasma pneumoniae antigens. Although the presence of secretory antibodies to *Mycoplasma pneumoniae* may translate into resistance to infection as suggested by Brunner and Chanock [75], their specificity of protection has been questioned [76].

Local secretory antibodies coat bacteria including *Streptococcus salivarius* and *mutans* and, in vivo, appear to inhibit their adherence to oroepithelial cells and teeth, thereby assisting in their disposal from the oral cavity. Local vaccination can be shown to increase salivary antibodies to specific microorganisms while intestinal vaccination with *Streptococcus mutans* was protective against dental carries [77]. In humans, oral immunization with such strains resulted in the appearance of antibodies in both saliva and tears [78]. Recent studies have supported the efficacy of shared mucosal immune reactivity by indicating that IgA in rat tears originates from local synthesis and not from serum transfer [79].

Secretory IgA also excludes the entry of many chemicals, bacterial byproducts, and inhaled and ingested materials of all kinds, including potential carcinogens that contact mucosal surfaces. The effectiveness of the immunized gut and lung to exclude antigens, increase goblet cell mucus secretion, and enhance local antigen retention and breakdown by intestinal and pancreatic enzymes has been demonstrated [35].

A number of other related, but nonimmunologic, factors may also contribute to mucosal defense. These include the establishment of indigenous nonpathogenic flora, as well as synergistic defense mechanisms involving secretory products found in quantity in all mucosal secretions such as lysozyme, lactoferrin, and peroxidase [50].

Functional aspects of IgA

Once the epithelial barrier is breached, antigen gaining access through the mucosa may form complexes with specific IgA2 and be secreted directly through the gut epithelium or enter the circulation to be transported to other mucosal tissues or the liver and from there back into the external secretions. Whether the IgA itself, the antigen, or the IgA2 -containing immune complex in the bile remains antigenic is not known. At the time of the 1914–1918 War, however, Besredka produced effective oral immunization against shigellosis and typhoid in man using killed organisms in a bile cocktail. The ox bile used may have been effective because it may have increased antigen binding or uptake by bowel mucosal cells or increased immunogenicity because of its acid-neutralizing and mucolytic properties [35].

The transcellular transportation of dimeric IgA–antigen complexes may offer additional advantages. Incompletely digested molecules, microbial metabolites or toxins or other potentially harmful substances may be subject to additional proteolysis or detoxification in the liver that could be especially important when their access is increased in mucosal inflammatory conditions. In addition, the uptake of IgA2 or its immune complexes by remote secretory mucosal tissues may provide passive immunity to those sites or modified antigenic drive to promote local active immunity to current environmental antigens [35]. Dimeric IgA–antigen complexes might also regulate subsequent immune reactivity by a variety of mechanisms including the induction of systemic tolerance, thereby avoiding systemic immunity or potentially damaging inflammatory reactions [36, 39].

The association of several clinical abnormalities including IgA nephropathy, Henoch-Schönlein purpura, and dermatitis herpetiformis with increased circulating or localized polymeric IgA immune complexes may reflect defective transport mechanisms. Thus, as in dermatitis herpetiformis patients known to have faulty IgG receptor function, a similar abnormality of IgA cellular receptors may be discovered [60, 80] in these conditions.

In addition to epithelial cells and hepatocytes, a number of cells that participate in or regulate immunologic and inflammatory reactions possess receptors for IgA and IgA–antigen complexes. These IgA-binding cells include polymorphonuclear leukocytes, monocytes, and lymphocytes. Of this latter group, some lymphocytes bind polymeric IgA and SC while IgA-immunoregulatory T(alpha)-lymphocytes residing in GALT and spleen also possess IgA receptors [81].

Although secretory IgA is not an opsonin and does not directly stimulate phagocytosis, serum IgA has been shown to activate blood monocyte killing of bacteria. It remains for a similar activity of secretory IgA to be demonstrated on mucosal leukocytes. It is now clear, however, that liver Kupffer cells and other resident phagocytic cells bear receptors for IgA as they do for complexed IgG [23].

Systemic immune tolerance after mucosal challenge

Oral or bronchial challenge with a variety of antigens and sensitizing agents has been shown to result in mucosal immunity accompanied by partial or profound systemic unresponsiveness. This has become known as the Sulzberger-Chase phenomenon even though 150 years ago the American Indians are credited with ingesting poison-ivy leaves to prevent subsequent contact dermatitis [82]. Depending upon the dose and mode of antigen presentation as well as the means used to test suppressed immune reactivity, several mechanisms of tolerance induction have been described. T-cells capable of suppressing IgG and IgM antibody production at first appear in the Peyer's patches and subsequently localize in the MLN and the spleen. Cells similarly affecting IgA production are not noted after antigen challenge although T-cell IgE antibody suppressors are found. In addition, IgG1 antigen-specific antibody that suppresses subsequent systemic IgG and IgM plaque-forming cell generation may be found in the serum after oral challenge, while macrophage-derived prostaglandin-induced suppression has also been noted [83, 84]. The interplay of these suppressive and regulatory mechanisms results in the sparing of systemic immune reactivity. Concurrently, a spectrum of mucosally derived regulator and effector cells is generated. These include IgA plasma cell precursors that selectively migrate from the site of antigen challenge to localize in other mucosal tissues.

The outcome of oral immunization depends on a number of factors including the form of the antigen, its dose, and frequency of immunization as well as the age and strain of the recipient and its previous exposure to the antigen [85–89]. In adult experimental animals, several groups have shown that feeding antigen alone (i.e., without systemic challenge) does not result in a systemic antibody response or increased elimination of subsequently injected protein antigen (e.g., human serum albumin or ovalbumin) from the circulation [86, 89, 90]. Although antigen clearance was not significantly affected, Hanson et al. [85] noted very small increases in antigen binding in the serum. Similarly, Devey and Bleasdale [90] observed small latticed serum immune complexes and the absence of immune complex disease in disease-prone mice fed antigen before the commencement of daily antigen injections. Unfortunately, the isotype and subclass of the circulating complexed immunoglobulin(s) were not identified.

A number of immunologic mechanisms have been identified in the induction of adult oral tolerance. These include the generation of antigen-specific T-suppressor and T-suppressor-inducer cells, the formation of circulating antigen–antibody complexes, and antibodies directed against the antigen-binding idiotopes of antibodies [91]. It is well known that immunologic tolerance is readily induced in neonates when antigen is given parenterally. One might, therefore, have expected oral tolerance to be more profound in antigen-fed neonates. However, this is not the case. Indeed, Strobel and Ferguson [91] have shown that systemic tolerance or priming for immune reactivity is related to the age at which antigen is first encountered. In these experiments carried out in mice, it was found that, after an antigen feed (ovalbumin) in the neonatal period, immunologic and digestive immaturity led to a net gain in T-helper-cell activity which prevented the induction of systemic hyporesponsiveness and resulted in both humoral and cell-mediated immune responses. It could be suggested that the relative immaturity of the immunologic mechanisms involved could account for the priming effects of oral antigen on neonates. Three features of neonatal immunity argue against this explanation, however: fetuses respond to antigenic stimuli, fetal and neonatal lymphoid cells can act as adult cells when transferred to adults, and neonates (but not adults) have a population of antigen nonspecific suppressor T cells [92]. Other features relating to the immaturity of neonatal digestive and absorptive functions may be key elements in the failure of oral protein antigens to induce systemic hyporeactivity. The increased permeability of the neonatal gut, the immunochemical properties of neonatally digested antigens, and immature hepatic processing of immunogenic and/or tolerogenic antigen fragments have been cited as possibilities in this regard [91].

THE STRUCTURE, ORIGIN, PRODUCTION, AND REGULATIONS OF IgA

Structural and chemical properties of IgA

Serum IgA consists mainly of 7S molecules composed of two heavy and two light chains arranged as in IgG. Approximately 10–20% is normally composed of 10S dimers or larger aggregates [50]. On the other hand, in secretions, 7S IgA constitutes only a minor fraction while the heavier polymeric forms predominate (80–90%). Secretory IgA is composed of a 10S IgA dimer (300,000 daltons) in which the two monomers are linked by a 15,000-dalton "joining chain" or J chain that is disulfide-linked to the penultimate cysteine of the C-terminal octapeptide of the heavy chains [93]. The J chain becomes incorporated into IgA prior to secretion of the dimer from the plasma cell. Regardless of the size of the IgA polymer, there is only one J chain connecting two subunits. The remaining polymer subunits in larger IgA aggregates are connected by inter-heavy-chain disulfide bridges [94]. J chains are found in only trace amounts in IgA polymers isolated from normal human serum [95], suggesting that the small amounts of normally occurring polymeric serum IgA are aggregates rather than true polymers.

In many species of mammals, including man, subclasses of IgA are recognized. In humans, differences in heavy-chain structure give rise to IgA1 and IgA2. Two variants of the IgA2 subclass exist. One variant lacks disulfide bonds between the heavy and light chains, the molecule being held together only by noncovalent forces. Interchain bonds are present in the other IgA2 variant and in all IgA1 molecules. Most IgA is synthesized by plasma cells located at mucosal surfaces. Indeed, more than half of all immunoglobulin-producing cells may be synthesizing IgA, and Heremans has suggested that it is produced at a higher rate than other immunoglobulins [96]. Measurements of immunoglobulin concentrations in saliva, tears, and a number of other external secretions indicate that IgA significantly exceeds IgG and IgM. For example, in parotid saliva and duodenal fluids, IgA is present in concentrations of 12 and 30 mg%, respectively. This is compared with approximately 0.03 and 10 mg% for IgG [50]. It has been estimated that there may be as many as 10^{10} IgA-producing cells for every meter length of gut [97].

The IgA2 produced by plasma cells in the intestinal mucosa may be either transported across the epithelium into the gut lumen or it may diffuse into the circulation or lymph where it binds to receptors on hepatocytes as it passes through the liver into the bile. Preceding its transport through the mucosal epithelial cells or hepatocytes, dimeric or J-chain-containing IgA polymers bind to the transmembrane glycoprotein (approximately 80,000 daltons) known as secretory component (SC). SC is synthesized within mucosal epithelial cells and hepatocytes (in some animals) and binds both by covalent and noncovalent interactions to polymeric IgA and IgM while they are being actively transported to the mucosal surface [52]. SC confers stability to secretory IgA so that it is especially well adapted to function in the protease-containing external secretions.

Origin of B-lymphocytes

Pluripotential stem cells present in adult bone marrow are generally accepted as the progenitors of B- and T-lymphocytes. Using a chromosomal marker, Wu and his colleagues [98] showed that both myeloid cells and thymocytes could arise from a common progenitor. More recent evidence supports that view and indicates that a single cell can give rise to myeloid cells and also to T- and B-lymphocytes [99].

The adult immune system is in a state of constant change, even in the absence of antigen administration, and each day receives large numbers of newly formed lymphocytes. The bone marrow is crucial to this continuous renewal, both in its regulation and because it is the direct source of B cells in normal animals and the indirect source of T cells, which are derived ultimately from stem cells that flow from the bone marrow to the thymus [99].

Most mature B cells have a relatively short half-life estimated to be between a few days and two weeks [100]. Since the mature B-cell repertoire must be continuously replenishing itself, the cells reflecting immune reactivity in the adult may bear little relationship to the B cells generated during the early phases of ontogency and neonatal development. Multiple B-cell subpopulations may be distinguished by functional differences in their responses to specific classes of thymus-dependent and thymus-independent antigens as well as the expression of cell surface markers [100]. It is perhaps also significant in the context of IgA nephropathy that secondary B cells differ from primary B cells in a number of ways, including their need for antigenic stimulation [101–103]. At the present time, it is not clear whether these differences reflect different B-cell lineages or different maturational states of the same lineage.

Molecular aspects of B-cell differentiation

Unstimulated populations of B-lymphocytes express little, if any, cytoplasmic J chain. After polyclonal activation with mitogens, however, there is a 100- to 200-fold increase in intracellular J chain that acts as a nucleating unit to promote the synthesis and exportation of pentameric IgM [104]. All Ig-secreting plasmacytoma cell lines, regardless of the Ig class produced, express large amounts of intracellular J chain. This suggests that one of the initial steps in B-cell differentiation is the activation of J chain synthesis by transcription of a previously silent gene. Once J chain is synthesized, it continues to be expressed during subsequent differentiative steps involving switches in heavy-chain class [105, 106]. It is also likely that another change occurring in B-cell differentiation involves the conversion of IgA from a membrane component to a soluble secreted product. Such a change has been described to occur in IgM-secreting B cells following the synthesis of an enzyme that catalyzes the disulfide crosslinking required for both IgM and IgA polymerization [107, 108]. A third feature of the stimulated B cell involves the amplification of protein synthesis. In lipopolysaccharide-stimulated mouse spleen cells, the intracellular levels of J chain and monomer IgM were shown to increase by orders of magnitude within four days. This constituted a gain exceeding many times that accounted for by cell division, nor was amplification limited to secreted products only [104, 109]. Further analysis of these early steps in the differentiation to secretory plasma cells suggests that a complex cascade of membrane interactions is set in motion by the binding of surface antibody receptors that initiates the production of secretory Ig mRNA and the binding of T-cell factors that trigger the expression of J chain [110–112].

Immunoglobulin class switch

A striking feature of the immune system is that a lymphocyte clone can switch the class of immunoglobulin that it expresses while maintaining the same V (variable) region and therefore the same antigen-binding specificity. This suggests that a single variable heavy-chain region can associate sequentially with different C (constant) heavy-chain regions within one cell or cell lineage.

Genetic and amino acid sequencing studies have established that there is a gene family for each of the two light chains (kappa and lambda) and a third for the various types of immunoglobulin heavy chains (μ, δ, γ_3, γ_1, γ_{2b}, $\gamma_{2\alpha}$, ε, and α in the mouse) [113]. Specific C_H genes are deleted in mouse myeloma DNAs, producing different immunoglobulin classes. The picture of the C_H gene order on the chromosome predicted by this deletion profile has been substantiated by subsequent studies by molecular cloning and nucleotide sequence determination [114]. The C_H gene order is $5'$–V_H–D–J_H–$C\mu$–$C\delta$–$C\gamma3$–$C\gamma1$–$C\gamma2b$–$C\gamma2\alpha$–$C\varepsilon$–$C\alpha$–$3'$ [115]. Analyses comparing genomic libraries of myeloma and embryonic (germline) H chain genes have suggested that the complete H chain gene is created by at least two types of DNA rearrangement. The first joins the three separate segments V_H, D, and J_H into one piece. This combination expresses the completed variable (V) gene as a μ chain because the $C\mu$ gene is closest to the J_H segment. The second DNA rearrangement joins S regions that are located at the $5'$ side of each C_H gene. The S-S recombination then brings the completed V_H gene adjacent to another C_H gene by the deletion of an intervening DNA segment [114].

Many B cells, including mucosal IgA-producing cell precursors, express more than one surface isotype [116]. Most commonly, double heavy-chain bearers carry μ and δ associated with the same V_H antigen-binding region. This is thought to occur as a result of RNA-splicing mechanism that allows the simultaneous synthesis of the μ and δ mRNAs [117]. The final differentiative step of IgA secretion by plasma cells may involve a similar mRNA differential splicing step followed by a DNA deletion linking the V_H and C regions. The factors that influence the various differentiative steps involved in antibody isotype secretion are not clear at this time. However, isotype-specific T cells and their immunoregulatory and potentiating products are emerging as important participants as determinants of the immunoglobulin class switch.

SELECTIVE CIRCULATION AND LOCALIZATION OF MUCOSAL LYMPHOCYTES

Many of the cellular differentiation and migration pathways that eventually lead to IgA synthesis have been determined [40]. Mucosal lymphoid follicles are found in two forms: aggregates and solitary. The aggregates are seen in the intestine Peyer's patches or other gut associated lymphoid tissues, GALT, and in the lungs (bronchus-associated lymphoid tissues, BALT). Both in the gut and the lungs, these tissues have similar functions and morphological features. They are covered by a specialized lymphoepithelium that selectively pinocytoses and phagocytoses material from the luminal environment. The follicles are primarily populated with IgA antibody-producing precursors. Under the influence of antigenic stimulation, these cells migrate to the mesenteric lymph nodes (MLN), the thoracic duct (TD), and the circulation. They eventually take up residence in the gut lamina propria where they

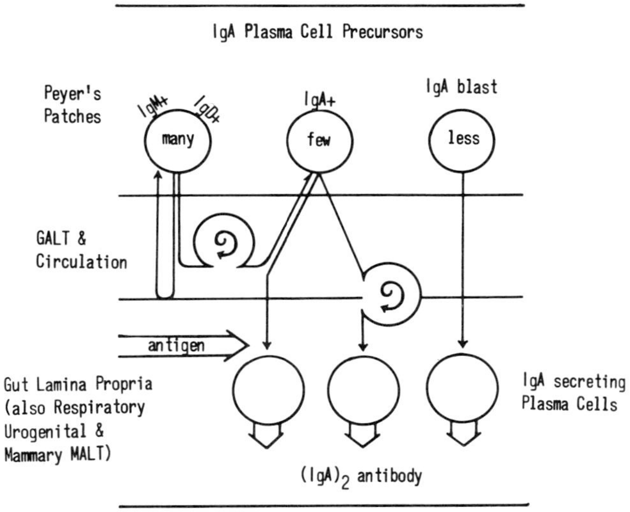

Figure 10-1. Most of the IgA precursors present in the Peyer's patches are IgM-IgD double-bearing lymphocytes. IgA-bearing cells are present in smaller numbers and there are very few IgA blasts.

IgA-bearing cells either (a) mature into IgA blasts that migrate directly to the gut lamina propria via the MLN, TD, and blood, or (b) continue recirculating through GALT until they contact antigens in the gut lamina propria where they divide and differentiate into IgA plasma cells.

The IgM-IgD cells may differentiate, in the course of their continuing migration through GALT, TD, blood, and spleen, to express surface IgA. They then recirculate or mature as already described for Peyer's patch IgA-bearing cells. Others may remain in a resting state and continue in the recirculating pool of GALT cells. It is clear that a proportion of IgA plasma cell precursors circulate to mucosal associated urogenital, respiratory, and mammary lymphoid tissues.

secrete IgA2 [40]. Although it was earlier suggested that it was IgA-bearing cells in the Peyer's patches that gave rise to the majority of IgA plasma cells in the gut lamina propria [118, 119], Tseng [116] has demonstrated that the precursors are actually IgM-IgD double-bearing resting lymphocytes resident in the Peyer's patches and MLN. It was also found that, although the IgA-bearing cells do serve as precursors, they have a very low repopulation efficiency (see figure 10-1).

Mucosal immunity is characterized by site-specific responses of a variety of activated lymphocytes and the subsequent sparing or down-regulation of systemic immunity to antigenic substances that gain access through mucosal surfaces. This regional division of immune reactivity is generated and reflected by the selective patterns of IgA plasma cell precursor migration and maturation as well as the mucosal generation of antigen- and isotype-specific and nonspecific immunoregulatory and effector T cells [25, 34].

Cebra and his colleagues [120, 121] proposed that Peyer's patches are a special tissue that favorably generate and accumulate IgA precorsor B cells by a process of extensive cell division without maturation. In this scheme, committed cells in Peyer's patches undergo immunoglobulin heavy-chain switching from μ to α. Tseng [116] supports this view and also extends this IgA precursor cell development process to the tissues through which migration occurs prior to the localization of IgA plasma cells in the gut lamina propria.

Most of the IgA precursor B cells present in the Peyer's patches are IgM-IgD double-bearing resting lymphocytes. Smaller numbers of IgA-bearing cells are also present as are a few IgA lymphoblasts that migrate directly to the gut lamina propria via the MLN, thoracic duct (TD), and blood. The IgA-bearing cells either mature into IgA blasts or continue circulating through the gut-associated lymphoid tissues until they contact antigen in the gut lamina propria, where they divide and differentiate into IgA-producing plasma cells.

The majority population of resting B cells, bearing both IgM and IgD on their surfaces, may differentiate as they migrate through GALT, TD, blood, and spleen to express surface IgA. They then recirculate or mature as described in figure 10-1. Others that remain resting continue their recirculating patterns in the pool of GALT cells. Since IgA-bearing and IgA blast cells obtained from GALT have been shown to selectively localize to other mucosal sites remote from the gut where they originally encountered antigen [34], it is clear that the patterns of migrating cells include mucosal lymphoid tissues of the urogenital and respiratory tracts as well as perhaps the mammary glands [34, 65].

The IgG-containing cells in the gut lamina propria may possibly also be derived from precursors located in the Peyer's patches. The mucosal IgG precursors probably exhibit the same relatively selective patterns of migration and localization displayed by mucosal IgA precursors [40].

The mucosal presentation of antigen may result in the generation of a number of T-cell-mediated immune reactions including delayed-type hypersensitivity, cytotoxic T-cell effectors, and the production of T-cell-derived lymphokines such as macrophage migration inhibition factor [35]. Compartmentalization of T-cell subsets has been found in bowel mucosa. Those lymphocytes distributed superficial to the epithelial basement membrane, intraepithelial lymphocytes (IEL), tend either to express surface antigens or morphologic features that mark them as T-cytotoxic or suppressor cells or natural killer cells that express cytotoxic potential [39].

In addition to those containing or secreting immunoglobulins, small lymphoid cells expressing surface characteristics common to T-helper or inducer cells are found in the lamina propria [39] as well as other areas of mucosal associated lymphoid tissues involved in immunoglobulin production.

In the normal intestinal lamina propria, such helper cells are balanced by the presence of functionally active suppressor cells. However, in disease states, such as inflammatory bowel disease or in patients with IgA nephropathy, the suppressor population is either reduced in number or functionally diminished in activity [13, 122–125].

Although open to considerable variation in the face of antigen challenge and inflammatory responses, intestinal mucosal small lymphocytes tend to repopulate selectively the sheep intestine and (to a lesser extent) the lungs [34]. It has also been found that MLN and TD immunoblasts tend to localize in the lamina propria and villous epithelium of normal small intestine as well as in (antigen-free) fetal gut isografts placed under the kidney capsule [34, 40]. Only if the intestine is markedly inflamed, as occurs, for example, with *Trichinella spiralis* in mice, do peripheral lymph node T blasts localize to any extent in the intestine [39]. It is thought that exposure to environmental microorganisms is highly significant in the development of GALT and BALT lymphoid cell behavior [39, 40, 126].

When activated, mucosal T cells may affect the functional integrity of the gut epithelium and the proliferation of crypt cells [36] and contribute to the partial villous atrophy that occurs in nematode infections in rats or is induced by *T. spiralis* or *Giardia muris* in mice and man [39]. Whether similar reactions occur in inflammatory bowel diseases including the gluten enteropathies remains a likely possibility.

Mucosal immunoregulation: IgA synthesis and secretion

Many studies over the past 15 years have determined that interacting networks or circuits of immune regulators control immunoglobulin synthesis and secretion. The elements active in those networks include direct antibody feedback, T suppressors, T helpers, and "helper-like" T contrasuppressors, as well as T suppressor-inducers [126–131]. Immunoregulation mediated by those populations of T cells can also, for the most part, be reproduced by T-cell-derived soluble factors [132].

Prior to specific antigen presentation to the intestinal mucosa, thymus-dependent helper (T alpha) cells specific for IgA-precursor lymphoblasts are found in Peyer's patches. These stimulatory cells are capable of migration to the draining mesenteric lymph nodes, but apparently not to the spleen [21, 40]. These T helpers operate by causing class-specific effects on B-cell DNA-switching events [130, 131] and in some respects appear similar to the IgE regulatory T cells described by Katz et al. [133] and Ishizaka [134]. It is notable that these "IgA class-specific switch T cells" located in Peyer's patches do not result in the terminal differentiation of B cells. This finding is in keeping with the small number of IgA plasma cells found in Peyer's patches [116]. There is, apparently, another population of GALT T-helper cells that operate on postswtich IgA B cells that may not be class specific, and Michalek and her colleagues [126] have produced two clones of Peyer's patch T cells that are capable of inducing small amounts of IgG and IgM while predominately helping IgA secretion. The switch signals produced by T-helper cells could involve the induction or activation of Ig class-specific enzymes active in the DNA-switching mechanisms described by Koshland [104].

T cells capable of suppressing IgA production have also been described in Peyer's patches and spleen [81] before antigen stimulation, but not after oral antigen challenge when the T-alpha-helper cells predominate. In addition, the cleavage of transmembrane secretory component may regulate the rate of IgA secretion while free or antigen-complexed IgA may control its own synthesis, and IgA has been shown to regulate SC synthesis in vitro [36]. It is also possible that IgA fragments, resulting from the action of IgA1 protease secreted by some microorganisms, may cause a local depression of IgA synthesis, the resultant amount produced being insufficient to control infection. A more detailed discussion of IgA regulation has been presented elsewhere [125–132].

Mucosal immunoregulation: systemic immunity following oral administration of antigen

Systemic tolerance or hyporeactivity to orally administered sheep erythrocytes in adult mice is mediated by T-suppressor-cell [126]. Using the same model, Mattingly [135] has shown that the cell of GALT that initiates the suppression circuit migrates from GALT to the spleen shortly after contacting antigen. The first cellular element in this circuit appears to be a T suppressor-inducer that, upon migration to the spleen, causes the generation or expression of a T-suppressor-cell population. This pattern of cell migration and cellular interaction among T cells must exist to result in orally induced tolerance.

Further studies by Michalek et al. [126] have drawn attention to a potentially important relationship between GALT immunoregulatory cells and the microflora of the bowel. It was found that T suppressors in GALT are extremely sensitive to the bacterial endotoxin lipopolysaccharide (LPS) and require stimulation by LPS to maintain a regulatory cell population that is responsible to systemic tolerance.

These results help to explain how a very good local antibody response can take place at the site of mucosal antigen presentation while suppressor cells are being induced. The GALT T-suppressor-inducer cells described by Mattingly have no suppressive capacity in the absence of splenic T suppressor cells. The LPS T suppressors also express their inhibitory capabilities outside GALT. Thus, the cells of the Peyer's patches, MLN, and lamina propria as well as other mucosal sites can produce antibody at the same time as these T-suppressor and suppressor-inducer populations are being formed for migration to the spleen while having no impact on the local immune response. In apparent balance to these systemically migrating T-cell down-regulators, Michalek et al. [126] have also described a GALT contrasuppressor circuit consisting of T inducers and contrasuppressor T cells that are resistant to LPS in normal mice.

Mucosal immunoregulation: IgA nephropathy

A detailed analysis of mucosal immunoregulatory lymphocyte subsets has not yet been reported. However, Rothschild and Chatenoud [123] have indicated that patients with IgA nephropathy had an increased OKT4–OKT8 ratio of T-helper–T-suppressor–cytotoxic cells that was suggestive of a suppressor cell deficiency in the peripheral blood. Although there was no overall increase in IgA in vitro production by cells from IgA nephropathy patients when compared with control renal patients, a special feature was an intense enhancement after OKT8 depletion in some IgA nephropathy patients. No clear-cut functional correlation between peripheral blood lymphocyte ratios and mitogen-induced IgA synthesis could be noted in this study, but the results of Bene et al. [122] indicating an imbalance in the numbers of IgA- and IgG-secreting cells in the tonsils of IgA nephropathy patients is in keeping with the hypothesis favoring a mucosal origin for the mesangial IgA present in their kidneys. This, in conjunction with the demonstration of decreased IgA-specific suppressor T-cell activity in patients with IgA nephropathy by Sakai et al. [136, 137], indicates that further analyses of mucosal immunoregulatory cell subpopulations are warranted.

HEPATIC TRANSPORT OF MUCOSALLY DERIVED IgA

Because of the association between mucosally derived IgA in the mesangium of patients with IgA nephropathy and impaired liver function, it is important to review the origins and transport of biliary IgA. Investigating IgG, IgM, and IgA natural antibodies to *Lactobacillus* and *Staphylococcus* in blood, bile, and lymph following rat thoracic duct cannulation or occlusion, Manning et al. [44] calculated that 50% of thoracic duct lymph IgA entering the blood is secreted in the bile. These workers also proposed that the major part of biliary IgA is derived from intestinal lymphoid tissues and that a portion of the remainder, as well as part of biliary IgG and IgM, results from local synthesis. These conclusions supported earlier work by Reynolds et al. [138] showing that 50% of thoracic duct lymph IgA injected intravenously into rats was rapidly transported into the bile. Additional sources of biliary immunoglobulins other than those carried in the thoracic duct have been proposed and in humans it has been estimated by Delacroix et al. that half of the biliary IgA may be of local origin [54]. Further recent studies on the appearance of specific antibodies in rat bile after injected antigen challenge have suggested the involvement of other lymphoid tissues including intrathoracic lymph nodes and the spleen [139–141].

An alternative route has been suggested by Renston et al. [142], in which IgA directly enters the venous drainage of the gut and reaches the liver via the portal vein without first entering the systemic circulation. However, this was tested by Manning and his associates [44] by thoracic duct ligation. Although the IgA concentration in the portal circulation increased, it was not sufficient to halt the decline of biliary IgA levels. In addition, it was shown that approximately 95% of thoracic duct lymph IgA is newly synthesized and that 50% of the lymph IgA arriving in the blood is subsequently removed by the liver.

The remaining 50% of IgA not transported to bile could be added to the serum pool of IgA, removed from the circulation by various mucosal sites (thereby augmenting the sharing of IgA plasma cells from one mucosal site to another), or IgA may be degraded by the liver. Although the bulk of evidence reviewed by Jones et al. [143] does not support this latter alternative as a major degradative pathway, recent evidence of biliary apoprotein fraction IgA fragments bound to bile cholesterol and phosphatidylcholine [144, 145] leaves the significance of IgA catabolism in the liver open to further question.

SPECULATION ON THE ETIOLOGY AND PATHOGENSIS OF IgA NEPHROPATHY

The strong association between circulating polymeric IgA and IgA-containing immune complexes and the severity of IgA nephropathy has been well reviewed [13, 17]. It is the polymeric nature of mesangial IgA deposits that has led to consideration of abnormalities of mucosal immunoglobulin synthesis that might be related to the pathogenesis of the disease. In brief, alterations in T immunoregulatory cell subpopulations associated with MALT have supported the view that abnormal control of IgA synthesis or secretion may play a pathogenetic, if not etiologic, role. It has also been suggested that the continuous or recurrent overproduction of polymeric IgA is likely to reflect the responses of secondary B cells to chronic antigen exposure or inflammation [101–103]. Indeed, in vitro findings indicate that specific abnormalities of intestinal mucosal and peripheral blood B-cell immunoglobulin synthesis occur in patients with ulcerative colitis and Crohn's disease [124, 125], and increased levels of IgA in pharyngeal washings that correlated with serum IgA were found in IgA nephropathy patients [146].

There is considerable evidence to indicate that the genetically controlled production of low-affinity antibody complexes produced in response to chronic antigen challenge induces glomerulonephritis [125, 147–149] and that chronic mucosal challenge leads to IgA-complex deposition in the mesangium [1].

The relatively high incidence of upper respiratory tract infections and tonsillitis suggests that the antigens playing a role in the etiology and/or maintenance of IgA nephropathy should perhaps be sought among the viruses often found in the oral cavity and in the nasopharynx. Nagy and her coworkers [61] examined the antibody titers of IgA nephropathy patients and controls against four viruses of the herpes group. In their study, elevated serum antibodies to HSV and cytomegalovirus antigens were more frequently found, but the effort to demonstrate HSV-associated antigen in the glomeruli of IgA nephropathy patients failed. This may have been due to technical difficulties; however, a direct etiologic relationship between herpes viruses and all patients with the disease was thought unlikely.

Other studies have indicated that IgA antibodies may be reactive against a variety of apparently endogenous antigens. Polymeric IgA rheumatoid factor has been associated with Sjögren's syndrome [150] and infectious endocarditis [151]. In addition, IgA antiidiotypic antibodies have been described in some IgA nephropathy patients [13]. Thus, intact IgA antibody or antigenic determinants on fragments or idiotopes of IgA may serve as either antibody or antigen in immune complex formation.

IgA eluted from renal biopsy specimens obtained from patients with IgA nephropathy has been shown to bind specifically to autologous kidney or tonsil cells [152]. This finding supports the possibility that local antigens of the upper respiratory tract might play a role in IgA-mediated renal disease. Additional demonstrations of antibodies to a variety of exogenous antigens including respiratory pathogens and dietary proteins in the serum of IgA nephropathy patients as well as occasional associations with mucosal inflammatory conditions raise questions relating to increases in antigen entry and defective mucosal immunoregulatory mechanisms.

There is, however, an apparent inconsistency in the mucosal associated theory of IgA nephropathy pathogenicity. For although the IgA subclass is well represented in mucosal secretions, it is either not present or relatively underrepresented in nephritic mesangial deposits [13, 17]. It appears that IgA2 may be particularly well suited to maintaining its molecular integrity in the face of proteolytic enzymes produced by a number of pathogenic microorganisms. The preferential secretion of IgA2 may therefore have a selective advantage for the individual. Thus, although IgA-secreting plasma cells in mucosal associated tissues such as the gut lamina propria may secrete both IgA1 and IgA2, it is possible that the dimeric IgA2–J-chain complex has a higher rate of enterocyte SC-mediated transport relative to IgA1. Less IgA2 would therefore be available as circulatory polymers or as immune complexes for mesangial deposition in IgA nephropathy. In this case, the relative concentrations of the IgA subclasses in mucosal secretions would not reflect serum levels of polymeric IgA or their immune complexes. The same situation would also apply if there were differential uptake, transport, or catabolism of the two IgA subclasses by the liver.

Mucosal surfaces are the sites of unavoidable recurrent or chronic antigenic stimulation related to the products of commensal and pathogenic organisms as well as foods and environmental debris. Clearly the sequelae that follow from systemic immune reactions to such a situation (e.g., ever-increasing levels of broad affinity antibody-producing and memory clones, antigenic competition, circulating nephritogenic IgG complexes, anaphylaxis, and a network of antiidiotypic antibodies that might eventually leave the system tolerant and defenseless) are better avoided. One way of circumventing this situation is the mucosal production of IgA that may decrease the flow of many substances through the mucosae, and thereby avoid systemic immune reactivity. The subsequent removal of mucosally derived IgA antigen immune complexes by the liver may be an important step in this process. It serves to remove potential feedback inhibitory IgA2 and IgA2 immune complexes and avoid the generation of anti-idiotypic antibodies that might defeat continuing surveillance. In addition, the transport of polymeric IgA and its immune complexes back into the bowel via the bile may serve to extract additional energy from nutrients by subjecting incompletely digested molecules (marked by their retention of recognizable antigenic determinants) to subsequent passages through the gut.

However, in this cycle of IgA from mucosal surfaces to the lumen of the bowel via the liver, it cannot be assumed that the IgA2 transport vehicle is not subject to a certain amount of wear and tear. Despite the protection from proteolysis afforded IgA by SC, a proportion of IgA molecules could be damaged in the process. It is suggested that these effete IgA molecules might be absorbed as antigenically recognizable fragments and elicit the generation of responding IgA2 antibody-forming cells in GALT. Since polymeric IgA immune complexes are preferentially deposited in the mesangium in conditions of antigen or antibody excess, it is not difficult to imagine that these IgA2 anti-IgA (fragment) complexes could be nephritogenic. Under these circumstances, mesangial deposits would appear to stain with anti-IgA2 reagents and perhaps for few other antigens.

In support of such an hypothesis, Lafont and coworkers [145] have shown that the apoprotein fraction of human bile lipoprotein complex consists of acidic polypeptide and IgA fragments. The IgA fragments of apobile lipoprotein complex in the liver arise from a fraction of circulating IgA. After hepatocyte uptake, this IgA fraction is deviated from the normal pathways toward the lysosomes where it is partially degraded and excreted into the bile along with other lysosomal contents.

Once in the intestinal lumen, the bile apoprotein fractions bound to phosphatidylcholine are poor substrates for pancreatic phospholipase A_2 and are not readily hydrolyzed [144, 145]. Evidence suggests that these phosphatidylcholine-associated IgA fragments may be absorbed by enterocytes as immunogenic determinants. These findings lead to further avenues of inquiry linking idiopathic IgA nephropathy with liver and/or gut-associated abnormalities.

The secretion of mucosal associated polymeric IgA, its binding to absorbed antigen, the circulation of IgA2 immune complexes, liver processing, and

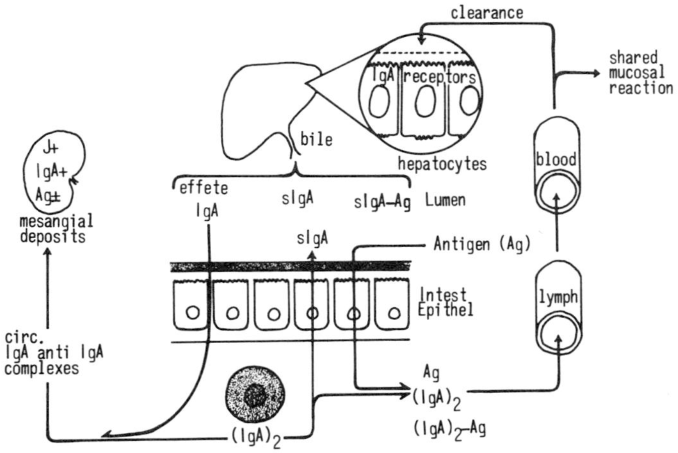

Figure 10-2. Endogenous or exogenous antigens presented at mucosal surfaces such as the intestinal epithelium may meet IgA that has been transported to the luminal surface via secretory component (SC) binding to enterocyte or dimeric IgA2 and Ag circulate via the thoracic duct and blood to other mucosal tissues that then share in immune reactivity by being antigen driven or by the local uptake of IgA2. Alternatively, a large proportion is cleared by the liver where Ag may be processed and the IgA2 and IgA2–Ag complexes transported through hepatocytes via a variety of potential IgA receptors to the bile.

Some of the IgA is diverted to hepatocyte lysosomes and reaches the bile as IgA fragments bound to bile cholesterol and phosphatidylcholine. IgA in this form is protected from pancreatic enzyme hydrolysis and may be antigenic. Upon reaching the lamina propria, these fragments or other effete IgA molecules may combine with locally produced IgA2 to form nephritogenic IgA2 anti-IgA fragment immune complexes.

eventual formation of (IgA) anti-effete IgA nephritogenic complexes are illustrated in figure 10-2.

In addition to the generation of IgA anti-IgA immune complexes, further speculation about the causes of IgA nephropathy should not overlook possible parallels with recent evidence for the in situ origin of poststreptococcal glomerulonephritis [153]. In those studies, Lange and associates indentified a cytoplasmic protein antigen, endostreptosin, derived from group A streptococci that preferentially localizes on the subendothelial side of the glomerular basement membrane. Shortly after the onset of symptoms, the antigen was no longer detected in the GBM or in the mesangium because the antigenic sites were saturated with patients' complement-binding antibodies. The cytoplasmic location of the antigen within the pathogenic streptococcus could easily lead to erroneous conclusions following serologic evaluations of host immune reactivity, while the apparently specific renal localization pattern of endostreptosin offers an example for the examination of other mucosal associated antigenic substances.

In conclusion, IgA nephropathy has been viewed in the context of mucosal IgA, and it relates to protective immunity as well as selective and regulatory reactions that tend to maintain mucosal and systemic homeostasis. Particular aspects of mucosally generated immunoregulation and hepatic IgA transport, clearance, and catabolism as well as chronic antigen challenge that might contribute to pathogenicity have been emphasized. Additional speculation concerning IgA anti-effete IgA immune complex formation and glomerular-localizing antigen in poststreptococcal glomerulonephritis has been discussed.

REFERENCES

1. Woodroffe AJ, Lomax-Smith JD: Pathogenetic mechanisms of IgA nephropathy from studies of experimental models. In: Robinson RR (ed) Nephrology I. New York: Springer-Verlag, 1984, pp 645–651.
2. Ward DM, Spiegelberg HL, Wilson CB: Persistence of IgA aggregates in the glomerular mesangium in mice [abstr]. Kidney Int 16:801, 1979.
3. Egido J, Sancho J, Rivera F, Sanchez-Crespo M: Handling of soluble IgA aggregates by the mononuclear phagocytic system in mice: comparison with IgG aggregates. Immunology 46:1–7, 1982.
4. Rifai A, Small PA, Teague PO, Ayoub EM: Experimental IgA nephropathy. J Exp Med 150:1161–1173, 1979.
5. Emancipator SN, Gallo GR, Lamm ME: Experimental IgA nephropathy induced by oral immunization. J Exp Med 157:572–582, 1983.
6. Lamm M: The secretory immune system in experimental IgA nephropathy. Contrib Nephrol 1984.
7. Isaacs K, Miller F, Lane B: Experimental model for IgA nephropathy. Clin Immunol Immunopathol 20:419–426, 1981.
8. Isaacs KL, Miller F: Antigen size and charge in immune complex glomerulo nephritis. Am J Pathol 111:298–306, 1983.
9. Van Marck EAE, Deelder AM, Gigase PLJ: Effect of partial portal vein ligation on immune glomerular deposits in *Schistosoma mansoni* infected mice. Br J Exp Pathol 58:412–417, 1977.
10. Melvin T, Burke B, Michael AF, Kim Y: Experimental IgA nephropathy in bile duct ligated rats. Clin Immunol Immunopathol 27:369–377, 1983.
11. Portis JL, Coe JE: Deposition of IgA in renal glomeruli of mink affected with Aleutian disease. Am J Pathol 96:227–236, 1979.
12. Hall RP, Strachura I, Cason J, Whiteside TL, Lawley T: IgA-containing circulating immune complexes in patients with IgA nephropathy. Am J Med 74:56–63, 1983.
13. Egido J, Sancho J, Blasco R, Lozano L, Hernando L: Immunologic aspects of IgA nephropathy in humans. In: Robinson RR (ed) Nephrology I. New York: Springer-Verlag, 1984, pp 652–664.
14. Conley ME, Cooper MD, Michael AF: Selective deposition of immunoglobulin A in immunoglobulin A nephropathy, anaphylactoid purpura nephritis and systemic lupus erythematosis. J Clin Invest 66:1432–1436, 1980.
15. Tomino Y, Sakai M, Miura M, Endoh M, Nomoto Y: Detection of polymeric IgA in glomeruli from patients with IgA nephropathy. Clin Exp Immunol 49:419–425, 1982.
16. Valentijn RM, Radl I, Haaiman JJ, Vermeer BJ, Weening JJ, Kauffmann RH, Daha MR, Van Es LA: Circulating and mesangial secretory component-binding IgA-1 in primary IgA nephropathy. Kidney Int 26:760–766, 1984.
17. Clarkson AR, Woodroffe AJ, Bannister KM, Lomax-Smith JD, Aarons I: The syndrome of IgA nephropathy. Clin Nephrol 21:7–14, 1984.
18. Haaijman JJ, Deen C, Krose CJM, Zijlstra JJ, Coolen J, Radl J: Monoclonal antibodies in immunocytology: jungle full of pitfalls. Immunol Today 5:56–58, 1984.

19. Peppard J, Orlans E, Payne AWR, Andrew E: The elimination of cirulating complexes containing polymeric IgA by excretion in the bile. Immunology 42:83–89, 1981.
20. Lemaitre-Coelho I, Jackson GDF, Vaerman J-P: High levels of secretory IgA and free secretory component in the serum of rats with bile duct obstruction. J Exp Med 147:934–939, 1978.
21. Orlans E, Peppard J, Reynolds J, Hall J: Rapid active transport of immunoglobulin A from blood to bile. J Exp Med 147:588–592, 1978.
22. Socken DJ, Jeejeebhoy KN, Bazin H, Underdown BJ: Identification of secretory component as an IgA receptor on rat hepatocytes. J Exp Med 150:1538–1548, 1979.
23. Sancho J, Gonzalez Ed, Rivera F, Escanero JF, Egido J: Hepatic and kidney uptake of soluble monomeric and polymeric IgA aggregates. Immunology 52:161–167, 1984.
24. Sancho J, Egido J, Sanchez-Crespo M, Blasco R: Detection of monomeric and polymeric IgA containing immune complexes in serum and kidney from patients with alcoholic liver disease. Clin Exp Immunol 47:327–335, 1982.
25. Egido J, Sancho J, Lorento F, Fontan G: Inhibition of neutrophil migration by serum from patients with IgA nephropathy. Clin Exp Immunol 49:709–716, 1982.
26. Sato M, Morekawa K, Koshikawa S: Attachment of polymorphonuclear leukocytes to glomeruli in IgA nephropathy. Clin Immunol Immunopathol 29:111–118, 1983.
27. Wilton JMA: Suppression by IgA of IgG-mediated phagocytosis by human polymorphonuclear leucocytes. Clin Exp Immunol 34:423–428, 1978.
28. Goldman M, Rose LM, Hochmann A, Lanbert PH: Deposition of idiotype–anti-idiotype immune complexes in renal glomeruli after polyclonal B cell activation. J Exp Med 155:1385–1399, 1982.
29. Roitt I: Essential immunology. London: Blackwell, 1980.
30. Egido J, Sancho J, Rivera F, Hernado L: The role of IgA and IgG immune complexes in IgA nephropathy. Nephron 36:52–59, 1984.
31. Doi T, Kanatsu K, Sekita K, Yoshida H, Nagai H, Hamashima Y: Circulating immune complexes of IgG, IgA, and IgM classes in various glomerular diseases. Nephron 32:335–341, 1982.
32. Woodroffe AJ, Clarkson AR, Seymour AE, Lomax-Smith JD: Mexangial IgA nephritis. Springer Semin Immunopathol 5:321–332, 1982.
33. Tomasi TB, Bienenstock J: Secretory immunoglobulins. In: Dixon FJ Jr, Kunkel HG (eds) Advances in immunology. New York: Academic Press, 1968, pp 1–96.
34. Bieninstock J, Befus AD: Mucosal immunology. Immunology 41:249–270, 1980.
35. Allardyce RA, Bienenstock J: The mucosal immune system in health and disease, with an emphasis on parasitic infection. Bull WHO 62:7–25, 1984.
36. Castro GA: Immunological regulation of epithelial function. Am J Physiol 243:G321–329, 1982.
37. Bienenstock J: Cellular and secretory aspects of the gastrointestinal tract. Clin Immunol Allergy 2:5–14, 1982.
38. Bienenstock J, McDermott MR, Befus AD: The significance of bronchus-associated lymphoid tissue. Bull Eur Physiopathol Respir 18:153–177, 1982.
39. Befus AD, Bienenstock J: Factors involved in symbiosis and host resistance at the mucosal–parasite interface. Prog Allergy 31:76–177, 1982.
40. Bienenstock J: Review and discussion of homing of lymphoid cells to mucosal membranes: the selective localization of cells in mucosal tissues. In: Strober W, Hanson LA, Sell KW (eds) Recent advances in mucosal immunity. New York: Raven, 1982, pp 35–43.
41. Roux ME, McWilliams M, Phillips-Quagliata JM, Weisz-Carrington P, Lamm ME: Origin of IgA-secreting plasma cells in the mammary gland. J Exp Med 146:1311–1322, 1977.
42. McDermott MR, Bienenstock J: Evidence for a common mucosal immunologic system. I. Migration of B immunoblasts into intestinal, respiratory and genital tissues. J Immunol 122:1892–1898, 1979.
43. McDermott MR, Clark DA, Bienenstock J: Evidence for a common mucosal immunologic system. II. Influence of the estrous cycle on B immunoblast migration into genital and intestinal tissues. J Immunol 124:2536–2539, 1980.
44. Manning RJ, Walker PG, Carter L, Barrington PJ, Jackson GDF: Studies on the origins of biliary immunoglobulins in rats. Gastroenterology 87:173–179, 1984.

45. Virella G, Montgomery P. Lemaitre-Coelho I: Transport of oligomeric IgA of systemic origin into external secretions. Adv Exp Med Biol 107:241–251, 1978.
46. Hall WH, Manion RE, Zinneman HH: Blocking serum lysis of *Brucella abortus* by hyperimmune rabbit immunoglobulin A. J Immunol 107:41–46, 1971.
47. Griffiss JM: Bactericidal activity of meningococcal antisera: blocking of IgA of lytic antibody in human convalescent sera. J Immunol 144:1179–1784, 1975.
48. Griffiss JM, Bertram MA: Serum IgA and susceptibility to meningococcal disease. Clin Res 24:344A, 1976.
49. Bellamy IEC, Nielsen NO: Immune-mediated emigration of neutrophils into the lumen of the small intestine. Infect Immun 9:615–619, 1974.
50. McNabb PC, Tomasi TB: Host defence mechanisms at mucosal surfaces. Annu Rev Microbiol 35:477–496, 1981.
51. Eidelman S: Intestinal lesions in immune deficiency. Hum Pathol 7:427–434, 1976.
52. Brandtzaeg P, Prydz H: Direct evidence for an integrated function of J chain and secretory component in epithelial transport of immunoglobulins. Nature 311:71–73, 1984.
53. Solari R, Krehenbuhl J-P: The biosynthesis of secretory component and its role in the transepithelial transport of IgA dimer. Immunol Today 6:17–20, 1985.
54. Delacroix DL, Hodgson HJF, McPherson A, Dive C, Vaerman J-P: Selective transport of polymeric immunoglobulin A in bile. J Clin Invest 70:230–241, 1982.
55. Mulks MH, Plaut AG: IgA protease production as a characteristic distinguishing pathogenic from harmless Neisseriaceae. N Engl J Med 299:973–976, 1978.
56. Labib RS, Calvanico NJ, Tomasi TB: Studies on extracellular proteases of *Streptococcus sanguis*: purification and characterization of a human IgA1 specific protease. Biochim Biophys Acta 526:547–559, 1978.
57. Mulks MH, Koinfeld SJ, Plaut AG: Specific proteolysis of human IgA by *Streptococcus pneumoniae* and *Haemophilus influenzae*. J Infect Dis 141:450–456, 1980.
58. Plaut AG, Gilbert JV, Wistar R: Loss of antibody activity in human immunoglobulin A exposed extracellular immunoglobulin A proteases of *Neisseria gonorrhoeae* and *Streptococcus sanguis*. Infect Immun 17:130–135, 1977.
59. Kilian M, Mestecky J, Kulhavy R, Tomana M, Butler W: IgA1 proteases from *Haemophilus influenzae, Streptococcus pneumoniae, Neissesia meningitis*, and *Streptococcus sanguis*: comparative immunochemical studies. J Immunol 124:2596–2600, 1980.
60. Allison RD: An evaluation of the potential for dietary proteins to contribute to systemic disease. Prepared for Bureau of Foods, Food and Drug Administration, Department of Health and Human Services, Washington DC, 1982.
61. Nagy J, Uj M, Szücs G, Trinn C, Burger T: Herpes virus antigens and antibodies in kidney biopsies and sera of IgA glomerulonephritic patients. Clin Nephrol 21:259–262, 1984.
62. Bariety J, Richer D, Appay MD, Grassetete J, Callard P: Frequency of intraendothelial "virus like" particles: an electron microscopy study of 376 human renal biopsies. J Clin Pathol 26:21–24, 1973.
63. Waldman RH, Wigley FM, Small PA Jr: Specificity of respiratory secretion antibody against influenza virus. J Immunol 105:1477–1483, 1970.
64. Morcin B: Immunity against parainfluenza-3 virus in cattle: immunoglobulins in response to vaccination. Z Immun Forsch 144:63–74, 1972.
65. Allardyce RA, Shearman DJC, McClelland DBL, Marwick K, Simpson AJ, Laidlaw RB: Appearance of specific colostrum antibodies after clinical infection with *Salmonella typhimurium*. Br Med J 3:307–309, 1974.
66. Goldblum RM, Ahlstedt S, Carlsson B, Hanson LA, Jodal U, Lindin-Janson G, Sohl-Akerlund A: Antibody forming cells in human colostrum after oral immunization. Nature 257:797–799, 1975.
67. Hanson LA, Carlsson B, Cruz JR, Garcia B, Holmgren J, Khan SR, Lindblad BS, Svennerholm AM, Svennerholm B, Urrutia J: Immune response in the mammary gland IN: Ogra PL, Dayton DH (eds) Immunology of breast milk. New York: Raven, 1979, pp. 145–157.
68. Fubara ES, Freter R: Protection against enteric bacterial infection by secretory IgA antibodies. J Immunol 111:395–403, 1972.

69. Wu AL, Walker WA: Immunological control mechanism against cholera toxin: interference with toxin binding to intestinal receptors. Infect Immun 14:1034–1042, 1976.
70. Sheelagh L, Soulsby EJL: The role of IgA immunoglobulins in the passive transfer of protection to *Taenia taeniaformis* in the mouse. Immunology 34:939–945, 1978.
71. Loftness TJ, Erlandsen SL, Wilson ID, Meyer EA: Occurrence of specific secretory immunoglobulin A in bile after inoculation of *Gardia lamblia* trophozoites into rat duodenum. Gastroenterology 87:1022–1029, 1984.
72. Svanborg Edén C, Hanson LA, Jodal U, Lindberg U, Sohl Akerlund A: Variable adherence to normal human urinary tract epithelia cells of *Escherichia coli* strains associated with various forms of urinary tract infection. Lancet 2:490–492, 1976.
73. Hanson LA, Ahlstedt S, Carlsson B, Kaijser B, Larsson P, Mattsby Maltzes I, Sohl Akerlund A, Svanborg Edén C, Svennerholm AM: Secretory IgA antibodies to enterobacterial virulence antigens, their induction and possible relevance in secretory immunity and infection. Adv Exp Med Biol 107:167–176, 1978.
74. Kaijser B, Larsson P, Olling S: Protection against ascending *Escherichia coli* pyelonephritis and significance of local immunity. Infect Immun 20:78–81, 1978.
75. Brunner H, Chanock RM: A radio immuno precipitation test for the detection of *Mycoplasma pneumoniae* antibody. Proc Soc Exp Biol Med 143:97–105, 1973.
76. Waldman RH, Lee JD, Polly SM, Dorfman A, Fox EN: Group A streptococcal M protein vaccine: protection following immunization via the respiratory tract. Dev Biol Stand 28:429–434, 1975.
77. Michalek SM, McGhee JR, Mestecky J, Arnold RR, Bozzo L: Ingestion of *Streptococcus mutans* induces secretory immunoglobulin A and carries immunity. Science 192:1238–1240, 1975.
78. Mestecky J: Structural aspects of human polymeric IgA. Ricerca Clin Lab [Suppl 3] 6: 87–92, 1976.
79. Sullivan DA, Allansmith MR: Source of IgA in tears of rats. Immunology 53:791–799, 1984.
80. Bienenstock J, Befus AD: Some thoughts on the biologic role of IgA. Gastroenterology 84:178–185, 1983.
81. Elson CO, Heck JA, Strober W: T cell regulation of murine IgA synthesis. J Exp Med 149:632–643, 1979.
82 Bienenstock J: The derivation, distribution and function of intestinal mucosal lymphocytes. Monogr Allergy 17:233–249, 1981.
83. Chalon MP, Milne RW, Vaerman JP: In vitro immunosuppressive effect of serum from orally immunized mice. Eur J Immunol 9:747–751, 1979.
84. Mattingly JA, Eardley DD, Kemp JD, Gershon RH: Induction of supressor cells in rat spleen: influence of microbial stimulation. J Immunol 122:787–790, 1979.
85. Hanson DG, Vaz NM, Maia LCS, Lynch JM: Inhibition of specific immune responses by feeding protein antigens. J Immunol 123:2337–2343, 1979.
86. Swarbrick ET, Stokes CR, Soothill JF: Abosrption of antigens after oral immunization and the simultaneous induction of specific systemic tolerance. Gut 20:121–125, 1979.
87. Challacombe SJ, Tomasi TB: Systemic tolerance and secretory immunity after oral immunization. J Exp Med 152:1459–1472, 1980.
88. Titus RG, Chiller JM: Orally induced tolerance: definition at the cellular level. Int Arch Allergy Appl Immunol 65:323–338, 1981.
89. Stokes CR, Swarbrick ET, Soothill JF: Genetic differences in immune exclusion and partial tolerance to ingested antigens. Clin Exp Immunol 52:678–684, 1983.
90. Devey ME, Bleasdale K: Antigen feeding modifies the course of antigen-induced immune complex disease. Clin Exp Immunol 56:637–644, 1984.
91. Strobel S, Ferguson A: Immune responses to fed protein antigens in mice. 3. systemic tolerance or priming is related to age at which antigen is first encountered. Paediatr Res 18:588–594, 1984.
92. Murgita RA, Wigzell H: Regulation of immune functions in the fetus and newborn. Prog Allergy 29:54–133, 1981.
93. Inman FP, Mestecky J: The J chain of polymeric immunoglobulins. Contemp Top Mol Immunol 3:111–141, 1974.

94. Koshland ME: Structure and function of the J chain. Adv Immunol 20:41–69, 1975.
95. Radl J, Swart ACW, Mestecky J: The nature of the polymeric serum IgA in man. Proc Soc Exp Biol Med 150:482–484, 1975.
96. Heremans JF: The secretory immune system: critical reappraisal. In: Neter N, Milgrom F (eds) The immune systems and infectious diseases. London: Karger, 1975, pp 376–385.
97. Heremans JF: Immunoglobulin A in the antigens, vol 2. Sela M (ed). New York: Academic Press, 1974, pp 365–522.
98. Wu AM, Till JE, Siminovitch L, McCulloch EA: Cytological evidence for a relationship between normal hematopoietic colony-forming cells and cells of the lymphoid system. J Exp Med 127:455–464, 1968.
99. Shrader JW: Stem cell differentiation in the bone marrow. In: Inglis JR (ed) B lymphocytes today. New York: Elsevier, 1982, pp 12–18.
100. Klimnam NR, Wylie DE, Teal JM: B cell development. In: Inglis JR (ed) B lymphocytes today. New York: Elsevier, 1982, pp 8–11.
101. Pierce SK, Klinman NR: Allogeneic carrier-specific enhancement of hapten-specific secondary B-cell responses. J Exp Med 144:1254–1262, 1976.
102. Klinman NR, Press JL: The B cell specificity repertoire: its relationship to definable subpopulations. Transplant Rev 24:41–83, 1975.
103. Teal JM, Lafrenz D, Klinman NR, Strober W: Immunoglobulin class commitment exhibited by B lymphocytes separated according to surface isotype. J Immunol 126:1952–1957, 1981.
104. Koshland ME: Presidential address: molecular aspects of B cell differentiation. J Immunol 131:i–ix, 1983.
105. McHugh Y, Yagi M, Koshland ME: The use of J and μ chain analyses to assign lymphoid cell lines to various stages in B cell differentiation. In: Klinman N, Mosier D, Scher I, Vitetta E (eds) B lymphocytes in the immune response: functional, developmental and interactive properties. New York: Elsevier/North Holland, 1981, pp 467–483.
106. Kaji H, Parkhouse RME: Intracellular J chain in mouse plasmacytomas secreting IgA, IgM and IgG. Nature 249:45–47, 1974.
107. Roth RA, Mather EL, Koshland ME: Intracellular events in the differentiation of B lymphocytes to pentamer IgM synthesis. In: Vogel H, Pernis B (eds) Cells of immunoglobulin synthesis. New York: Academic Press, 1979, pp 141–156.
108. Roth RA, Koshland ME: Indentification of a lymphocyte enzyme that catalyses pentamer immunoglobulin M assembly. J Biol Chem 256:4633–4639, 1981.
109. Roth RA, Koshland ME: Role of disulfide interchange enzyme in immunoglobulin synthesis. Biochemistry 20:6594–6599, 1981.
110. Parker DC, Wadsworth DC, Schneider GB: Activation of murine B lymphocytes by anti-immunoglobulin is an inductive signal leading to immunoglobulin secretion. J Exp Med 152:138–150, 1980.
111. Melchers F, Anderson J, Lernhardt W, Schreier MH: H-2 unrestricted polyclonal maturation without replication of small B cells induced by antigen-activated T cell help factors. Eur J Immunol 10:679–685, 1980.
112. Nakanishi K, Howard M, Muraguchi A, Farrar J, Takatsu K, Hamaoka T, Paul WE: Soluble factors involved in B cell differentiation: identification of two distinct T cell-replacing factors (TRF). J Immunol 130:2219–2224, 1983.
113. Adams JM: The organisation and expression of immunoglobulin genes. In: Inglis JR (ed) B lymphocytes today. New York: Elsevier, 1982, pp 21–29.
114. Honjo T: The molecular mechanisms of the immunoglobulin class switch. In: Inglis JR (ed) B lymphocytes today. New York: Elsevier, 1982, pp 36–39.
115. Liu CP, Tucker PW, Mushinski JF, Blattner FR: Mapping of heavy chain genes for mouse immunoglobulins M and D. Science 209:1348–1353, 1980.
116. Tseng J: A population of resting IgM-IgD double-bearing lymphocytes in Peyer's patches: the major precursor cells for IgA plasma cells in the gut lamina propria. J Immunol 132:2730–2735, 1984.
117. Maki R, Roeder W, Traunecker A, Sidman C, Wabe M, Raschika W, Tonegawa S: The ole of DNA rearrangement and alternative RNA processing in the expression of immunoglobulin delta genes. Cell 24:353–365, 1981.

118. Jones PP, Craig SW, Cebra JJ, Herzenberg LA: Restriction of gene expression in B lymphocytes and their progeny. II. Commitment to immunoglobulin heavy chain isotype. J Exp Med 140:452–469, 1974.
119. Jones PP, Cebra JJ: Restriction of gene expression in B lymphocytes and their progeny. III. Endogenous IgA and IgM on the membrane of different plasma cell precursors. J Exp Med 140:966–976, 1974.
120. Cebra JJ, Gearhart PJ, Halsey JF, Hurwitz JL, Shahin RD: Role of environmental antigens in the ontogeny of secretory immune response. J Reticuloendothel Soc 28:61s–71s, 1980.
121. Cebra JJ, Cebra ER, Clough ER, Fuhrman JA, Komisar JL, Schweitzer PA, Shahin RD: IgA commitment: model for B cell differentiation and possible roles for T cells in regulating B-cell development. Ann NY Acad Sci 30:25–38, 1983.
122. Bene MC, Faure G, Hurault de Ligny B, Kessler M, Duheille J: Quantitative immunohistomorphometry of the tonsillar plasma cells evidences and inversion of the immunoglobulin A versus immunoglobulin G secreting cell balance. J Clin Invest 71:1342–1347, 1983.
123. Rothschild E, Chatenoud L: T cell subset modulation of immunoglobulin production in IgA nephropathy and membranous glomerulonephritis. Kidney Int 25:557–564, 1984.
124. Sieber G, Herrmann F, Zeitz M, Teichmann H, Rühl H: Abnormalities of B-cell activation and immunoregulation in patients with Crohn's disease. Gut 25:1255–1261, 1984.
125. Danis VA, Harries AD, Heatley RV: In vitro immunoglobulin secretion by normal human gastrointestinal mucosal tissues, and alterations in patients with inflammatory bowel disease. Clin Exp Immunol 56:159–166, 1984.
126. Michalek SM, McGhee J, Kujons H, Colwell DE, Eldridge JH, Wannemuehler MJ, Koopman WJ: The IgA response: inductive aspects, regulatory cells, and effector functions. Ann NY Acad Sci 409:48–71, 1983.
127. Green DR, Gold J, St Martin S, Gershon R, Gershon RK: Microenvironmental immunoregulation: possible role of contrasuppressor cells in maintaining immune responses in gut-associated lymphoid tissues. Proc Natl Acad Sci USA 79:889–892, 1982.
128. Green DR, St Martin S: Suppression and contrasuppression in the regulation of gut associated immune responses. Ann NY Acad Sci 409:284–291, 1983.
129. Cebra JJ, Cebra ER, Clough ER, Fuhrman JA, Komisar JL, Schweitzer PA, Shahin RD: IgA commitment: models for B cell differentiation and possible roles for T cells in regulating B cell development. Ann NY Acad Sci 409:25–38, 1983.
130. Elson CO, Weiserbs DB, Ealding W, Machelski E: T-helper cell activity in intestinal lamina propria. Ann NY Acad Sci 409:230–237, 1983.
131. Kawaniski H, Strober W: Regulatory T cells in murine Peyer's patches directing IgA-specific isotype switching. Ann NY Acad Sci 409:243–257, 1983.
132. Mayer L, Fu Sm, Kunkel HG: IgA specific T-cell factor produced by a human T-T hybridoma. Ann NY Acad Sci 409:238–242, 1983.
133. Katz DH, Zuraw BL, Chen P, Cohen PA, O'Hair CM: Human IgE antibody synthesis in vitro. In: Kerr JW, Ganderton MA (eds) Proceedings of the 11th international congress of allergology and clinical immunology. London: Macmillan, 1983, pp 377–383.
134. Ishizaka K: Isotype specific regulation of IgE-binding factors. In: Kerr JW, Ganderton MA (eds) Proceedings of the 11th international congress of allergology and clinical immunology. London: Macmillan, 1983, pp 367–370.
135. Mattingly JA: Immunologic suppression after oral administration of antigen. III. Activation of suppressor-inducer cells in the Peyer's patches. Cell Immunol 86:46–52, 1984.
136. Sakai H, Nomoto Y, Arimori S: Decrease of IgA specific suppressor T cell activity in patients with IgA nephropathy. Clin Exp Immunol 38:243–248, 1979.
137. Sakai H, Endoh M, Tomino Y, Nomoto Y: Increase of IgA- specific helper Tα cells in patients with IgA nephropathy. Clin Exp Immunol 50:77–82, 1982.
138. Reynolds J, Gyure L, Andrew E, Hall JG: Studies of the transport of polyclonal IgA antibody from blood to bile in rats. Immunology 39:463–467, 1980.
139. Spencer J, Gyure LA, Hall JG: IgA antibodies in the bile of rats. III. The role of intrathoracic lymph nodes and the migration pattern of their blast cells. Immunology 48:687–693, 1983.

140. Dahlgren U, Ahlstedt S, Andersson J, Hedman L, Hanson LA: IgA antibodies in rat bile are not solely derived from thoracic duct lymph. Scand J Immunol 17:569–574, 1983.
141. Jackson GDF, Walker PG: The transient appearance of IgM antibodies in the bile of rats injected with *Salmonella enteritidis*. Immunol Lett 7:41–45, 1983.
142. Renston RH, Jones AL, Christiansen WD, Hradek GT, Underdown RJ: Evidence for a vesicular transport mechanism in hepatocytes for biliary secretion of immunoglobulin A. Science 208:1276–1278, 1980.
143. Jones AL, Renston RH, Burwen SJ: Uptake and intracellular deposition of plasma-derived proteins and apoproteins by hepatocytes. Prog Liver Dis 7:51–69, 1982.
144. Nalbone G, Lairon D, Charbonnier-Augeire M, Vigne JL, Leonardi J, Chabert C, Hauton JC, Verger R: Pancreatic phospholipase A_2 hydrolysis of phosphatidylcholines in various physicochemical states. Biochim Biophys Acta 620:612–625, 1980.
145. Lafont H, Lechene de la Porte P, Vigne JL, Chanussot F, Nalbone G, Lairon D, Charbonnier-Augeire M, Hauton JC: Immunohistochemical localization of the apoproteins of the bile lipoprotein complex in the human intestine. Digestion 28:164–169, 1983.
146. Tomina Y, Endoh M, Kaneshige H, Nomoto Y, Sakai H: Increase of IgA in pharyngeal washings from patients with IgA nephropathy. Am J Med Sci 286:15–21, 1983.
147. Devey ME, Steward MW: The induction of chronic antigen–antibody complex disease in selectively bred mice producing either high or low affinity antibody to protein antigens. Immunology 41:303–311, 1980.
148. Steward MW, Collins MJ, Stanley C, Devey ME: Chronic antigen–antibody-complex glomerulonephritis in mice. Br J Exp Pathol 62:614–622, 1981.
149. Devey ME, Bleasdale K, Collins M, Steward MW: Experimental antigen–antibody complex disease in mice: the role of antibody levels, antibody affinity and circulating antigen–antibody complexes. Int Arch Allergy Appl Immunol 68:47–53, 1982.
150. Elkon KB, Delacroix DL, Gharavi AE, Vaerman JP, Hughs GRV: Immunoglobulin A and polymeric IgA rheumatoid factors in systemic sicca syndrome: partial characterization. J Immunol 129:576–581, 1982.
151. Elkon KB, Inman RD, Culhane L, Christinal CL: Induction of polymeric IgA rheumatoid factor in infective endocarditis. Am J Med 75:785–789, 1983.
152. Tomino Y, Endoh M, Nomoto Y, Sakai H: Specificity of eluted antibody from renal tissues of patients with IgA nephropathy. Am J Kidney Dis 1:276–281, 1982.
153. Lange K, Seligson G, Cronin W: Evidence for the in situ origin of poststreptococcal glomerulonephritic glomerular localization of endostreptosin and the clinical significance of the subsequent antibody response. Clin Nephrol 19:3–10, 1983.

11. THE ROLE OF POLYMERIC IgA IN THE PATHOGENESIS OF IgA NEPHROPATHY

JESUS EGIDO

Primary IgA nephropathy is characterized by the presence of IgA at the mesangium level accompanied or not by other immunoglobulins in the absence of systemic liver disease. A similar immunofluorescence pattern has been observed in an array of diseases involving mucosal surfaces and the term *syndrome of IgA nephropathy* has been suggested [1].

Since IgA plays an important role in mucosal immunity, presumably serving as an immunologic barrier to the penetration of macromolecules and microorganisms into the body [2], it is thought that the IgA deposited in the mesangium has a mucosal origin.

In a simplified view it has been classically assumed that mucosal IgA-positive cells produce predominantly dimeric or polymeric IgA, while bone marrow and various nodes secrete predominantly monomeric IgA (m-IgA) [3]. For that reason, several authors have studied the nature of mesangial and serum IgA in patients with IgA nephropathy. Although the issue remains unsettled, in this chapter we attempt to show that certain evidence exists supporting a role for polymeric IgA (p-IgA) in the pathogenesis of this disease [4].

SERUM IgA

In most studies, high serum IgA levels have been found in 50–70% of patients with IgA nephropathy. No correlation between IgA levels and any clinical, histologic, and immunologic features has been observed. Furthermore, for unknown reasons, serum IgA tends to be lower in patients with renal failure and even high levels of IgA have been associated with a favorable course. These data suggest that only some of the circulating IgA may be pathogenic (reviewed by Egido et al. [5]).

Although the possibility of an abnormal IgA was suggested by Lagrue et al. [6] and Berger et al. [7], our group was the first to publish detailed biochemical characteristics of IgA in this nephropathy [8, 9]. Of 15 patients with this disease, 11 had an increased proportion of serum IgA in 9S–21S fractions on 5–40% sucrose density-gradient ultracentrifugation. The serum treated by acid pH only partially reduced this proportion in forms between 13S and 21S. However, the reduction with dithiotreitol and the affinity of the high molecular weight IgA for human secretory component (SC) as well as the detection of J chain on urea alkaline polyacrylamide electrophoresis are compatible with the presence of a large amount of polymeric forms, partially as immune complexes (IC), in the serum of patients with IgA nephropathy. Elevations of serum polymeric IgA have also been found in other forms of nephritis with mesangial IgA deposits such as Henoch-Schönlein purpura and alcoholic cirrhosis [10, 11]. In fact this last disease is the one in which higher levels were observed [11]. As will be discussed later, this could be due to the combination of two factors: the increased production of p-IgA and its slow elimination by the liver.

Our initial data on IgA nephropathy have been confirmed by some authors [12, 13], but not by others [14, 15] (table 11-1). The possibility that the elevation of p-IgA in IgA nephropathy is a consequence of a general increase in the total IgA has been raised by Newkirk et al. [16] and Berger [17]. The Canadian group found that 36% of 30 patients studied by the secretory-binding assay had elevated p-IgA expressed in absolute values (0.35 ± 0.05 mg/ml) in relation to normal subjects (0.13 ± 0.02; $p < 0.005$), but there were no differences when expressed as percentage of the total IgA. The levels of p-IgA found by Berger were 0.043 ± 0.16 g/liter in patients and 0.17 ± 0.7 g/liter in controls ($p < 0.001$), but the level of p-IgA was correlated with the level of total serum IgA ($p < 0.001$). However, recently Valentijn et al. [12] have found in 12 patients with a positive anti-IgA inhibition binding assay an increase in the mean range of polymeric IgA and in the mean polymer–monomer ratio in relation to controls, excluding therefore the possibility of proportional changes between the amounts of polymeric and monomeric IgA in serum. In the three patients with a negative anti-IgA inhibition binding assay, the polymer–monomer ratio for IgA did not differ from that of controls. Since the mean (± SD) polymer–monomer ratio for IgA2 found in 15 patients with IgA nephropathy did not present differences with those found for controls, the authors suggested that these patients had elevated serum levels exclusively of dimeric–polymeric IgA1 [12]. These results can explain, at least partially, the discrepancy found on this topic in the literature: the different assays in the detection of p-IgA may

Table 11-1. Studies on serum levels of polymeric IgA in IgA nephropathy

Authors[a]	Method	Serum levels	Correlation with total serum levels	Ref.
Lopez Trascasa et al. (1979–1980)	Ultracentrifugation and SC binding	Elevated (73%)	No	9, 10
Woodroffe et al. (1980)	Column chromatography and ultracentrifugation	Normal	—	14
Lesavre et al. (1982)	SC-binding assay	Normal	—	15
Newkirk et al. (1983)	SC-binding assay	Elevated (36%)	Yes	16
Valentijn et al. (1984)	SC-binding assay in column fractions	Elevated IgA1[b]	No	12
Bernasconi et al. (1984)	SC-binding assay	Elevated (52%)	No	13
Berger (1984)	Cross-immuno-electrophoresis	Elevated	Yes	17
Feehally (1984)	High-performance liquid chromatography	Elevated	Not mentioned	18

[a]( ) Percent of patients studied.
[b]Expressed only in mean ± SD.

also be important. Thus, recently Bernasconi et al. [13], by using a secretory component solid-phase assay, found that 13 (52%) out of 25 of patients had elevated levels of p-IgA and, as in our initial description, there was no correlation between the levels of p-IgA and total serum IgA. (table 11-1). The normal p-IgA values observed in some patients by several groups may also be due to the intermittent nature of p-IgA production. Thus, we and Feehally [18] have seen an increase in serum dimeric and polymeric IgA in relapse that is not present in remission.

CLINICAL SIGNIFICANCE OF POLYMERIC AND MONOMERIC IgA-IMMUNE COMPLEXES

Several pieces of evidence suggest that circulating immune complexes (IC) may play a role in the deposition of IgA in patients with IgA nephropathy: first, the mesangial location of IgA in a granular pattern, second, the presence of electron-dense deposits in the mesangium, and third, the recurrence of IgA dense deposits in renal allografts. Initially most methods used to study circulating IC were designed to detect IgG. Since IgA is the predominant immunoglobulin deposited in the kindeys of these patients, the existence of techniques able to detect IgA IC seemed necessary. Our group initially showed the presence of such complexes in these patients by sucrose density-gradient ultracentrifugation at physiologic and acid pH values [9]. However, the practical limitation of this laborious assay to study a large amount of patients was evident.

During the last few years, several groups have demonstrated in patients

Table 11-2. Circulating immune complexes in IgA nephropathy

Class of IC[a]	Patients (66)[b]	Sera (136)
Polymeric IgA IC	30%	20%
Monomeric IgA IC	39%	26%
Multimeric IgA IC	55%	46%
IgG IC	46%	35%

[a]Raji cell assay.
[b]Numbers in parentheses indicate the number of sera of patients studied. Patients with at least one positive value were considered as having immune complexes.

with IgA nephropathy the presence of circulating IgA IC by different techniques, such as Raji cell assay, conglutinin-binding assay, anti-IgA inhibition assay, or other less specific methods (reviewed by Egido et al. [5, 19]). All these assays, however, do not distinguish p-IgA from m-IgA IC. Taking into account that p-IgA is found in the mesangium of these patients, the existence of a technique permitting the study of these two classes of IC seemed necessary. Based upon the specific binding of the secretory component for p-IgA, we developed a method that enables us to differentiate both classes of IC [20]. Following our preliminary results in 31 patients [21], the number has now been enlarged to 66. With this assay, 55% of patients had multimeric IgA (polymeric and monomeric IgA similtaneously) IC, 30% had p-IgA IC, and 39% had m-IgA IC on at least one determination (table 11-2). The intermittent nature of their appearance is clearly noted when sequential examinations are performed.

Although several groups, including our own [22], have found a certain correlation between the bouts of macroscopic hematuria, or the persistence of microhematuria, and the presence of multimeric IgA IC in the circulation (reviewed by Egido et al. [5]), it is interesting to note that, in this large series of 66 patients, a significant correlation was found only with polymeric IgA IC ($p < 0.025$), but none with either m-IgA IC or multimeric IgA IC (figure 11-1). In this sense only one patient without hematuria (more than four RBC per high-power field) had p-IgA IC. Thus, according to these results, p-IgA IC are almost exclusively found in patients with hematuria.

The importance of the presence of dimeric or polymeric IgA in the circulating IC in relation to the clinical activity of the nephritis has also been confirmed recently by Valentijn et al. [12]. Thus, 12 (80%) of the 15 patients with IgA nephropathy had IC determined by the anti-IgA inhibition binding assay with a molecular weight of dimeric IgA and a binding to free SC. This macromolecular IgA was present in eight out of 12 patients with persistent hematuria during the follow-up and, in the other four patients, only in those samples taken during hematuria. It is also important that the presence of these complexes distinguishes between patients with primary IgA nephropathy and those with other renal diseases presenting with hematuria, while

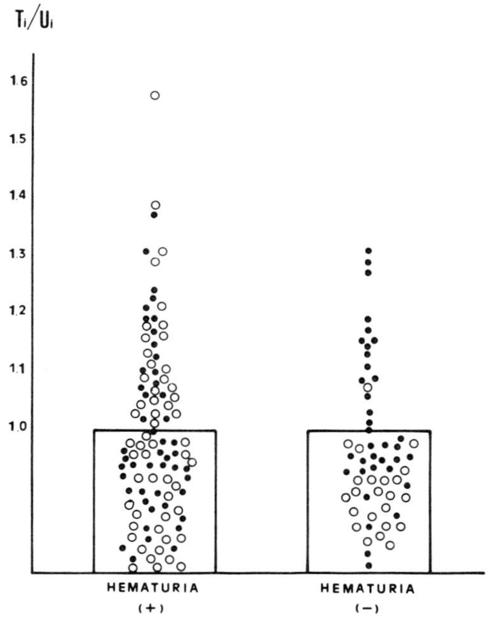

Figure 11-1. Relationship between the presence and levels of monomeric IgA immune complexes (●) and polymeric IgA immune complexes (○) and the existence of hematuria: (●) p = NS; and (○) $p < 0.025$.

complexes determined with the C1q-binding assay or the conglutinin-binding assay did not [12]. Apparent discrepancy was observed by Lesavre et al. [15], who found that IgA IC determined by conglutinin-binding assay was present in two main forms in the sera of patients with IgA nephropathy: high molecular weight IgA complex (400,000–800,000 daltons) and predominantly m-IgA. Since IgA IC of high molecular weight were also found in patients with SLE, they suggested that the large amount of conglutinin-binding m-IgA was rather specific for IgA nephropathy [15]. It is possible, however, that the method employed is critical for the detection of IC of different sizes [22]. Thus, recently Doi et al. [23] observed, according to ultracentrifugation analysis, that conglutinin-binding IgA IC were found mostly in the fractions containing m-IgA, whereas anti-C3d-binding IgA IC were found in fractions between 21S and 7S.

Already in the first described model of experimental IgA nephropathy, p-IgA was observed to be critical for renal deposition of complexes and induction of nephritic histologic changes. IC formed either in vivo or in vitro with m-IgA failed to induce glomerulonephritis [24]. The reason for the apparently major nephritogenic potential of p-IgA IC is not known. Recently Rifai et al. [25] approached this problem by injecting into mice IC prepared with m-IgA or p-IgA. Immunofluorescence studies showed that only p-IgA IC deposited in the kidneys. Also, electron-dense deposits in the glomeruli were observed in mice receiving p-IgA IC. According to the analysis of the IC size, the authors believe that multivalent p-IgA is nephritogenic because it forms predominantly large-latticed IC. In contrast, monovalent mIgA forms only small-latticed complexes that persist in the circulation without glomerular deposition. When large-latticed m-IgA IC were prepared, by covalent cross-linking m-IgA with a specific affinity-labeling antigen, deposition in the kidneys in a pattern similar to p-IgA IC was seen [25].

The size of IgA complexes in patients with IgA nephropathy has been studied only by some groups and in a small number of patients. Most authors agree that they are of small (7–13S) or intermediate (13–17S) size (review by Egido et al. [5, 19]). Although these differences could be due to the fact that different assays can detect IC of a specific size, it is also possible that it depends on the presence of p-IgA IC, m-IgA IC, or both. However, we have observed that in some samples having exclusively m-IgA IC, detected by the technique described in our laboratory [20], a macromolecular IgA, with a size between 13 and 17S, but without binding to SC, was detected in ultracentrifugation studies. Further studies are needed in this field to clarify the compostion of that macromolecular monomeric IgA. In this sense, circulating IC containing both IgA and IgG were detected in sera of IgA nephropathy patients with a significantly higher frequency as compared with healthy individuals [26]. It is also possible that m-IgA rheumatoid-factor-like activity can be detected in these patients as well as IC-containing idiotypes–antiidiotypes [27]. These results are in agreement with the classic view that poorly soluble immune complexes of intermediate size, one million molecular weight or greater, tend to localize exclusively within the glomerular mesangium, resulting in mesangial glomerulonephritis. The theoretically greater affinity or avidity of p-IgA could also be important since it has been shown that intravenous injection to mice of soluble complexes of high avidity resulted in a purely mesangial localization of the complexes [28].

It is also possible that, besides the size, other characteristics of IgA, e.g., charge, may be important for their deposition at the mesangial level. Thus, Monteiro et al. [29] have shown that the eluted IgA from kidneys of patients with IgA nephropathy was predominantly anionic with a pI ranging from 4.5 to 5.6. Since mesangial IgA was mainly composed of p-IgA and dimeric IgA, representing 64% of the total eluted IgA [29], one can indirectly assume that deposited p-IgA is also more anionic than m-IgA.

The possibility cannot be excluded that circulating macromolecular IgA, alone or forming part of nonimmunologic complexes, may be the source of mesangial deposits. In this sense, it is known that many serum proteins (albumin, $\alpha 1$ microglobulin, apolypoproteins, and others) can bind to IgA. Recently a surface receptor specific for human IgA on group-B streptococci possessing the Ibc protein antigen (common to many strains) has been

Table 11-3. Studies on the presence of polymeric IgA at the mesangium level

Authors	SC binding	J chain	Ref.
Egido et al. (1980)	16/20	5/5	10
Bene et al. (1982)	15/15	15/15	35
Tomino et al. (1982)	ND[a]	7/10[b]	36
Donini et al. (1982)	ND	18/27	37
Komatsu et al. (1983)	ND	8/8	38
Lomax-Smith et al. (1983)	1/10	10/11[c]	33
Waldherr et al. (1983)	4/10	15/15	39
Valentijn et al. (1984)	12/14	9/9	12

[a]ND, not done
[b]These authors also demonstrated polymeric IgA measured by sucrose density-gradient ultracentrifugation in renal eluates.
[c]Four of them without IgM deposits.

described [31]. Surprisingly, no IgA IC were found in the serum of some patients with IgA nephropathy having macrohematuria following tonsillectomy (unpublished observations).

NATURE OF MESANGIAL IgA

The nature and origin of the IgA deposited in the renal mesangium in patients with IgA nephropathy have been the subject of controversy during the last few years. Because this disease often follows infections of the upper respiratory tract, it seems likely that the source of IgA is in the external secretions. However, several studies have failed to reveal glomerular location of secretory IgA in IgA nephropathy [32, 33]. This is not surprising since this IgA normally circulated in blood in minimal amounts, increasing only when an abnormality in the permeability of the intestinal mucosa exists. By contrast, taking into account that p-IgA is increased in blood in these patients, our group looked for its presence in the kidney, based upon the affinity of the secretory component for the p-IgA and the presence of J chain [10]. This technique has been successfully applied by Brandtzaeg [34] to study immune cells in the intestinal epithelium and circulating B cells. Thus, 16 out of 20 patients studied presented criteria of p-IgA at the mesangium level. As IgM can also bind the SC, cases with these Ig were excluded. Furthermore, the distribution pattern of the binding of SC in the mesangium was identical to that observed for IgA. The presence of J chain was also visualized as spots in the areas presenting IgA. The treatment of cryostat sections with 6 *M* urea in glycine–HCl buffer produced sometimes a better demonstration of J chain, probably because this method unfolds Ig polymers exposing J-chain determinants [34].

From our initial work [10], several authors have also studied the nature of mesangial IgA either in kidney sections (table 11-3) or in renal eluates [12, 33, 35–39]. Most of these studies have confirmed the presence of p-IgA in the

Table 11-4. The subclasses of IgA deposited in the renal glomeruli

Author	Antiserum class	IgA1	IgA2	Ref.
André et al. (1980)	Polyclonal	5/10	10/10	42
Conley et al. (1980)	Monoclonal	10/10	0/10	43
Tomino et al. (1982)	Monoclonal	15/15	2/15	36
Waldherr et al. (1983)	Monoclonal	14/14	0/14	39
Hall et al. (1983)	Monoclonal	5/5	0/5	44
Lomax-Smith et al. (1983)	Monoclonal	10/11	2/11	33
	Polyclonal	10/11	9/11	33
Murakami et al. (1983)	Polyclonal	17/17	7/17	45
Valentijn et al. (1984)	Monoclonal	12/13	0/13	12

mesangium, though some discrepancies still exist. The employment of antisera with different specificities, the diversity in the fixation techniques of kidney sections, and their treatment under various conditions capable or not of exposing binding sites of p-IgA for SC and J-chain determinants, might account for these differences. Because codeposition of IgM (also possessing SC-binding affinity and J chain) with IgA is not infrequently found in the renal mesangium, it is possible to be sure of the presence of p-IgA in relatively few patients with IgA nephropathy. For these reasons, elution studies are important. Thus, IgA in the eluates of renal biopsy specimens in three out of five patients examined by Tomino et al. [36] were found in sediment predominantly as 9–11S using sucrose density-gradient analysis. This peak of protein was completely adsorbed with antihuman IgA or antihuman J-chain antisera. Monteiro et al. [29] have recently shown that about 70% of IgA eluted from kidney biopsies of ten patients with IgA nephropathy have characteristics of true p-IgA. Also about 55% of the IgA eluted from autopsy kidneys from patients with IgA deposits secondary to alcoholic liver disease have a molecular weight comprised of 9-12S [11]. The percentage of eluted p-IgA was, in each patient, higher than that observed in serum, suggested a special predisposition of this Ig to deposit in the mesangium. It is important to note that IgA in polymeric forms has also been demonstrated in the mesangium of mice with experimentally induced IgA nephropathy [40, 41] (Gonzalez, unpublished observations).

Since around 90% of serum IgA belongs to the IgA1 subclass, while IgA from the external secretions is equally represented by IgA1 and IgA2, some authors studied the subclasses of the IgA deposited in the mesangium in an attempt to establish the mucosal origin of this IgA. In this sense, preliminary results afforded conflicting data, probably caused by the employment of polyclonal and monoclonal antisera (table 11-4). Thus, André et al. [42], using polyclonal antisera, found that glomerular IgA deposits consist predominantly of IgA2. By contrast, Conley et al. [43], using monoclonal antibodies, have shown predominantly IgA1. Recently, other authors [12,

36, 39, 44], also employing monoclonal antibodies, have confirmed that the glomerular IgA in this disease is mostly IgA1 and polymeric. Furthermore, one of these authors [12] has shown that circulating IC contained polymeric IgA1. Recent data, however, support the idea that polymeric IgA has an equal distribution between the IgA1 and IgA2 subclasses [46] and that, in order to know about the polymeric nature of IgA, it is probably more appropriate to use its ability to bind the SC and/or to look for the J chain (once the presence of IgM has been excluded). The reasons why IgA1 predominates over IgA2 in the glomerular mesangium of patients with IgA nephropathy are not known.

In summary, although a majority of authors agree that mesangial IgA is in a great percentage polymeric, the coexistence of m-IgA indicates that m-IgA IC alone, or IgA-Ige IC, might also be important in provoking glomerular injury. It is possible, however, that the persistence or disappearance of IgA IC at the mesangium level may be governed by, among other factors, the molecular form of IgA. In this sense, though the blood clearance of monomeric or p-IgA IC or immune aggregates of the same size was similar [47, 48], aggregated p-IgA was deposited in larger amounts and persisted longer in the kidney than aggregated m-IgA [48].

INCREASED PRODUCTION OF POLYMERIC IgA AND Tα-CELL ABNORMALITIES

The high concentration in serum of polymeric IgA in patients with IgA nephropathy compared with normal subjects [9] could be due a priori to an increase in synthesis or to a defect in IgA clearance by the mononuclear phagocytic system, chiefly by the liver. Although IgA from the external secretions is almost exclusively polymeric [2], in sharp contrast to IgA from human serum, recently it has been demonstrated that mitogen-stimulated B-lymphocytes from peripheral blood of normal individuals produce IgA predominantly in a polymeric form [49]. Therefore we examined the percentage of polymeric IgA-producing cells based upon the ability of this immunoglobulin to bind SC. The percentage of these cells was significantly higher in 42 patients than in controls (64 ± 21 vs 44 ± 27) after seven days of culture (figure 11-2). The true nature of polymeric IgA released by these cells was confirmed by their ability to bind secretory component, the existence of covalent structures, and the decrease of the larger forms of IgA after reduction and alkylation. Furthermore, since some patients have, at least on several occasions, normal percentages of p-IgA lymphocytes, we looked for a relation with the clinical history. Thus lymphocytes from patients with IgA nephropathy, having episodes of macroscopic hematuria, produce more polymeric IgA than those without these bouts (figure 11-3). These results could afford immunologic support to the hypothesis that two subentities within adult primary IgA nephropathy exist based upon clinical history, HLA-DR, and Gm allotypes [51].

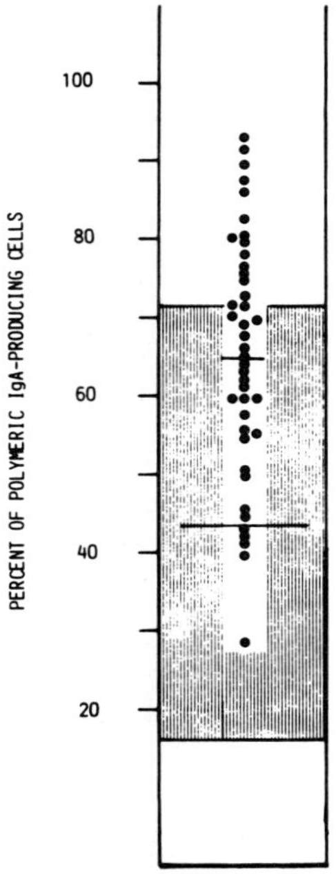

Figure 11-2. Percentages of PWM-stimulated blood lymphocytes from patients with IgA nephropathy simultaneously binding SC and IgA compared with controls. The *dashed area* represents the mean ± 2 SD of control values ($n = 29$): $p < 0.025$.

Taking into account the association of bouts of macrohematuria with upper respiratory tract infections, we speculated that lymphocytes originating from secretory tissues in these patients could produce high amounts of polymeric IgA following bacterial or viral infections, just as occurred in pokeweed-stimulated blood lymphocytes in vitro. In this sense, we have recently shown that tonsil lymphocytes obtained from tonsillectomy specimens also synthesized more polymeric IgA than control subjects suffering from chronic tonsillitis (figure 11-4) [52]. The finding of a significant decrease of polymeric IgA synthesis by blood lymphocytes two years after tonsillectomy in seven patients (figure 11-5) suggests that tonsils could be an important source of this polymeric IgA [53].

Following the original demonstration by Lum et al. [54] of the existence of T cells in human peripheral blood with Fc receptors for IgA (Tα cells), Sakai et al. [55] found, by three different methods, that these cells are significantly increased in patients with IgA nephropathy. Although the functions of Tα cells have not been fully determined, several studies have shown that they have IgA-specific helper activity in vitro [56]. In this sense, it has been suggested that the increased levels of Tα cells in patients with IgA nephro-

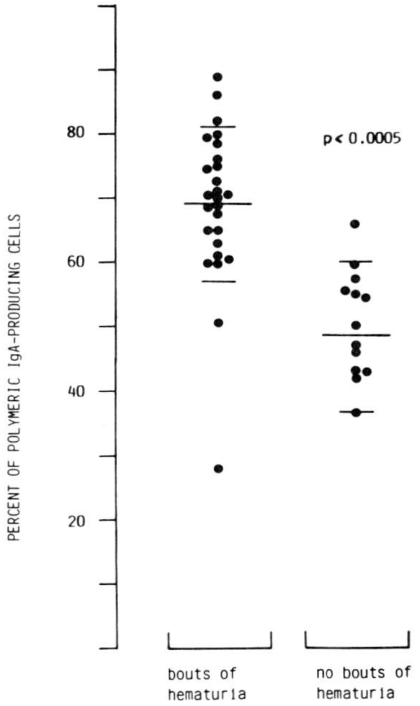

Figure 11-3. Percentages of polymeric IgA-producing lymphocytes in patients with or without bouts of hematuria.

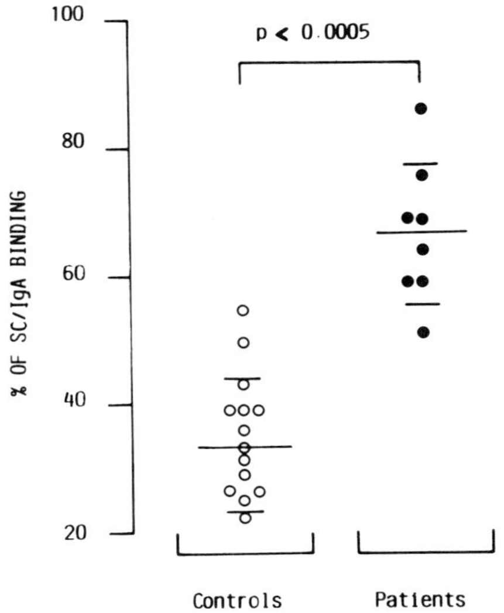

Figure 11-4. Percentages of tonsil lymphocytes producing polymeric IgA in patients and controls.

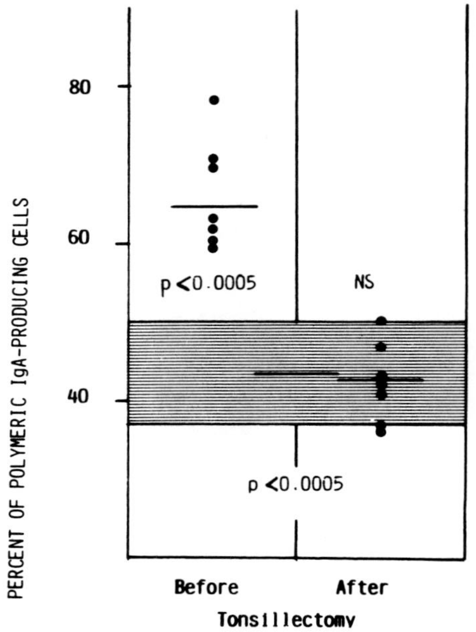

Figure 11-5. Percentages of blood lymphocytes producing polymeric IgA in patients with IgA nephropathy before and after tonsillectomy. The *shaded area* represents the mean ± 2 SD.

pathy may be responsible for the increased synthesis of IgA in such patients [55]. However, since the number of Tα cells is augmented in mice with IgA-secreting myelomas, a phenomenon closely linked to the high serum levels of polymeric IgA, the increased number of Tα cells found in these patients may simply reflect the increased p-IgA concentration. Recently we have seen a close correlation between the percentage of p-IgA-producing lymphocytes and the percentage of Tα cells (figure 11-6). Furthermore, the addition of serum fom patients with IgA nephropathy to lymphocyte cultures of normal subjects induced a significant increase in the production of IgA when compared with that induced by control serum (unpublished observations). However, the cell expression of these receptors was not increased in these patients following incubation with mouse myeloma IgA (MOPC 315), probably indicating that they were already expressed in vivo on the cells of these patients [57].

All these data suggest that the increase in the percentage of Tα cells could be a secondary phenomenon, the fundamental abnormality being the abnormal production of p-IgA. Further studies on the effect of polymeric IgA on the expression of receptors for the Fc of IgA (FcR) and the function of Tα cells are needed to clarify the alterations of IgA synthesis in patients with IgA nephropathy [50, 58].

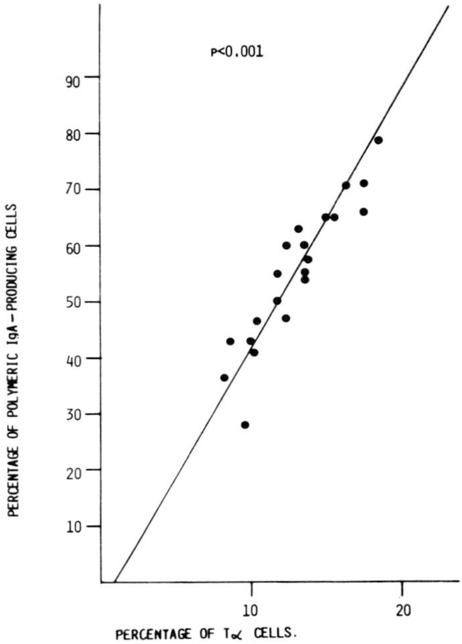

Figure 11-6. Correlation between the percentage of polymeric IgA-producing cells and the percentage of Tα cells in patients with IgA nephropathy. *Each point* represents a subject.

POLYMERIC IgA, THE MONONUCLEAR PHAGOCYTIC SYSTEM, AND THE LIVER

The finding only intermittently of circulating immune complexes in this nephropathy could be due to a temporal formation and/or a defect in their blood clearance. In this sense, a reduction in the ability of the mononuclear phagocyte system to cope with circulating complexes has been considered of great importance in the pathogenesis of glomerulonephritis in man. Soluble immune complexes, as opposed to those formed with particulate antigens, are chiefly eliminated by the liver. Those composed of IgA also have some differences in their clearance with respect to those composed of IgG. Thus, IgA immune aggregates (akin to immune complexes) injected into mice clear from the circulation more slowly than do IgG immune aggregates, and their catabolism by the liver cells and macrophages is also slower [59]. Polymeric IgA immune complexes are removed by the liver through the secretory component on the hepatocytes, at least in rodents [60]. Our group has recently demonstrated that both polymeric and monomeric IgA complexes are also eliminated through the Fc receptors of the hepatocytes and Kupffer cells [61, 62]. All these studies are in agreement with the high prevalence of IgA deposits in the glomerular mesangium of patients with alcoholic cirrhosis, probably due to a decrease in the hepatic clearance of immune complexes [11]. In fact, this has been clearly demonstrated in mice with experimental cirrhosis of the liver [61]. Blood retention of IgA has been observed in rats with ligated bile ducts and with liver damage. Although a similar mechanism has not been demonstrated in man, the existence in serum of large amounts of p-IgA in patients with liver dysfunction suggests a role for the human liver in IgA clearance.

Taking into account the theoretic difficulties in measuring blood clearance of labeled IgA aggregates or IC in man and the specific hepatobiliary transport by IgA of circulating antigens entering through the mucosal surface [63], we studied the elimination of IgA IC formed physiologically after ingestion of food containing a large amount of protein. In patients with IgA nephropathy, there was a continuing rise in p-IgA IC which persisted above the normal range at 24 h. In normal subjects, they disappeared within 4–6 h of protein ingestion, suggesting the existence in patients of a specific defect in clearance of these complexes [64].

Recently it has been demonstrated that the splenic components of reticulophagocytic function, as measured by the clearance of IgG-coated cells, is impaired in most patients with IgA nephropathy [65, 66]. Sato et al. [67] also found depressed phagocytic activity of polymorphonuclear leukocytes (PMN) in these patients. Also, in dermatitis herpetiformis, another linked IgA disease in which deposits of p-IgA are seen in the skin lesions [68], a diminution of the Fc function of the mononuclear phagocytic system has been demonstrated [69]. Although the reasons for this phenomenon are not clear, it is possible that the p-IgA could diminish the IgG Fc receptor function of the mononuclear phagocytic system [70]. Thus, in patients with IgA nephropathy, a good correlation between serum levels of polymeric IgA and the presence of circulating IgA IC has been found [22]. Furthermore, serum from patients with IgA nephropathy, having higher levels of p-IgA, is capable of inhibiting the directional migration and phagocytosis of PMN from control subjects [71]. In preliminary experiments, the number of Fc receptors for p-IgA seems to be slightly impaired in PMN from these patients in relation to those of control subjects (González, unpublished observations). Although the origin of the clearance defects is not known, an alternative explanation is that the IgG IC or the IgA-IC, frequently found in patients with IgA nephropathy, provoke a blockade of the Fc receptors.

In an experimental model of IgA nephropathy induced by dextran, a delayed clearance of p-IgA aggregates, in relation with the nonimmunized animals, was observed, probably due to a diminution of the Fc receptors for IgA in the hepatocytes [72]. Since the levels of serum IgA increase during immunization, we speculate that p-IgA, alone or forming part of IC, saturates these receptors, increasing in turn the levels of p-IgA IC and therefore resulting in deposition at the mesangium level.

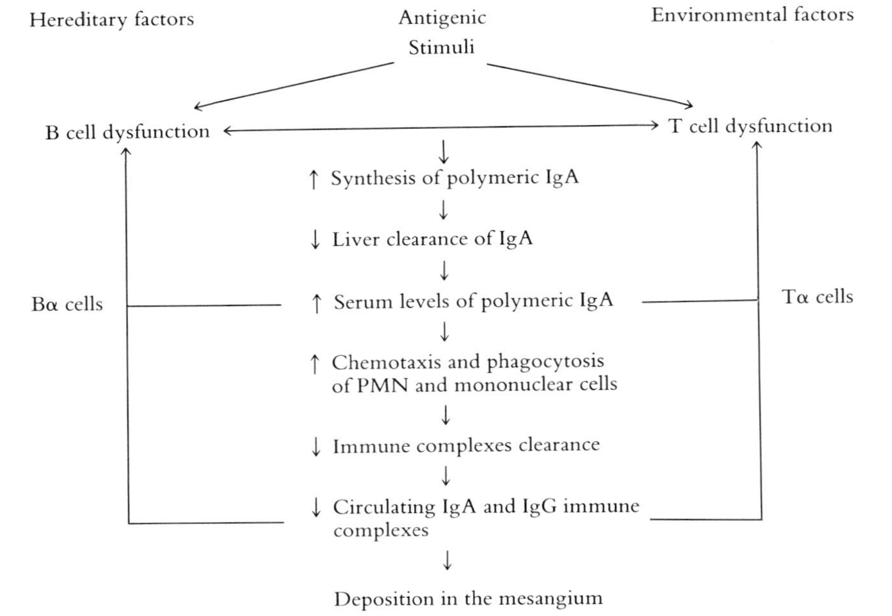

Figure 11-7. Schematic working hypothesis on the role of polymeric IgA in IgA nephropathy.

TENTATIVE HYPOTHESIS ON THE PATHOGENETIC ROLE OF p-IgA IN IgA NEPHROPATHY (figure 11-7)

Patients with IgA nephropathy with a certain background of hereditary and environmental factors have an increased synthesis of p-IgA (probably IgA1) following viral, bacterial, or dietary stimuli. This p-IgA saturates the liver receptors for this Ig with subsequent augmentation in the serum levels. Polymeric IgA also induces the expression of FcαR on T-cell lymphocytes which, from the functional point of view, could act for unknown reasons as helper or suppressor cells on the synthesis of total IgA. The diminution of chemotaxis and phagocytosis of PMN and monocytes by p-IgA would facilitate the persistent circulation and renal deposition of IC.

Although in this schematic working hypothesis, every step does not need to be certainly true, we think that there is some evidence in the literature as shown in this chapter suggesting a pathogenetic role for p-IgA in IgA nephopathy.

More basic studies about the sites and the mechanisms of synthesis of p-IgA [73] are needed in order to advance knowledge of the pathogenesis of this common and peculiar nephritis.

ACKNOWLEDGMENTS

This work has been supported by grants from the Fondo de Investigaciones Santiarias de la Seguridad Social, Comision Asesora de Investigacion Cientidica y Tecnica y Fundacion Inigo Alvarez de Toledo. We thank Rosario de Nicolas and Liselotte Gulliksen for excellent technical and secretarial assistance. The author is also indebted to colleagues J. Sancho, L. Lozano, R. Garcia Hoyo, E. González, P. Hernando, and J. González Cabrero for assistance in preparation of this chapter.

REFERENCES

1. Clarkson AR, Woodroffe AJ, Bannister KM, Lomax-Smith JD, Aarons I: The syndrome of IgA nephropathy. Clin Nephrol 21:7–14, 1984.
2. Bienenstock J, Befus AD: Some thoughts on the biologic role of immunoglobulin A. Gastroenterology 84:178–185, 1983.
3. Kutteh WH, Prince SJ, Mestecky J: Tissue origins of human polymeric and monomeric IgA. J Immunol 128:990–995, 1982.
4. Egido J, Sancho J, Blasco R, Hernando L: Le rôle de l'IgA polymerique dans la pathogenie de la néphropathie à IgA. Néphrologie 4:99–101, 1983.
5. Egido J, Sancho J, Blasco R, Hernando L: Immunopathogenetic aspects of IgA nephropathy. Adv Nephrol 12:103–137, 1983.
6. Lagrue G, Hirbec G, Fournel M: Glomérulonéphritis à dépôts d'IgA: étude des IgA sériques. J Urol Nephrol 80:385–389, 1974.
7. Berger J. Yaneva H, Nabarra B, Barbanel C: Recurrence of mesangial deposition of IgA after renal transplantation. Kidney Int 7:232–245, 1975.
8. Lopez-Trascasa M, Egido J, Sancho J, Hernando L: Evidence of high polymeric IgA levels in serum of patients with Berger's disease: its modification with phenytoin treatment. Proc Eur Dial Transplant assoc 16:513–519, 1979.
9. Lopez Trascasa M, Egido J, Sancho J, Hernando L: IgA glomerulonephritis (Berger's disease): evidence of high serum levels of polymeric IgA. Clin Exp Immunol 42:247–254.
10. Egido J, Sancho J, Mampaso F, Lopez Trascasa M, Sanchez Crespo M, Blasco R, Hernando L: A possible common pathogenesis of the mesangial IgA glomerulonephritis in patients with Berger's disease and Schönlein-Henoch syndrome. Proc Eur Dial Transplant Assoc 17:660–666, 1980.
11. Sancho J, Egido J, Sanchez Crespo M, Blasco R: Detection of monomeric and polymeric IgA containing immune complexes in serum and kidney from patients with alcoholic liver disease. Clin Exp Immunol 47:327–335, 1982.
12. Valentijn RM, Radl J, Haaijman JJ, Vermeer BJ, Weening JJ, Kauffmann RH, Daha MR, Van Es LA: Circulating and mesangial secretory component-binding IgA-1 in primary IgA nephropathy. Kidney Int 26:760–766, 1984.
13. Bernasconi P, Sinico RA, Fornasieri A, Castiglione A, D'Amico G: IgA-immune complexes and polymeric IgA in IgA nephropathy. In: Mucosal Immunity, J.P. Revillard, C. Voisin, N. Wierzbicki (eds) pp. 298–299, Paris, 1984.
14. Woodroffe AJ, Gormly AA, McKenzie DE, Wooton AM, Thompson AJ, Seymour AE, Clarkson AR: Immunologic studies in IgA nephropathy. Kidney Int 18:366–374, 1980.
15. Lesavre Ph, Digeon M, Bach JF: Analysis of circulating IgA and detection of immune complexes in primary IgA nephropathy. Clin Exp Immunol 48:61–69, 1982.
16. Newkirk MM, Klein MH, Katz A, Fisher MM, Underdown BJ: Estimation of polymeric IgA in human serum: an assay based on binding of radiolabeled human secretory component with applications in the study of IgA nephropathy, IgA monoclonal gammapathy, and liver disease. J Immunol 130:1176–1181, 1983.
17. Berger J: IgA mesangial nephropathy 1968–1983. Contrib Nephrol 40:4–6, 1984.
18. Feehally: Discussion on immune system abnormalities in idiopathic IgA nephropathy in "IgA mesangial nephropathy." Contrib Nephrol 40:142, 1984.

19. Egido J, Sancho J, Blasco R, Lozano L, Hernando L: Immunologic aspects of IgA nephropathy in humans. In: Robinson RR (ed) Nephrology, vol 1: proceedings of the 9th international congress on nephrology. New York: Springer-Verlag, 1984, pp 652–664.
20. Sancho J, Egido J, Gonzalez E: A simplified method for determining polymeric IgA-containing immune complexes. J Immunol Methods 60:305–317, 1983.
21. Egido J, Sancho J, Hernando P, Gonzalez J, Hernando L: The presence of specific IgA immune complexes in IgA nephropathy. Contrib Nephrol 40:85–87, 1984.
22. Egido J, Sancho J, Rivera F, Hernando L: The role of IgA and IgG immune complexes in IgA nephropathy. Nephron 36:59–66, 1984.
23. Doi T, Kanatsy K, Sekita K, Yoshida H, Nagai H, Hamashima Y: Detection of IgA class circulating immune complexes bound to anti C3d antibody in patients with IgA nephropathy. J Immunol Methods 69:95–104, 1984.
24. Rifai A, Small PA, Teague PO, Ayurb EM: Experimental IgA nephropathy. J Exp Med 150:1161–1173, 1979.
25. Rifai A, Millar K, Verani R: IgA molecular form nephritogenicity correlates immune complex formation and glomerular deposition. Kidney Int 27:221 A, 1985.
26. Czerkinsky C, Crago SS, Koopman WJ, Jackson S, Schrohenloher RE, Galla J, Mestecky J: The occurrence of circulating IgA-IgG immune complexes in IgA nephropathy. In: Mucosal Immunity, J.P. Revillard, C. Voisin, N. Wierzbicki (eds) pp. 295–297, Paris, 1984.
27. González Cabrero J., Egido J, Sancho J, Moldenhauer F.: Presence of shared idiotypes in serum and immune complexes in patients with IgA nephropathy. Clin Exp Immunol 1987 (in press).
28. Germuth FG, Rodriguez E, Lorelle CA, Trump EI, Milano L, Wise OL: Passive immune complex glomerulonephritis in mice: models for various lesions found in human disease. I. High avidity complexes and mesangiopathic glomerulonephritis. Lab Invest 41:360–365, 1979.
29. Monteiro RC, Halbwachs-Mecarelli L, Berger J, Lesavre P: Characteristics of eluted IgA in primary IgA nephropathy. Contrib Nephrol 40:107–111, 1984.
30. Border WA: Role of antigen and antibody charge in immune complex disease. In: Robinson RR (ed) Nephrology, vol 1: proceedings of the 9th international congress on nephrology, Los Angeles, pp 550–559.
31. Russel-Jones GJ, Gotschlich EC, Blake MS: A surface receptor specific for human IgA on group B streptococci possessing the Ibc protein antigen. J Exp Med 160:1467–1475, 1984.
32. Dobrin RS, Knudson FE, Michael AF: The secretory immune system and renal disease. Clin Exp Immunol 21:318–328, 1975.
33. Lomax-Smith JD, Zabrowarny LA, Howarth GS, Seymour AE, Woodroffe AJ: The immunochemical characterization of mesangial IgA deposits. Am J Pathol 113:359–364, 1983.
34. Brandtzaeg P: Characteristics of SC-IgA complexes formed in vitro. Adv Exp Med Biol 45:87–93, 1974.
35. Bene MC, Faure G, Duheille J: IgA nephropathy: characterization of the polymeric nature of mesangial deposits by in vitro binding of free secretory component. Clin Exp Immunol 47:527–534, 1982.
36. Tomino Y, Sakai M, Miura M, Endoh M, Nomoto Y: Detection of polymeric IgA in glomeruli from patients with IgA nephropathy. Clin Exp Immunol 49:419–425, 1982.
37. Donini V. Casanova S, Zimi N, Zucchelli P: The presence of J-chain in mesangial immune deposits of IgA nephropathy. Proc Eur Dial Transplant Assoc 19:655–661, 1982.
38. Komatsu N, Nagura H, Watanabe K, Nomoto Y, Kobayashi K: Mesangial deposition of J-chain-linked polymeric IgA in IgA nephropathy. Nephron 33:61–64, 1983.
39. Waldherr R, Seelig HP, Rambausek M, Andrassy K, Ritz E: Deposition of polymeric IgA1 in idiopathic mesangial IgA: glomerulonephritis. Klin Wochenschr 61:911–915, 1983.
40. Emancipator S, Gallo G, Lamm M: Experimental IgA nephropathy induced by oral immunization. J Exp Med 157:572–582, 1983.
41. Gallo GR, Emancipator SN, Lamm ME: Experimental cholestasis and deposition of glomerular IgA immune complexes. Contrib Nephrol 40:55–61, 1984.
42. André C, Berthoux C, André F, Guillon J, Genin C, Sabatier JC: Prevalence of IgA_2 deposits in IgA nephropathy: a clue for their pathogenesis. N Engl J Med 303:1343–1346, 1980.

43. Conley ME, Cooper MD, Michael AF: Selective deposition of immunoglobulin A1 in immunoglobulin A nephropathy, anaphylactoid purpura nephritis and systemic lupus erythematosus. J Clin Invest 66:1432–1436, 1980.
44. Hall RP, Stachura I, Cason J, Whiteside TL, Lawley TL: IgA-containing circulating immune complexes in patients with IgA nephropathy. Am J Med 74:56–63, 1983.
45. Murakami T, Furuse A, Hattori S, Kobayashi K, Matsuda J: Glomerular IgA1 and IgA2 deposits in IgA nephropathies. Nephron 35:120–123, 1983.
46. Delacroix DL, Liroux E, Vaerman JP: High proportion of polymeric IgA in young infant's sera and independence between IgA-size and IgA subclass distributions. J Clin Immunol 3:53–58, 1983.
47. Rifai A, Mannik M: Clearance kinetics and fate of mouse IgA immune complexes prepared with monomeric or dimeric IgA. J Immunol 130:1826–1832, 1983.
48. Sancho J, Gonzalez E, Rivera F, Escanero JF, Egido J: Hepatic and kidney uptake of soluble monomeric and polymeric IgA aggregates. Immunology 52:161–167, 1984.
49. Kutteh WH, Koopman WJ, Conley ME, Egan ML, Mestecky J: Production of predominantly polymeric IgA by human peripheral blood lymphocytes stimulated in vitro with mitogens. J Exp Med 152:1424–1427, 1980.
50. Egido J, Blasco R, Sancho J, Lozano L, Sanchez Crespo M, Hernando L: Increased rates of polymeric IgA synthesis by circulating lymphoid cells in IgA mesangial glomerulonephritis. Clin Exp Immunol 47:309–316, 1982.
51. Beukhof JR, Ockhnizen Th, Halie LM, Westra J, Belen JM, Donker AJM, Hoedemaeker Ph J, Van der Hem GK: Subentities within adult primary IgA nephropathy. Clin Nephrol 22:195–199, 1984.
52. Egido J, Blasco R, Lozano L, Sancho J, Garcia Hoyo R: Immunological abnormalities in tonsils of patients with IgA nephropathy inversion in the percentage of IgA versus IgG bearing lymphocytes and increased polymeric IgA synthesis. Clin Exp Immunol 57:101–106, 1984.
53. Lozano L, Garcia Hoyo R, Blasco R, Sancho J, Egido J. Effect of tonsillectomy on polymeric IgA synthesis by blood lymphocytes in patients with IgA nephropathy. Eur J Clin Invest 15, A40, 1985.
54. Lum LG, Muchmore AV, Keren D, Decker J, Koski I, Strober W, Blaese RM: A receptor for IgA on human T lymphocytes. J Immunol 122:65–69, 1979.
55. Sakai H, Endoh M, Tomino Y, Nomoto Y: Increase of IgA specific helper Tα cells in patients with IgA nephropathy. Clin Exp Immunol 50:77–82, 1982.
56. Endoh M, Sakai H, Nomoto Y, Tomino Y, Kaneshige H: IgA-specific helper activity of Tα cells in human peripheral blood. J Immunol 127:2612–2613, 1981.
57. Adachi M, Yodoi J, Masuda T, Takatsuki K, Uchino H: Altered expression of lymphocyte Fcα receptor in selective IgA deficiency and IgA nephropathy. J Immunol 131:1246–1251, 1983.
58. Egido J, Blasco R, Sancho J, Lozano L: T-cell dysfunctions in IgA nephropathy: specific abnormalities in the regulation of IgA synthesis. Clin Immunol Immunopathol 26:201–2 1983.
59. Egido J, Sancho J, Rivera F, Sanchez Crespo M: Handling of soluble IgA aggregates by the mononuclear phagocytic system in mice: a comparison with IgG aggregates. Immunology 46:1–7, 1982.
60. Peppard J, Orlans E, Payne AWR, Andrew E: The elimination of circulating complexes containing polymeric IgA by excretion in the bile. Immunology 42:83–89, 1981.
61. Sancho J, Gonzalez E, Egido J: Handling of IgA immune aggregates by liver cells. Contrib Nephrol 40:93–98, 1984.
62. Sancho J, Gonzalez E, Egido J: The importance of the Fc receptors for IgA in the recognition of IgA by mouse liver cells: its comparison with the carbohydrate and secretory component receptors. Immunology 57:37–42, 1986.
63. Russell MW, Brown TA, Claffin JL, Schroer K, Mestecky J: Immunoglobulin A mediated hepatobiliary transport constitutes a natural pathway for disposing of bacterial antigens. Infect Immun 42:1041–1048, 1983.
64. Sancho J, Egido J, Rivera F, Hernando L: Immune complexes in IgA nephropathy: presence of antibodies against diet antigens and delayed clearance of specific polymeric IgA immune complexes. Clin Exp Immunol 54:104–111, 1983.

65. Lawrence S, Pussell BA, Charlesworth JA: Mesangial IgA nephropathy: detection of defective reticulophagocytic function in vivo. Clin Nephrol 16:280–283, 1983.
66. Bannister KM, Hay J, Clarkson AR, Woodroffe AJ: Fc-specific reticulo-endothelial clearance in systemic lupus erythematosus and glomerulonephritis. Am J Kidney Dis 3:287–292, 1984.
67. Sato M, Kinugasa E, Ideura T, Koshikawa S: Phagocytic activity of polymorphonuclear leukocytes in patients with IgA nephropathy. Clin Nephrol 19:166–171, 1983.
68. Unsworth DJ, Leonard JN: IgA in dermatitis herpetiformis skin is dimeric. Lancet 27:479–481, 1982.
69. Lawley TJ: Reticuloendothelial system function, p 863. In: Katz SI (moderator) dermatitis herpetiformis: the skin and the gut. Ann Intern Med 93:857–869, 1980.
70. Wilton JMA: Suppression by IgA of IgG-mediated phagocytosis by human polymorphonuclear leukocytes. Clin Exp Immunol 34:423–428, 1978.
71. Egido J, Sancho J, Lorente F, Fontan G: Inhibition of neutrophil migration by serum from patients with IgA nephropathy. Clin Exp Immunol 49:709–716, 1982.
72. Gonzalez E, Sancho J, Gonzalez J, Blasco R, Garcia Hoyo R, Lozano L, Egido J, Hernando L: IgA nephropathy in mice: mechanisms involved in the deposition of IgA in the mesangium. Eur J Clin Invest 15:A46, 1985.
73. Moldoveanu Z, Egan ML, Mestecky J: Cellular origins of human polymeric and monomeric IgA: intracellular and secreted forms of IgA. J Immunol 133:3156–3162, 1984.

12. LYMPHOCYTE FUNCTION IN IgA NEPHROPATHY

HIDETO SAKAI

IgA nephropathy is now an accepted disease entity that is characterized by preponderant mesangial deposition of IgA [1, 2]. An increasing body of evidence suggests that the mesangial IgA deposits are likely to be either IgA polymers or IgA-dominant immune complexes [3, 4]. These IgA seem to circulate in the blood because of a frequent recurrence of this disease after renal allotransplantation [5, 6] and a rapid disappearance of IgA deposits in a grafted kidney from a donor with unsuspected IgA nephropathy [7]. The presence of such IgA in the circulation suggests an increased synthesis of IgA in patients with IgA nephropathy. Although the mechanism of immune regulation of IgA has not been fully elucidated, rapidly accumulating evidence indicates that the interaction of B and T cells plays a key role in the regulation of IgA, an isotype known to be highly T-cell specific [8]. The discussion on the altered lymphocyte function in this chapter is limited to *primary* IgA nephropathy because mesangial deposits of IgA are observed in various other diseases such as alcoholic cirrhosis [9].

INCREASED IN VIVO FUNCTION OF B CELLS

Mesangial IgA

The hallmark of IgA nephropathy is the mesangial deposition of IgA although it is not clear whether this IgA is responsible for the development of glomerular destruction. In order to elucidate the origin of the mesangial IgA, it is important to note that all abnormalities in the regulation of IgA should be related to the properties of IgA deposited in the glomeruli. The subclass of IgA in the mesangium of patients with IgA nephropathy has been a matter of controversy. André et al. [10], using rabbit antihuman $\alpha 1$ and $\alpha 2$ antisera, reported that glomerular IgA deposits consisted predominantly of IgA2. However, Conley et al. [11], using monoclonal hybridoma anti-IgA subclass antibodies, showed a predominance of IgA1. Subsequently, Tomino et al. [12], using both rabbit antihuman $\alpha 1$ and $\alpha 2$ antisera and monoclonal anti-IgA subclass antibodies, demonstrated the predominance of IgA1. Valentijn et al. [13] further supported the dominance of IgA1 using monoclonal mouse antibodies against human IgA1 or IgA2 subclasses. The reason for this geographic heterogeneity is presently unknown. The predominance of subclass in the mesangial IgA, however, does not imply the origin of that IgA. A relative increase of IgA2 has been noted in the external secretions [14, 15] but yet-to-be identified antigen(s) in this disease may stimulate either subclass of IgA. A majority of previous studies have failed to show secretory component and J chain in the glomeruli. However, more recent studies indicated the presence of J chain in the mesangial areas using the pretreatment of tissue sections with 6 *M* urea in glycine–HCl (pH 3.2) presumably due to exposure of the antigenic sites of the J chain [16] as well as the absorption of acid-eluted IgA with antihuman J chain antiserum [17]. The presence of mesangial IgM in some patients with IgA nephropathy might be responsible for the detection of the J chain, but the identical localization of the specific fixation of secretory component with that of mesangial IgA indicated that the majority of glomerular IgA is polymeric in patients with IgA nephropathy [13, 18]. The origin of polymeric IgA in humans is yet to be established, but Kutteh et al. [19] indicated that lymphoid tissues associated with secretory surfaces may provide a greater proportion of polymeric IgA than other lymphoid tissues.

Serum IgA

Elevation of serum IgA is frequently observed in patients with IgA nephropathy [20, 21] although there is no significant correlation between the levels of serum IgA and the degree of the severity of IgA nephropathy. On the other hand, there was a persistent elevation of serum IgA in many patients during the three year follow-up period [22]. Such persistent elevation of serum IgA may be related to the persistent deposition of IgA in the mesangial areas although a direct relationship between the serum and mesangial IgA remains to be established. The observation of high serum levels of polymeric IgA in patients with IgA nephropathy [23] is possibly related to these findings. Patients with IgA nephropathy showed an increased production of polyclonal IgA antibodies as reflected by a simultaneous increase of the IgA antiinfluenza virus antibody and the IgA rheumatoid factor [24]. IgA-dominant immune complexes have been observed in patients with IgA nephropathy by using sensitive techniques to detect circulating immune complexes with individual isotypes of immunoglobulins [3, 25]. Several investigators observed a positive correlation between the levels of circulating IgA-dominant immune complexes and the degree of clinical activities [3, 26, 27]. These observations suggest that many patients with IgA nephropathy show polyclonal activation of IgA synthesis. It is presently unknown whether such increase of polyclonal IgA is due to stimulation of some specific antigens and/or expression of some immunogenetic abnormalities.

INCREASED IN VITRO FUNCTION OF B CELLS

IgA-secreting cells

In vitro secretion of IgA into culture media by peripheral blood mononuclear cells (PBM) has been observed in patients with IgA nephropathy. There is a general agreement that *spontaneous* in vitro production of IgA by PBM without addition of mitogens is not observed in healthy adults. Some patients with IgA nephropathy, however, showed *spontaneous* IgA synthesis during the seven-day culture period without addition of mitogens [28]. Increased in vitro secretion of IgA by PBM from patients with IgA nephropathy was also observed in the other culture systems: table 12-1 shows our previous studies on IgA-specific suppressor T-cell activity, and the results obtained unexpectedly showed an increased production of IgA by the B-cell-rich fractions from a patient with IgA nephropathy [29]. The underlined figures in the table indicate that only B cells from a patient with IgA nephropathy (but not those from her identical twin sister or a healthy adult) showed increased in vitro secretion of IgA in cultures with concanavalin-A-induced suppressor T cells from the sister or the control adult. Feehally et al. [30] supported the *spontaneous* increase of in vitro secretion of IgA, i.e., increased IgA synthesis by PBM in cultures without addition of mitogens. On the other hand, Egido et al. [31] reported an increase of IgA secretion in pokeweed mitogen-stimulated cultures but not in unstimulated cultures in PBM from patients with IgA nephropathy. Cosio et al. [32] reported negative results in either mitogen-stimulated or unstimulated cultures.

It is difficult to compare the results from studies on cell cultures in various laboratories because of heterogeneity in not only culture systems but also populations of patients examined. At least one of the groups described above [30] showed a positive correlation between the increase in *spontaneous* in vitro IgA synthesis and the episodes of relapse of clinical symptoms in patients with IgA nephropathy. IgA-secreting cells can be identified by staining of cytoplasmic IgA with the fluorescein- or rhodamine-conjugated $F(ab')_2$ portion of IgG obtained from heavy-chain-specific antihuman IgA antisera.

Table 12-1. Suppressor activity of T cells and T-cell supernatant (TCS) in a patient with IgA nephropathy and her identical twin sister.

Donor of B cells	Donor of T cells	Donor of TCS	IgG (ng/2 × 10^6 cells)	IgA (ng/2 × 10^6 cells)	IgM (ng/2 × 10^6 cells)
Patient	Patient	—	300	>2500	320
Patient	—	Patient	260	>2500	410
Patient	Sister	—	520	750	390
Patient	—	Sister	250	1030	140
Patient	Control	—	340	1210	340
Patient	—	Control	880	2010	910
Sister	Sister	—	260	400	280
Sister	—	Sister	450	520	480
Sister	Patient	—	250	>2500	380
Sister	—	Patient	170	ND	420
Sister	Control	—	740	520	430
Sister	—	Control	1550	630	550
Control	Control	—	620	710	550
Control	—	Control	ND[a]	630	590
Control	Patient	—	150	2010	340
Control	—	Patient	20	>2500	450
Control	Sister	—	1550	490	410
Control	—	Sister	460	740	710

[a]ND, not done. Modified from Sakai et al. [29].

There was a significant increase of cytoplasmic IgA-positive cells in cultures of B-cell-enriched fraction of PBM with and without addition of helper T cells in patients with IgA nephropathy [33]. Immunohistopathologic studies on tonsils demonstrated that the number of dimeric IgA-secreting plasma cells was increased in patients with IgA nephropathy [34]. This observation on the tonsils was then confirmed by Egido et al. [35], who showed an increase of polymeric IgA-producing cells in the tonsils of patients with IgA nephropathy.

It is tempting to speculate on the mucosal origin of the increased IgA in the circulation of patients with IgA nephropathy, because the increase of IgA-producing cells was also observed in patients associated with scleritis. Nomoto et al. [36] first described that approximately 15% of patients with IgA nephropathy eventually developed scleritis. The emergence of scleritis was then confirmed by Hurault de Ligny et al. [37], who showed that approximately 18% of French patients developed scleritis. The French group subsequently biopsied the region of scleritis in a patient with IgA nephropathy and observed numerous dimeric IgA-secreting lymphoplasmacytic perivascular infiltrates [38]. The same group reported an association of episcleritis with hematuria in the same patient. These observations further support the hypothesis of the mucosal origin of the increased IgA in the circulation of patients with IgA nephropathy although further studies are warranted to elucidate the pathologic significance of the increased IgA in the circulation.

IgA-bearing cells

It is generally accepted that immunoglobulin-bearing cells are precursors of immunoglobulin-secreting cells in vivo and in vitro. Isotypes of the cell surface immunoglobulins reflect switching of premature to mature B cells. In human B cells, it is now becoming clear that single switches from μ to expression of another heavy chain are the rule [39] just like the order of the variable-region gene complex on chromosome 12 in mice. IgA-bearing B cells are thus relatively mature B cells that transform to IgA-secreting B cells after stimulation by antigens or mitogens under the yet-to-be clarified interaction with T cells and monocytes. It has been a matter of controversy as to whether IgA-bearing lymphocytes are increased in the peripheral blood of patients with IgA nephropathy. Nomoto et al. [40] observed an increase of peripheral blood IgA-bearing lymphocytes in patients with IgA nephropathy, and Sakai et al. [41] subsequently reported that such increase of IgA-bearing lymphocytes occurred not only in patients but also in some of the family members of these patients. Feehally et al. [30] also observed an increase of IgA-bearing lymphocytes in the majority of patients with IgA nephropathy. On the other hand, Cosio et al. [32] and Fiorini et al. [42] did not observe such increase of peripheral blood IgA-bearing lymphocytes. The reason for this dichotomy is presently unknown. However, it is likely that not only the heterogeneity of the methods utilized for the quantification of IgA-bearing lymphocytes but also the difference of the patient populations examined in various laboratories might lead to the different conclusions. At least one of the groups [30] described above noted that the amount of IgA-bearing lymphocytes was increased during the period of relapse but remained within normal limits during the period of remission in their patients with IgA nephropathy. Although the origin of the increased IgA-bearing lymphocytes is yet to be identified, two recent reports [34, 35] showed a marked increase of IgA-bearing lymphocytes in the tonsils of patients with IgA nephropathy.

It is interesting to note that there was a striking similarity in the distribution patterns of immunoglobulin-bearing lymphocytes in the peripheral blood [40] and the tonsils [35]. Figure 12-1 shows the two patterns obtained from each laboratory. Although the dates and the locations of these two studies were completely different, there were common distribution patterns in the amounts of lymphocytes bearing each isotype of immunoglobulins, i.e., increase of IgA-bearing lymphocytes and decrease of IgG-bearing lymphocytes. It is well established that IgA-bearing lymphocytes migrate from the intestinal mucosa to the tonsils via the circulation [43, 44], but it is still to be confirmed whether that migration pathway is the same in

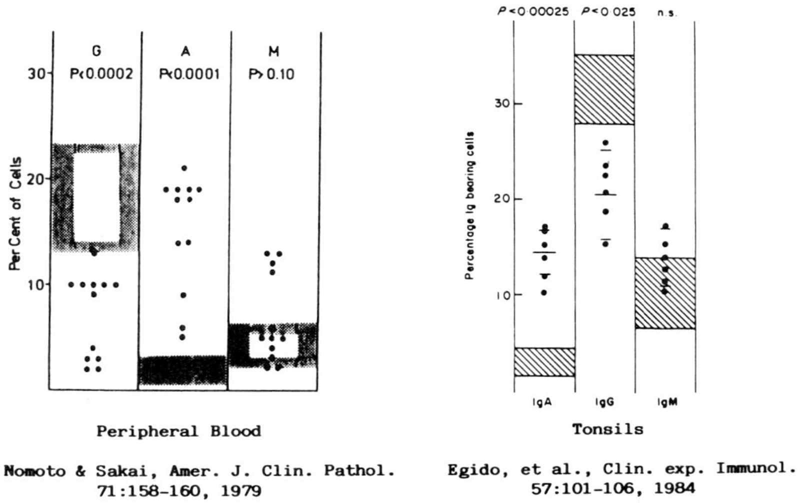

Figure 12-1. Distribution patterns of immunoglobulin-bearing cells in peripheral blood (**left**) and tonsils (**right**) in patients with IgA nephropathy Modified from Nomoto et al. [40] and Egido et al. [35].

the reverse fashion. The similarity of the distribution patterns of immunoglobulin-bearing lymphocytes in the peripheral blood and the tonsils, however, suggests that the reverse fashion of the migration of IgA-bearing lymphocytes might occur in patients with IgA nephropathy.

It should be noted that the migration of IgA-bearing lymphocytes from mucosal lymphoid tissues to the circulation might not be a continuous, but a pulsative, phenomenon because the patients with increased IgA-bearing lymphocytes in the tonsils did not show an increase of same cells in the peripheral blood at the time of the examination [35]. Further studies are required to elucidate the pathologic significance of these increased IgA-bearing lymphocytes in both lymphoid tissues and the peripheral blood of patients with IgA nephropathy.

DECREASED ACTIVITY OF IgA-SPECIFIC SUPPRESSOR T CELLS

IgA-specific suppressor T cells

In contrast to B-cell functions, T-cell functions in humans can not be determined in vivo because of the small amounts of T-cell products, i.e., lymphokines. Therefore, all T-cell functions in humans have been determined in vitro. In vivo correlates of all T-cell functions determined in patients and healthy persons remain to be clarified in the future. However, the increased activity of IgA-producing B cells in patients with IgA nephropathy suggests the possibility of either decreased IgA-specific suppressor

T-cell activity and/or increased IgA-specific helper T-cell activity. Results from recent studies indicate that both suppressor and helper T cells are altered in patients with IgA nephropathy. Sakai et al. [29] first described the decreased activity of IgA-specific suppressor T cells in patients with IgA nephropathy.

Table 12-1 demonstrates that, not only concanavalin-A (Con A)-stimulated T cells, but also column-purified supernatants of these Con-A-stimulated T-cell cultures suppressed in vitro production of IgA from pokeweed mitogen (PWM)-stimulated B cells. This IgA-specific suppressor T-cell activity was markedly decreased in patients with IgA nephropathy and thus allowed to produce larger amounts of IgA in the B-cell cultures. In contrast to the decreased IgA-specific suppressor T-cell activity in a patient with IgA nephropathy, T cells obtained from an identical twin sister of that patient showed normal activity of the IgA-specific suppression. These results indicate that IgA-specific suppressor T-cell activity is transmitted by some soluble factor(s), presumably lymphokine(s), and that the decrease of IgA-specific suppressor T-cell activity in patients with IgA nephropathy is not genetically defined. Parallel studies [29] showed that there was a significant inverse relationship between the degree of the decrease in IgA-specific suppressor T-cell activity and the levels of either serum IgA and/or IgA-bearing lymphocytes in the peripheral blood of patients with IgA nephropathy. This inverse relationship may indicate that the decrease of IgA-specific suppressor T-cell activity is a result of the increased activity of IgA-producing B cells.

The finding of the decreased activity of IgA-specific suppressor T-cell activity was supported by Egido et al. [45], who subsequently showed that the decrease of IgA-specific suppressor T-cell activity was also observed in some of the family members of these patients [46]. Although the study on identical twins denied the immunogenetic control on IgA-specific suppressor T cells [29], the decreased activity of such T cells in family members [46] indicates that some familial factors may be involved in the altered IgA immunity in patients with IgA nephropathy.

Altered lymphocyte function in families

Reports of the emergence of IgA nephropathy in identical siblings are relatively rare [47, 48]. However, analysis of family history suggests the multiple emergence of patients with IgA nephropathy in some closely inbred families [49, 50]. Although there is no common agreement with regard to the deviation of HLA antigens [51], there have been several reports showing altered lymphocyte functions in some family members of patients with IgA nephropathy. These alterations include an increase of IgA-bearing peripheral blood lymphocytes [41], emergence of a cold-reacting antinuclear factor [52], increased spontaneous synthesis of IgA by cultured PBM [53], an increase in the percentage of polymeric IgA-producing cells in PWM-stimulated cultures [46], and loss in the suppression of IgA synthesis induced by PBM exposed to a high dose of Con A [46]. Although the activity of IgA-specific suppressor T cells seems to be out of genetic control, it is likely that some aspects in the immunologic sequelae in patients with IgA nephropathy are affected by some familial factors. Elucidation of these familial factors may shed light on the pathogenesis of IgA nephropathy.

INCREASE OF IgA-SPECIFIC HELPER T CELLS

OKT_4^+ cells

Regulatory T-cell subsets control both the intensity and the isotype of cellular and humoral immune responses in many species. In humans, the activity of regulatory T cells is determined by in vitro regulation of immunoglobulin production in PWM-stimulated PBM. Previously, the most popular methods to identify regulatory T cells in humans was to detect the cell surface receptors for the Fc fragment of IgG and IgM [54]. A new probe of monoclonal antibodies directed against specific cell surface antigens of human T cells is now available commercially. The most widely used ones among these monoclonal antibodies are the OKT series, including OKT3 which binds to 95% of total T cells, OKT4 which detects the majority of helper T cells, and OKT8 which recognizes most suppressor/cytotoxic T cells in humans [55]. There have been several reports showing the deviation of T-cell subsets in patients with IgA nephropathy using the OKT monoclonal antibodies, and the authors observed a common denominator of an increased ratio of $OKT4^+/OKT8^+$ [56–58]. Although there were some differences among the investigators with regard to the absolute number of $OKT4^+$ and $OKT8^+$ cells in the patients, the increased ratio of $OKT4^+/OKT8^+$ suggests the dominance of helper T cells against suppressor T cells in patients with IgA nephropathy. It is premature to conclude, however, that the dominance of the cell surface marker for helper T cells reflects the involvement of helper T cells in the increased IgA synthesis in vivo. So far there has been no firm evidence to indicate the positive correlation between the degree of the increase of $OKT4^+/OKT8^+$ ratio and the levels of serum IgA and/or IgA-dominant immune complexes in patients with IgA nephropathy.

$T\alpha$ cells

Human T cells are known to have receptors for the Fc portion of various isotypes of immunoglobulins. Functional correlates of these receptors have been analyzed during the past ten years, and it is recognized that T cells with Fc-IgG receptors represent the majority of suppressor cells and those with Fc-IgM receptors show helper activity in B-cell differentiation in vitro. Human T cells bearing receptors for Fc-IgA were reported by Lum et al. [59, 60] and Gupta et al. [61, 62]. The Fc-IgA receptors have also been recognized on B cells [63] and monocytes [64], but the functional correlates of these cells including Fc-IgA bearing T cells remain to be elucidated. Induction of Fc-IgA receptors on mouse spleen cells required addition of polymeric IgA both in vivo and in vitro [65, 66], and these cells with Fc-IgA receptors showed in vitro suppressor effect on B cells when cultured with polymeric IgA [65, 67] while cells from mouse Peyer's patches with Fc-IgA receptors demonstrated an IgA-specific in vitro helper effect on B cells when cultured without addition of polymeric IgA [68].

Studies on the function of T cells with receptors for Fc-IgA (Tα cells) in humans have been performed without addition of polymeric IgA in vitro. Previously, Tα cells in the peripheral blood from healthy adults were regarded as polyclonal helper T cells [60]. This study used a technique of rosette formation to concentrate Tα cells, but rosette formation is known to result in the contamination of non-rosette-forming cells. Subsequent studies using a cell sorter provided highly concentrated populations of Tα cells, and it was shown that peripheral blood Tα cells in healthy adults were IgA-specific helper T cells when cultured with B cells without addition of polymeric IgA [69]. Studies on patients with IgA nephropathy showed a significant increase of peripheral blood Tα cells in such patients [33, 70]. These Tα cells seemed to be increased in vivo because of the extremely short time required for the induction of these cells in vitro [66]. There was an increase in the absolute number of Tα cells in patients with IgA nephropathy because the per cell activity of the IgA-specific in vitro helper effect was not different between patients and healthy adults [33]. The type of the cell surface markers on Tα cells is different between mice and humans. Tα cells from mouse spleens showed $Lyt1^{-}2^{+}$ [65] while those from human peripheral blood showed predominantly $OKT4^{+}$ and a few $OKT8^{+}$ [71]. The dominance of the OKT4 antigen on Tα cells may indicate that the majority of these cells are helper T cells. However, the presence of Tα cells with OKT8 antigen suggests that Tα cells are heterogeneous cell populations. Studies on the pathologic significance of Tα cells in patients with IgA nephropathy are warranted.

SUMMARY

A rapidly accumulating body of evidence indicates that patients with IgA nephropathy show altered lymphocyte functions related to an increased production of IgA, presumably polymeric IgA1. Some family factors may be involved in the development of such increase in IgA production. It is likely that the main aberration of cellular immunity in patients with IgA nephropathy is the alteration of B cells which subsequently induces the aberration of T-cell functions. These altered T-cell functions, however, may amplify the production of IgA from B cells and thus contribute to the modification of the clinical course of IgA nephropathy.

ACKNOWLEDGMENT

A part of this work was supported by grants from the Ministry of Education and the Ministry of Health of Japan.

REFERENCES

1. Berger J, Hinglais N: Les Dépôts intercapillaires d'IgA-IgG. J Urol (Paris) 74:694–695, 1968.
2. McCoy RC, Abramowsky CR, Tisher CC: IgA nephropathy. Am J Pathol 76:123–144, 1974.
3. Digeon M, Lesavre Ph, Bach JF: Analysis of circulating IgA and detection of immune complexes in primary IgA nephropathy. Clin Exp Immunol 48:61–69, 1982.
4. Woodroffe AJ, Clarkson AR, Seymour AE, Lomax-Smith JD: Mesangial IgA nephritis. Springer Semin Immunopathol 5:321–332, 1982.
5. Berger J, Yaneva H, Nabarra B, Barbanel C: Recurrence of mesangial deposition of IgA after renal transplantation. Kidney Int 7:232–241, 1975.
6. Cameron JS, Turner DR: Recurrent glomerulonephritis in allografted kidneys. Clin Nephrol 7:47–54, 1977.
7. Berger J: IgA mesangial nephropathy 1968–1983. In: D'Amico G, Minetti L, Ponticelli C (eds) IgA mesangial nephropathy. Basel: S Karger, 1984 p 4.
8. Elson CO: T cells specific for IgA switching and for IgA B-cell differentiation. Immunol Today 4:189–190, 1983.
9. Clarkson AR, Woodroffe AJ, Bannister KM, Lomax-Smith JD, Aarons I: The syndrome of IgA nephropathy. Clin Nephrol 21:7–14, 1984.
10. André C, Berthoux FC, André F, Gillon J, Genin C, Sabatier J-C: Prevalence of IgA_2 deposits in IgA nephropathies: a clue to their pathogenesis. N Engl J Med 303:1343–1346, 1980.
11. Conley ME, Cooper MD, Michael AF: Selective deposition of immunoglobulin A_1 in immunoglobulin A nephropathy, anaphylactoid purpura nephritis, and systemic lupus erythematosus. J Clin Invest 66:1432–1436, 1980.
12. Tomino Y, Endoh M, Nomoto Y, Sakai H: Immunoglobulin A_1 in IgA nephropathy. N Engl J Med 305:1159–1160, 1981.
13. Valentijn RM, Radl J, Haaijman JJ, Vermeer BJ, Weening JJ, Kauffmann RH, Daha MR, Van Es LA: Circulating and mesangial secretory component-binding IgA-1 in primary IgA nephropathy. Kidney Int 26:760–766, 1984.
14. Vaerman JP, Heremans JF, Laurell CB: Distribution of αchain subclasses in normal and pathological IgA-globulins. Immunology 14:425–432, 1968.
15. Delacroix DL, Dive C, Rambaud JC, Vaerman JP: IgA subclasses in various secretions and in serum. Immunology 47:383–385, 1982.
16. Komatsu N, Nagura H, Watanabe K, Nomoto Y, Kobayashi K: Mesangial deposits of J-chain linked polymeric IgA nephropathy. Nephron 33:61–64, 1983.
17. Tomino Y, Sakai H, Miura M, Endoh M, Nomoto Y: Detection of polymeric IgA in glomeruli from patients with IgA nephropathy. Clin Exp Immunol 49:419–425, 1982.
18. Bene MC, Faure G, Duheille J: IgA nephropathy: characterization of the polymeric nature of mesangial deposits by in vitro binding of free secretory component. Clin Exp Immunol 47:527–534, 1982.
19. Kutteh W, Prince SJ, Mestecky J: Tissue origins of human polymeric and monomeric IgA. J Immunol 128:990–995, 1982.
20. Lague G, Hirbec G, Fournel M, Intrator L: Glomérulonéphrite mesangiale à dépôts d'IgA: étude des immunoglobulins sériques. J Urol (Paris) 80:385–392, 1973.
21. Whitworth JA, Leibowitz S, Kennedy MC: IgA and glomerular disease. Clin Nephrol 5:33–36, 1976.
22. D'Amico G: Idiopathic mesangial IgA nephropathy. In: Bertani T, Remuzzi G (eds) Glomerular injury. Milan: Wichtig Editore, 1983, pp 205–228.
23. Trascasa ML, Egido J, Sancho J, Hernando L: IgA glomerulonephritis (Berger's disease): evidence of high serum levels of polymeric IgA. Clin Exp Immunol 42:247–254, 1980.
24. Endoh M, Suga T, Miura M, Tominò Y, Nomoto Y, Sakai H: In vivo alteration of

antibody production in patients with IgA nephropathy. Clin Exp Immunol 57:564–570, 1984.
25. Hall RP, Stachura I, Cason J, Whiteside TL, Lawley TJ: IgA-containing circulating immune complexes in patients with IgA nephropathy. Am J Med 74:56–63, 1983.
26. Woodroffe AJ, Gormly AA, McKenzie PE, Wootton AM, Thompson AJ, Seymour AE, Clarkson AR: Immunologic studies in IgA nephropathy. Kidney Int 18:366–374, 1980.
27. Coppo R, Basolo B, Martina G, Rollino C, De Marchi M, Giacchino F, Mazzucco G, Messina M, Piccoli G: Circulating immune complexes containing IgA, IgG and IgM in patients with primary IgA nephropathy and with Henoch-Schönlein nephritis. Correlation with clinical and histologic signs of activity. Clin Nephrol 18:230–239, 1982.
28. Endoh M: Increase in lymphocytes with Fc receptors for IgA and rates of spontaneous IgA synthesis in patients with IgA nephropathy. Jpn J Nephrol 26:1179–1185, 1984.
29. Sakai H, Nomoto Y, Arimori S: Decrease of IgA-specific suppressor T cell activity in patients with IgA nephropathy. Clin Exp Immunol 38:243–248, 1979.
30. Feehally J, Brenchley PE, Coupes BM, Beattie TJ, Mallick NP, Postlethwaite RJ: IgA immune system activation in IgA nephropathy during macroscopic haematuria. In: Robinson RR (ed) Proceeding of the 9th international congress on nephrology, Los Angeles, 1984, p 278A.
31. Egido J, Blasco R, Sancho J, Lozano L, Sanchez-Crespo M, Hernando L: Increased rates of polymeric IgA synthesis by circulating lymphoid cells in IgA mesangial glomerulonephritis. Clin Exp Immunol 47:309–316, 1982.
32. Cosio FG, Lam S, Folami AO, Conley ME, Michael AF: Immune regulation of immunoglobulin production in IgA-nephropathy. Clin Immunol Immunopathol 23:430–436, 1982.
33. Sakai H, Endoh M, Tomino Y, Nomoto Y: Increase of IgA specific helper Tα cells in patients with IgA nephropathy. Clin Exp Immunol 50:77–82, 1982.
34. Bene MC, Faure G, Hurault de Ligny B, Kessler M, Duheille J: Immunoglobulin A nephropathy: quantitative immunohistomorphometry of the tonsillar plasma cells evidences an inversion of the immunoglobulin A versus immunoglobulin G secreting cell balance. J Clin Invest 71:1342–1347, 1983.
35. Egido J, Blasco R, Lozano L, Sancho J, Garcia-Hoyo R: Immunological abnormalities in the tonsils of patients with IgA nephropathy: inversion in the ratio of IgA:IgG bearing lymphocytes and increased polymeric IgA synthesis. Clin Exp Immunol 57:101–106, 1984.
36. Nomoto Y, Sakai H, Endoh M, Tomino Y: Scleritis and IgA nephropathy. Arch Intern Med 140:783–787, 1980.
37. Hurault de Ligney B, Sirbat D, Bene MC, Faure G, Kessler M: Scleritis associated with glomerulonephritis. Nephron 35:207, 1983.
38. Bene MC, Hurault de Ligny B, Sirbat D, Faure G, Kessler M, Duheille J: IgA nephropathy: dimeric IgA-secreting cells are present in episcleral infiltrate. Am J Clin Pathol 82:608–611, 1984.
39. Kuritani T, Cooper MD: Human B cell differentiation. I. Analysis of immunoglobulin heavy chain switching using monoclonal anti-immunoglobulin M, G, and A antibodies and pokeweed mitogen-induced plasma cell differentiation. J Exp Med 155:839–851, 1982.
40. Nomoto Y, Sakai H, Arimori S: Increase of IgA-bearing lymphocytes in peripheral blood from patients with IgA nephropathy. Am J Clin Pathol 71:158–160, 1979.
41. Sakai H, Nomoto Y, Arimori S, Komori K, Inouye H, Tsuji K: Increase of IgA-bearing peripheral blood lymphocytes in families of patients with IgA nephropathy. Am J Clin Pathol 72:452–456, 1979.
42. Fiorini G, Fornasieri A, Sinico R, Colasanti G, Gibelli A, Corneo R, D'Amico G: Lymphocyte populations in the peripheral blood from patients with IgA nephropathy. Nephron 31:354–357, 1982.
43. Strober W, Hanson LA, Swell KW (eds): Recent advances in mucosal immunity. New York: Raven, 1982, p 1.
44. McGhee JR, Mestecky J (eds): The secretory immune system. Ann N Y Acad Sci :1.
45. Egido J, Blasco R, Sancho J: Immunoregulation abnormalities in patients with IgA nephropathy. Ann N Y Acad Sci 409:817–818, 1983.
46. Egido J, Blasco RA, Sancho J, Hernando L: Immunological abnormalities in healthy relatives of patients with IgA nephropathy. Am J Nephrol 5:14–20, 1985.
47. Turkoff-Rubin NE, Cosini AB, Fuiler T, Rubin RH, Colvin RB: IgA nephropathy in HLA identical siblings. Transplantation 26:430–433, 1978.

48. Sabatier JC, Genin C, Assenat H, Colon S, Ducret F, Berthoux FC: Mesangial IgA glomerulonephritis in HLA identical brothers. Clin Nephrol 11:35–39, 1979.
49. Montoliu J, Darnell A, Torras A, Ercilla G, Valles M, Revert L: Familial IgA nephropathy. Arch Intern Med 140:1374–1375, 1980.
50. Julian BA, Quiggins PA, Thompson JS, Woodford SY, Gleason K, Wyatt RJ: Familial IgA nephropathy: evidence of an inherited mechanism of disease. N Engl J Med 312:202–208, 1985.
51. Egido J, Sancho J, Blasco R, Rivera F, Hernando L: Immunopathogenetic aspects of IgA nephropathy. Adv Nephrol 12:103–137, 1983.
52. Nomoto Y, Miura M, Suga M, Endoh M, Tomino Y, Sakai H: Cold reacting anti-nuclear factor (ANF) in families of patients with IgA nephropathy. Clin Exp Immunol 58:63–67, 1984.
53. Suga T: Enhanced IgA production in family members of patients with IgA nephropathy. Jpn J Nephrol (in press), 1986.
54. Moretta L, Mingari MC, Moretta A: Human T cell subpopulation in normal and pathologic conditions. Immunol Rev 45:163–193, 1979.
55. Reinherz EL, Schlossman SF: The differentiation and function of human T lymphocytes. Cell 19:821–827, 1980.
56. Chatenoud L, Bach M-A: Abnormalities of T-cell subsets in glomerulonephritis and systemic lupus erythematosus. Kidney Int 20:267–274, 1981.
57. Bannister KM, Drew PA, Clarkson AR, Woodroffe AJ: Immunoregulation in glomerulonephritis, Henoch-Schönlein purpura and lupus nephritis. Clin Exp Immunol 53:384–390, 1983.
58. Rothschild E, Chatenoud L: T cell subset modulation of immunoglobulin production in IgA nephropathy and membranous glomerulonephritis. Kidny Int 25:557–564, 1984.
59. Lum LG, Muchmore AV, Keren D, Decker J, Koski I, Strober W, Blaese RM: A receptor for IgA on human T lymphocytes. J Immunol 122:65–69, 1979.
60. Lum LG, Benveniste E, Blaese RM: Functional properties of human T cells bearing Fc receptors for IgA. I. Mitogen responsiveness, mixed lymphocyte culture reactivity, and helper activity for B cell immunoglobulin production. J Immunol 124:702–707, 1980.
61. Gupta S, Platsoucas CD, Good RA: Receptors for IgA on a subpopulation of human B lymphocytes. Proc Natl Acad Sci USA 76:4025–4028, 1979.
62. Gupta S, Good RA: Subpopulations of human T lymphocytes. XV. T lymphocytes with receptors for IgA(Tα), a distinct subpopulation of T lymphocytes: studies in patients with primary immunodeficiency disorders. Clin Exp Immunol 41:363–371, 1980.
63. Endoh M, Sakai H, Suga T, Miura M, Tomino Y, Nomoto Y: Increase of peripheral blood B cells with Fc receptor for IgA in patients with IgA nephropathy. Scand J Immunol 17:437–441, 1983.
64. Fanger MW, Shen L, Pugh J, Bernier GM: Subpopulations of human peripheral granulocytes and monocytes express receptors for IgA. Proc Natl Acad Sci USA 77:3640–3644, 1980.
65. Hoover RG, Dieckgraefe BK, Lynch RG: T cells with Fc receptors for IgA: induction of Tα cells in vivo and in vitro by purified IgA. J Immunol 127:1560–1562, 1981.
66. Yodoi J, Adachi M, Masuda T: Induction of Fcα on murine lymphocytes by IgA in vitro. J Immunol 128:888–894, 1982.
67. Muller S, Hoover RG: T cells with Fc receptors in myeloma: suppression of growth and secretion of MOPC-315 by Tα cells. J Immunol 134:644–647, 1985.
68. Kiyono H, Cooper MD, Kearney JF, Mosteller LM, Michalek SM, Koopman WJ, McGhee JR: Isotype specificity of helper T cell clones: Peyer's patch Th cells preferentially collaborate with mature IgA B cells for IgA responses. J Exp Med 159:798–811, 1984.
69. Endoh M, Sakai H, Nomoto Y, Tomino Y, Kaneshige H: IgA-specific helper activity of Tα cells in human peripheral blood. J Immunol 127:2612–2613, 1981.
70. Adachi M, Yodoi J, Masuda T, Takatsuki K, Uchino H: Altered expression of lymphocyte Fcα receptor in selective IgA deficiency and IgA nephropathy. J Immunol 131:1246–1251, 1983.
71. Suga T, Endoh M, Sakai H, Miura M, Tomino Y, Nomoto Y: Tα cell subsets in human peripheral blood. J Immunol 134:1327–1329, 1985.

13. ANIMAL MODELS OF IgA NEPHROPATHY

STEVEN N. EMANCIPATOR, GLORIA R. GALLO, and MICHAEL E. LAMM

The traditional goal of experimental pathology is to elucidate pathogenesis and pathophysiology, thereby promoting understanding of a disease process, more accurate prognostication, and logical therapeutic intervention. While total satisfaction of these objectives is rare, even partial attainment assists in patient management and offers hope for greater future fulfillment. Limitations inherent in the study of experimental models include species differences between patients and experimental animals and the nearly inevitable variance of the model from the human disease.

Developments in experimental IgA nephropathy have been relatively rapid, aided in part by insights gleaned from other glomerulonephritides, and the variety of model systems rivals the diversity of the clinical and pathologic manifestations in patients with IgA nephropathy. Each study has focused on specific issues, and the experiments have evolved in concert with increased comprehension of the clinical disease. At present, experimental models of IgA nephropathy are principally based on variations of classic serum sickness, parallel to immune-complex-mediated glomerulonephritis in general. Passive systems employ the intravenous injection of antibody of the IgA class and of appropriate antigen, either simultaneously as immune complexes or sequentially, allowing formation of immune complexes in the circulation. Successful simulation of a disease via this approach provides evidence that the disease may be immune complex in nature. Passive systems also serve as powerful tools for elucidating mechanisms of immune complex deposition, since the chemical and physical properties of the complexes can be regulated, including the ratio of antigen to antibody and, therefore, the size of the complex. The effects of size, charge, and other physicochemical properties of the complexes can be related to clinical and morphologic features in the experimental animals, allowing inferences to their roles in human disease. These maneuvers have proved effective in IgA nephropathy, as detailed below [1, 2].

Necessarily, the source of antibody, locale of stimuli, and dynamics of the natural disease are not apparent from passive models, but are approachable in active systems wherein experimental animals can be immunized with known antigens. However, the design and interpretation of active models with predominantly IgA antibody require some appreciation of the secretory immune system and its relation to systemic immunity.

IgA is the principal exocrine immunoglobulin and is uniquely adapted to serve as a barrier to penetration of mucosal surfaces by macromolecules and microorganisms [3]. The lamina propria of mucosal surfaces contains abundant plasma cells which synthesize IgA in response to mucosal antigenic stimulation. The highest concentration of plasma cells in the body is observed in the intestinal lamina propria, and the vast majority of such cells are IgA secretors. Intestinal plasma cells, not suprisingly, produce a major proportion of total body IgA [3, 4].

Mucosal IgA plasma cells are thought to arise from IgA-committed B-lymphocytes in organized lymphoid tissue anatomically related to the mucosa. The gut-associated lymphoid tissue (GALT) is the archetype of the mucosal immune system. IgA-committed lymphocytes in lymphoid aggregates (Peyer's patches), separated from the gut lumen by thin specialized epithelial cells (M cells), first contact antigen, whereupon they migrate to the draining lymph nodes in the mesentery. The cells continue to divide and differentiate within the mesenteric nodes, emigrate to the systemic circulation via the thoracic duct, and home to secretory mucosae throughout the body, where they complete their differentiation into IgA-secreting plasma cells [3]. Within the lamina propria, most of the IgA secreted is in the form of a dimer, composed of two subunits, each of which contains two heavy polypeptide chains and two light chains, joined together by a J (joining) chain. The remainder of the IgA is largely 7S immunoglobulin without J chain. The J-chain-linked dimer of IgA has two possible fates after being secreted into the interstitial fluid of the lamina propria. First, the overlying epithelial cells bear a receptor, called secretory component, for J-chain-linked immunoglobulin oligomers; binding of IgA to this cell surface secretory component results in the transport and secretion of the IgA, now covalently bound to a portion of the secretory component, onto the mucosal surface [5]. Second, the IgA that escapes such transport, including monomeric 7S IgA which cannot bind to secretory component, gains access to the general circulation.

Active models of IgA nephropathy, in which the deposited immunoglobulin is endogenous IgA synthesized by the experimental animal itself, frequently have used stimulation of the secretory immune system to promote a preferentially IgA immune response to prolonged exogenous antigenic stimulation [6–9]. Continued exposure to antigen at high doses can potentially surmount the antibody barrier in an immunized host. Penetrance of antigen in the face of an IgA immune response may promote the generation of soluble immune complexes containing IgA antibody within the mucosa. Such complexes could gain access to the circulation and deposit in glomeruli. An active model of IgA nephropathy that occurs spontaneously has been ascribed to altered localization of IgA plasma cells to sites where all of the IgA synthesized necessarily gains access to the circulation because secretion to a mucosal surface cannot occur; again, many weeks are required before significant glomerular deposits of IgA are observed [10].

The active models support the view that the secretory immune system is important in the genesis of primary IgA nephropathy, i.e., IgA nephropathy not associated with underlying disease. The active models also provide evidence for the similarities between IgA nephropathy and serum sickness-like glomerulonephritides, while underscoring the differences in dynamics.

Models of secondary IgA nephropathy, i.e., IgA glomerulonephritis associated with another anteceding disease process, have focused upon hepatobiliary abnormalities, which clinically may be associated with renal IgA deposits [11–13]. In these models, clearance of IgA immune complexes may be impaired, or exposure to antigen absorbed from the intestines may be enhanced consequent to portosystemic blood shunts. These models also support a role for the secretory immune system and illustrate similarities between IgA nephropathy and traditional serum sickness-like glomerulonephritides.

This chapter briefly reviews groups of experiments by describing the rationale, summarizing the data and conclusions, and commenting upon the advantages and limitations of each system. The individual experiments are integrated, and the interplay between clinical and experimental observations is delineated. Finally, selected prospects and priorities are discussed.

MODELS OF PRIMARY IgA NEPHROPATHY

The first model of IgA nephropathy employed antigen–antibody complexes of the hapten-specific mouse IgA myeloma protein MOPC-315 and dinitrophenyl hapten conjugated to bovine serum albumin (DNP-BSA) in mice [1]. At the time, the fundamental nature of the mesangial deposits in the human disease was unknown: there was no evidence in support of the view that the deposited IgA was an antibody component of immune complexes as opposed to nonspecifically aggregated IgA, nor had immune complexes been demonstrated in patients' sera. Indeed, it was widely believed that IgA was incapable of mediating immunologic injury. Rifai and colleagues demonstrated that injection of immune complexes of MOPC-315 IgA and DNP-BSA, or separate injections of MOPC-315 IgA and DNP-BSA, resulted in deposition of IgA antibody and DNP-BSA in the mesangium. Moreover, these investigators showed that similar deposits could result from injection of DNP-BSA alone into mice bearing the plasmacytoma MOPC-315. The degree of deposition observed was related to the dose and size (as determined by antibody–antigen ratio) of the complexes and, interestingly, required oligomeric antibody. Complexes prepared with dimeric or polymeric IgA regularly generated mesangial deposits, whereas monomeric IgA at the same dose and degree of antigen excess failed to deposit. Finally, these investigators demonstrated that IgA immune complexes could expand the mesangial matrix, observed as increased material reactive with periodic acid–Schiff's base in tissue sections, induce deposits of complement component C3, and, most significantly, elicit microhematuria. Thus, the authors had reproduced the clinical and pathologic findings most frequently observed in patients with IgA nephropathy. They proposed that the human disease is immune complex in nature, the antibody being predominantly of the IgA class [1].

With this evidence for a role of IgA immune complexes in a passive system, attention focused upon whether endogenous antibody synthesized in response to an exogenous antigen could generate immune complexes with predominantly IgA antibody that were capable of depositing in the glomerulus. This issue was resolved by two experimental approaches.

Isaacs and Miller exploited the known restriction in antibody class in the immune response to intraperitoneal immunization with polysaccharides such as dextran. Protracted intraperitoneal and intravenous immunization of aged mice over a period of 75 days led to immune deposits of predominantly IgA, with associated IgM and C3, along with generally mild mesangial proliferation, electron-dense deposits, and hematuria [6, 7].

This group of investigators continued studying dextran-IgA antidextran immune complex glomerulonephritis in the active system [7], and subsequently also in an analogous passive system [2]. The purpose of these studies was to assess the role of the size and charge of the complexes in the degree and pattern of glomerular deposits. Size was manipulated principally by using carefully characterized fractions of dextran; the antigen–antibody ratio was also controlled in the passive studies. Charge was altered by substitution of neutral dextran with amine (diethylaminoethyl-) or acid (sulfate), creating respectively cationic and anionic dextrans. In both active and passive models, the electrostatic charge and the size of the immune complexes proved to be significant variables, not only for the degree of deposition, but also for the glomerular compartment in which the deposits were located. With regard to the mesangium, large complexes containing the 500-kD antigen were more effective than small complexes at eliciting injury, and anionic dextrans were more noxious than cationic or neutral dextrans;

complexes with both attributes, large size and negative charge, promoted the most injury. Of interest was the enhanced complement deposition observed with anionic dextran and the correlation between complement deposition and cellular proliferation. However, clinical manifestations were not correlated with any of these differences since 5–10 erythrocytes per high-power field were present in urinary sediment from all experimental animals [2, 7].

A second approach to an active system was developed in our laboratories [8]. Cognizant of the special features of the secretory immune system, we hypothesized that enteric (mucosal) immunization might elicit a preferentially IgA response, a response that could generate immune complexes capable of depositing in the glomerulus. This scheme was consistent with the temporal association of onset of IgA nephropathy with infections of mucosal surfaces, presumably viral, that had been noted in clinical reports. In contrast to the earlier active model, this system seems to be independent of the nature of the antigen and does not require older animals. We used protracted oral immunization with a variety of protein antigens to stimulate the GALT. Beginning at eight weeks of immunization and peaking at 12–14 weeks, mice continuously exposed to any of several proteins responded with significant elevations in serum IgA antibody and mesangial deposits of IgA. Further analysis of the mesangial deposits revealed that the IgA did indeed include antibody that was specific for the protein used for immunization, and that specific antigen was also present. Because we easily demonstrated free antibody-binding sites, yet antigen was more difficult to demonstrate, we suggested that the deposits were in antibody excess. The deposits also contained J chain, indicating that at least a portion of the IgA was oligomeric. Mesangial IgG and IgM were not increased, nor were IgG or IgM antibodies detected in serum. We concluded that prolonged oral immunization not only can elicit an IgA predominant antibody response, but also can give rise to IgA immune deposits in the mesangium. The immunofluorescence findings and ultrastructural appearance of glomeruli in such mice closely resembled those from patients with IgA nephropathy. In this experimental system, however, there is neither glomerular proliferation nor deposition of C3, hematuria, or other clinical manifestations of nephritis [8].

Yet another murine model of primary IgA nephropathy has been described recently. Genin and colleagues have emphasized the role of genetic background in the genesis of an IgA immune response and IgA mesangial deposits [9]. These investigators used two substrains of C3H mice: HeJ and eB. In a relatively short-term active oral immunization system using horse spleen ferritin as antigen, the high IgA-producing substrain C3H/HeJ showed increased serum IgG and IgA, although the specific antibody was predominantly IgG and IgM. Specific IgA antibody was detected at low levels in both the high (C3H/HeJ) and low (C3H/eB) IgA-producing strains without significant differences. IgG and IgM were detected in the mesangium of immunized and nonimmunized mice of both substrains, with no apparent differences among the groups. Renal IgA deposits were rare and faint in nonimmunized mice of both substrains; in immunized mice, increased deposits of IgA were observed in the immunized C3H/HeJ high-IgA-producing mice, but not in the low-IgA-producing C3H/eB animals. Deposits of ferritin (the antigen) were not found, proteinuria and hematuria were absent, and complement deposits were not sought. These studies emphasize the importance of genetic factors, predicted from numerous clinical studies.

Further progress in developing models of IgA nephropathy was reported recently by Imai and colleagues, who described and characterized the only spontaneously occurring form of murine disease, in the ddY strain [10]. In contrast to the models already discussed, the glomerulopathy and glomerular immune deposits develop without the deliberate introduction of exogenous antigen. Mesangial changes and deposits are thought by the authors to result from increased IgA synthesis associated with retrovirus-induced tumors. While such synthesis may represent an immune response to the virus, the latency period (mice must be at least 40 weeks old) and the temporal relations between glomerular IgA deposits, sharp increases in serum IgA, and decrements in serum IgA with the onset of tumors of breast, lung, and lymphoid tissue suggest that the IgA deposits may not merely represent immune complexes of retrovirus and IgA antibody [10].

MODELS OF SECONDARY IgA NEPHROPATHY

Recognition of a secondary form of clinical IgA nephropathy stimulated several experimental studies designed to elucidate the nature of glomerular IgA associated with systemic diseases, particularly whether IgA immune complexes are present [11–13]. The findings are useful for comprehending secondary IgA nephropathy as well as for defining the relationship between primary and secondary disease and permitting additional refinement of our understanding of the pathogenesis of IgA nephropathy in general. The most prevalent clinical conditions associated with secondary glomerular deposits of IgA relate to hepatobiliary disease. Therefore, experiments have emphasized alterations of the hepatobiliary system to initiate renal disease. In fact, all the models of secondary IgA nephropathy reported to date have utilized either chemical cirrhosis or bile duct ligation. Other conditions associated with deposits of IgA, such as carcinomas of secretory epithelium, IgA myelomas, and dermatitis herpetiformis have not been modeled, although the ddY mouse model may ultimately be recognized as such [10].

Gormly et al. reported that, beginning five weeks after a sublethal dose of carbon tetrachloride, rats developed cirrhosis [11]; with the onset of cirrhosis there was an increasing frequency and prominence of glomerular IgA [11]. In the early phases, there were small amounts of C3; light-microscopic changes, hematuria, and proteinuria were not observed. However, animals with long-standing cirrhosis did develop more intense C3 deposits associated with mesangial proliferation. Serum IgA levels became elevated in parallel with the development of glomerular IgA deposits; serum immune complexes were also detected. Although the carbon tetrachloride might have elicited the IgA deposits by toxic effects on lymphoid cells, promoting heightened IgA synthesis and, secondarily, renal deposits, or by direct injury of glomeruli, the hepatocellular injury antedated the deposits, and elevated serum IgA and glomerular deposits developed only after the advent of cirrhosis.

The authors suggested that failure of removal of antigens derived from the gut flora or from the portal circulation by the injured liver promoted sensitization to these antigens. Alternately, impaired clearance of IgA immune complexes may have been responsible. Melvin et al. studied a model of extrahepatic cholestasis to determine whether biliary abnormalities could elicit a result similar to hepatocellular injury [12]. Interestingly, the findings in this system closely approximated the experimental cirrhosis system. Initially, rats had increased levels of IgA in serum and progressively more frequent and more intense mesangial IgA deposits, with some C3 but without urinary abnormalities. Over a period of weeks, deposits became more prominent, complement was present, and there was increasing expansion of mesangial matrix with equivocal proliferation. Secretory component was associated with glomerular deposits of IgA in bile-duct-ligated rats.

Both hepatocellular and biliary disease have thus been implicated in the genesis of secondary glomerular IgA deposits and the development of nephritis. Increased serum IgA and IgA mesangial deposits were ascribed to compromise of the secretory component-dependent transport of oligomeric IgA and immune complexes containing oligomeric IgA from blood to bile. It was not clear in these experiments whether the glomerular IgA represented immune complexes inadequately cleared from the blood, or whether the IgA was simply aggregated polymer, perhaps altered because of hepatocellular disease.

We pursued this last issue via a murine model with short-term bile duct ligation [13]. Using our active system of oral immunization [8] and a passive system modified from that described by Rifai et al. [1], we compared renal immunofluorescence findings in immunized and nonimmunized mice, and in mice passively administered immune complexes, with and without bile duct ligation. In the passive system, mice were given immune complexes of either MOPC-315 (IgA anti-DNP) and DNP conjugated bovine gamma globulin carrier (DNP-BGG) or TEPC-15 (IgA antiphosphorylcholine [PC]) and PC conjugated carrier bovine serum albumin (PC-BSA). Complexes were prepared with purified dimeric IgA myeloma protein and hapten carrier at fivefold antigen excess. The dose of complexes was adjusted so that no IgA or antigen was detectable by immunofluorescence after injection into normal mice in a pilot study. In half the animals, the common bile ducts were ligated three days prior to injection of immune complexes; the remaining animals underwent sham surgery. Ligated and sham-operated animals were also used as controls, given MOPC-315 or TEPC-15 intravenously, but with the irrelevant antigen (MOPC-315 with PC-BSA, or TEPC-15 with DNP-BGG). Generally, sham-operated animals failed to develop glomerular deposits of either IgA or antigen. Bile-duct-ligated mice given mixtures of antibody and irrelevant antigen had mesangial deposits of IgA, but failed to reveal the antigen in the renal deposits; thus, the deposited IgA was polyclonal endogenous IgA, not injected antibody. In contrast, mice with ligated bile ducts injected with immune complexes showed bright deposits of antigen as well as IgA. Since antigen was deposited only when injected with specific IgA and only in ligated mice, we concluded that bile duct ligation promoted or enhanced the deposition of immune complexes containing dimeric IgA antibody. J chain and secretory component were also demonstrated in ligated mice, and some IgM was observed. Complement deposits, mesangial proliferation, hematuria, and proteinuria were not present.

In the active system, deposits of the specific antigen used for oral immunization and specific antibody were more intense in ligated than in sham-operated mice; IgA, some IgM, J chain, and secretory component were deposited in nearly all ligated mice, immunized or not. Sham-operated immunized mice had less J chain than their ligated counterparts, in parallel with the IgA and specific antigen, but secretory component was not observed. None of the mice had urinary or light-microscopic changes or C3 deposits. Thus, the active system confirmed that bile duct ligation enhances the deposition of IgA immune complexes; we suggested that the IgA in ligated mice that had not been deliberately immunized was also the antibody component of immune complexes with unknown spontaneously occurring antigen(s). Based on the associated secretory component, we proposed that the enhanced deposition resulted in part from reflux of immune complexes containing the secretory form of IgA which is normally excreted via the bile into the duodenum [13].

INTERRELATIONSHIPS AMONG THE MODELS

The various models of IgA nephropathy are summarized in table 13-1. Despite distinct differences in approach and emphasis, all share certain features. Among the models of primary IgA nephropathy, the active ones elicit an immune response by antigenic stimulation of mucosa-associated lymphoid tissue such as Peyer's patches and mesenteric lymph nodes [6-9]. Save for the naturally occurring model described by Imai et al. [10] in which, like the human disease, the antigen is unknown, the models suggest an immune complex pathogenesis by demonstrating an antigen-specific serum antibody response and/or antigen in the glomerular immune deposits [6–9]. The deposits induced by oral immunization revealed specific antibody in the

Table 13-1. Models of IgA nephropathy

Antigen	Source of antibody	Conclusions	Ref.
DNP-BSA	Passively injected MOPC 315 myeloma protein	IgA immune complexes injected into mice recapitulate the clinical signs and immunopathologic features of the human disease. Size (antigen/antibody ratio) is an important determinant of glomerular deposition. J-chain linked oligomeric IgA is necessary for glomerular deposition.	1
Dextrans	Passively injected W3129 myeloma protein	Size and charge of IgA immune complexes are important factors in formation of glomerular deposits. The clinical signs and immunopathologic features of the human disease are reproduced in animals given IgA immune complexes.	2
Dextrans	Actively immunized (i.p. and i.v.)	Size and charge of IgA immune complexes are important factors in formation of glomerular deposits. The clinical signs and immunopathologic features of the human disease are reproduced in animals immunized to produce an IgA response, if antigenic challenge continues.	6, 7
Various proteins	Active oral immunization	Protracted oral immunization with a variety of antigens elicits an IgA immune response in gut, bronchi, and serum. Continued antigenic challenge results in the glomerular deposition of immune complexes of specific antibody and antigen at antibody excess. Deposition of "pure" IgA immune complexes in glomeruli is not accompanied by complement deposits, mesangial proliferation, or hematuria, although electron-dense deposits and immunofluorescent deposits are demonstrable. The glomerular deposits include J-chain-linked IgA oligomers.	8, 9
?	Endogeneous IgA from unknown source(s)	Mesangial IgA deposits are associated with the onset of retrovirus-induced tumors spontaneously occurring in ddY mice.	10
?	Endogenous IgA from unknown source(s)	Altered hepatobiliary function increases serum IgA levels. Altered hepatobiliary function promotes the deposition of IgA and C3 within mesangium, with concomitant proliferation. These immunopathologic changes are not associated with hematuria.	11, 12
Various proteins coupled with DNP and PC	Active oral immunization and passively injected MOPC 315 and TEPC 15 myeloma proteins	Cholestasis increases serum IgA levels. Cholestasis promotes the deposition of IgA within mesangium, perhaps with concomitant proliferation and C3 deposits. The immunopathologic changes are not associated with hematuria. The IgA deposits most likely represent IgA immune complexes, since enhanced deposition of such immune complexes is observed in bile-duct-ligated mice.	13

glomerulus as determined by antigen binding in conjunction with the specific antigen, indicative of immune complexes [8]. The passive systems are clearly induced by immune complexes [1, 2].

Several of the models, both active and passive, demonstrated J chain to be associated with the IgA deposits, or showed a dependence on oligomeric IgA for accumulation in the kidney [1, 8, 13]. In fact, J chain has been found whenever sought, and the polymeric nature of the IgA deposited is an important feature of the models. The significance of polymerization has been emphasized in the passive MOPC-315/DNP-BSA system by Rifai and Millard [14]. Immune complexes were prepared with purified MOPC-315 IgA, either as monomer or as dimer, and DNP_8 Ficoll. When the kinetics of clearance of injected complexes from the serum were studied, monomer and dimer complexes had nearly identical first phases, but there were profound differences in the second phases. The reason was established by examining the size of the complexes. As suggested by failure of the monomer to immunoprecipitate antigen, further experiments revealed that intact monomer antibody, although bearing two antigen-combining sites, failed to form cross-linked immune complexes. Thus Rifai et al.'s earlier work, confirmed by others and reconfirmed in this most recent study, is explained by failure of the monomer to form complexes of sufficient size to permit glomerular deposition. This fully conforms to the observations of Isaacs and Miller [2, 7] and further speaks for the role of immune complex lattices in the genesis of the natural disease. Rifai and Millard suggest that there is a general requirement for J-chain-linked oligomeric IgA for the formation of large lattices. These data are fully compatible with the prevalent finding of J chain in the IgA deposits in an active model [8, 13] and in the human disease as well [15, 16].

The models of secondary IgA nephropathy, perhaps as a result of their similar induction, are even more cohesive. Deposits of IgA are associated with minimal microscopic changes in glomeruli, modest or no C3 deposits, and no significant urinary abnormalities. All the studies ascribe the deposition to alteration in hepatobiliary clearance mechanisms [11–13], including reflux of secretory IgA complexes from bile to blood. Simple deposition of oligomeric IgA not bound to antigen consequent to increased serum levels cannot be excluded, but is regarded as a less likely possibility. Finally, Gormly et al. suggest a third mechanism: hepatobiliary abnormalities result in increased exposure to antigens absorbed from the gut, which in turn promotes a prominent polyclonal IgA immune response [11]. Renal disease would still result from impaired clearance of IgA immune complexes.

RELEVANCE OF MODEL SYSTEMS TO HUMAN DISEASE

Overall, the models are close approximations of the human disease [15]. In terms of immunopathology, there is an excellent correlation between the experimental findings and the disease: generally mild mesangial proliferation associated with electron-dense immune deposits containing predominantly IgA and often C3 are the most frequent findings in both murine models and primary IgA nephropathy in humans. In humans, the spectrum ranges from no changes by light microscopy (10%) to severe diffuse proliferative glomerulonephritis (5%); similarly, the murine models of Genin et al. [9] and Emancipator et al. [8] require immunofluorescence and electron microscopy to recognize an abnormality, whereas mice challenged with large anionic immune complexes in the system developed by Isaacs and Miller [2, 7] manifest severe proliferative nephritis. Urinary abnormalities, when observed in mice, consist principally of microhematuria, which is the most prevalent symptom among patients [15]. Finally, the mesangial deposits in mice develop best when large anionic immune complexes formed with J-chain-containing oligomeric IgA are present [1, 2, 6–8, 13]; the same features are observed in immune complexes eluted from patients' kidneys [17, 18].

There are, however, several issues raised by the differences among the models and between the models and patients. Most prominent are inconstancy of signs of nephritis in mice and lack of complement deposits in two of the models. Virtually all patients with primary IgA nephropathy have both urinary abnormalities and glomerular C3 deposits. Part of this discrepancy is resolved with recognition that the diagnosis of IgA nephropathy is made by renal biopsy, a procedure that is performed selectively on patients with urinary abnormalities suggestive of glomerulonephritis, whereas in experimental systems all subjects are studied morphologically. Additionally, the degree of mesangial proliferation and the intensity of complement deposition are closely related in all of the experimental models: little or no complement is deposited in the asymptomatic models of Emancipator et al., Genin et al., and Imai et al., whereas complement deposits and mesangial expansion are regularly present in hematuric mice in the models of Rifai et al. and Isaacs and Miller [1, 2, 6–10]. Isaacs and Miller, who used a size- and charge-graded system, observed differences in the degree of complement deposition in the different groups that correlated with differences in the degree of mesangial proliferation, but no quantifiable differences in hematuria [2, 7].

The variations in C3 localization among the models is of interest, particularly because deposits of C3, mesangial proliferation and hematuria tend to be associated in patients. In the system described by Rifai et al. [1], in which pure IgA antibody was injected and deposited, highly substituted DNP-BSA at antigen excess was most effective at eliciting hematuria, whereas 2–3 times as much antibody in complexes near equivalence was required with a less highly substituted antigen [1]. IgA, particularly murine IgA, is a poor complement-*fixing* antibody. Although complement *activation* via the alternative pathway is promoted by murine IgA immune complexes, the nascent C3b generated does not bind well to the complexes [19]; thus fluid-phase consumption of C3 is not followed by fixation of C3b to complexes, and the fluid-phase C3b decays, unable to generate C3 or C5 convertase. We agree with Rifai (personal communication) that human IgA is probably even less efficient at complement fixation or activation. The nucleophile DNP, when present in high concentration, is known to fix C3 by itself. Indeed, consumption of C3 by free DNP-BSA and DNP-BGG has been observed in our laboratory. Consumption is related to the degree of substitution: unsubstituted BSA or BGG, and lightly substituted DNP-BSA, have little effect on hemolytic C3 or total hemolytic complement in fresh rat serum (J. Broestl et al., unpublished). Thus, the nature of the antigen, in concert with IgA antibody, may be important in promoting C3 deposition and eliciting hematuria. This role of antigen in the promotion of glomerular C3 deposits should not be dismissed as artificial; it is conceivable that such a mechanism is operative in human disease.

In the dextran model, IgM as well as IgA antibody deposited [6, 7]. We have argued that admixture of antibody classes in predominantly but not purely IgA immune deposits somehow enhances complement deposition, perhaps by permitting fixation of nascent C3b to the complexes [20]. However, in a dextran–antidextran passive model using pure IgA antibody, immune complex deposits with C3 have been observed and these mice become quite ill (F. Miller, personal communication). Complexes prepared with pure IgA or IgM antibody localize poorly at best with no complement evident, and mice given IgG or IgM complexes do not become ill. These findings suggest that there may be a factor related to the IgA class of antibody which promotes glomerular deposition. With respect to complement deposition, either the IgA myelomas used by Miller (W3129 and J558) behave differently toward C3 than other IgA myelomas, or the dextran used as antigen can "capture" nascent C3b generated by the antibody more effectively than other antigens used to study complement activation by IgA immune complexes. We have observed no tendency for dextran itself to activate complement in vitro (unpublished). Curiously, enhanced deposition of C3 observed in association with dextran sulfate in the active dextran–antidextran system might be explicable by antigen-induced complement activation, as dextran sulfate alone does activate complement in vitro (J. Broestl et al., unpublished).

In the human, 75% of biopsied, and therefore symptomatic, patients have IgA and/or IgM codeposited in a mesangial pattern, and our experimental data associate IgG/IgM participation with C3 deposition and microhematuria in mice with predominantly IgA immune deposits [20]. Perhaps in the remaining 25% of patients, with only IgA immunoglobulin deposited, antigen promotes the "capture" of C3b, or even activates complement directly. It should be emphasized that the observed association of complement deposits and urinary manifestations in both mouse and man is not necessarily indicative of causality. Although activated complement components are generally biologically potent in a number of ways, there is currently no direct evidence implicating complement in the genesis of hematuria.

Another difference between the model systems and the human disease relates to the presence of secretory component together with IgA in the deposits in rodents with hepatobiliary abnormalities. Secretory component has only rarely been demonstrated in human glomeruli and is typically not found even in IgA nephropathy associated with hepatobiliary disease [15, 21, 22]. Thus, while in rodents the renal IgA deposits associated with hepatobiliary disease probably represent reflux of complexes containing secretory IgA from bile to blood, or misdirected secretion of such complexes into blood instead of bile by injured hepatocytes, some other mechanism may be operative in humans. Rifai and Mannik have shown that secretory component-dependent hepatobiliary transport of oligomeric IgA and IgA immune complexes accounts for only a small proportion of clearance of IgA complexes from the blood in mice and argue that this route might not be significant in humans either [23]. These investigators further demonstrated a receptor specific for IgA immune complexes on Kupffer cells, and proposed that hepatocellular injury and/or cholestasis could impair its function [24].

FUTURE INITIATIVES

In addition to the differences between the experimental models and human IgA nephropathy discussed above, there are others. In several instances the differences parallel major clinical questions. The human disease, it is now widely recognized, can progress to renal failure and end-stage kidney [15]; in rodents, progression, vascular sclerosis, and glomerulosclerosis have not been described, but, to our knowledge, have not been sought. Patients with IgA nephropathy frequently have synpharyngitic exacerbation, presumably related to viral infections of mucosae [15]; no virally induced model of IgA nephropathy has been reported. A variety of immunoregulatory abnormalities, including polyclonal B-cell activation, increased propensity to generate plasma cells which synthesize dimeric rather than monomeric IgA, increased T-helper and decreased T-suppressor activities (IgA specific or not), have been described in patients with IgA nephropathy [15]; the issue of immunoregulation has not been studied in the models. Several therapeutic regimens have been attempted in patients, but not in the models. On the other hand, IgA nephropathy is a relatively new disease, and so the models are still young. Future initiatives will likely include modifications of the models directed to addressing the just-mentioned issues.

CONCLUSION

Extrapolation of animal models to disease in patients must always be accompanied by caution. Yet, the models of IgA nephropathy described to date, particularly in conjunction with current clinical understanding, hold great promise. Taken collectively, the models enable us to conclude with fair assurance that events which increase the level of IgA-containing immune complexes, either by promoting an IgA immune response, as by mucosal immunization in the continued presence of antigen, or by impairing clearance of IgA immune complexes, as in hepatobiliary disease, can result in IgA immune deposits in glomeruli. Alteration in IgA synthesis or in immunoregulation may be operative in humans, but has not been demonstrated in experimental systems to date, although IgA-specific regulatory cells are well described [15]. There is a dose–response relationship in several models [1, 2, 13], which agrees with the correlation between IgA immune complex levels and disease activity in patients [15]. Since, in all experimental systems employing active immunization, antigen is present when antibody is also present, deposition of circulating immune complexes constitutes the likely mechanism.

In both humans and rodents, morphologic alterations and urinary abnormalities do not always accompany IgA immune deposits in glomeruli although C3 deposition is generally correlated with mesangial proliferation and hematuria [1, 2, 6–13, 15]. The pathogenesis of IgA nephropathy in rodents is immune complex in nature, but the mechanism(s) of injury can only be suggested. Implication of complement would be of great value, and this issue is under study in our laboratory. The molecular mechanisms underlying hematuria are even more remote. It is likely that those mechanisms which prove operative in hematuria in mice will also be operative in humans. Further study and modification of the models is certainly warranted.

Finally, the relationship of IgA nephropathy to other glomerulonephritides, at both the clinical and experimental levels, is noteworthy. In experimental systems [1, 2, 6–8, 13], and apparently in clinical situations as well [15, 17, 18], dose, size, and electrostatic charge of immune complexes are important determinants of the amount and distribution, mesangial versus capillary wall, of glomerular deposits. Symptoms and morphologic expression of injury are generally related to phlogogenic sequelae of the deposition of immune complexes. Indeed, symptoms and progression in IgA nephropathy are similar to those of glomerulonephritis associated with IgG or IgM with comparable histopathology [25]. IgA nephropathy has been distinguished from other glomerulonephritides in two respects: the class of the antibody and the more indolent course. Recognition of the special role IgA plays in the mucosal immune system has allowed the development of active models of IgA nephropathy, and has prompted an interpretation associating secretory sites with the spontaneous model. It is not surprising that IgA nephropathy is a common type of glomerulonephritis when one considers the vast opportunities for penetration of foreign (antigenic) materials into various mucosae. The route, duration, and degree of antigenic stimulation are important; factors that favor an IgA immune response must prevail over factors that favor an IgG/IgM response. The role of genetic control of the IgA immune response is clearly demonstrated in the work of Genin et al. [9], where the propensity to mount an IgA immune response predicts whether glomerular immune deposits develop. The numerous studies that implicate a genetic factor in the risk for disease in humans further suggest a direction to pursue, namely, the capacity for and tendency toward IgA immune responses.

The indolent progression of many cases of IgA nephropathy remains unexplained, but may reside in the route, duration, and dose of antigenic stimulation or involve other mechanisms set in motion concomitant with or consequent to stimulation of IgA antibody. Other things being equal, a preferentially IgA response would be expected to be less injurious in that IgA appears to be much less phlogogenic than other classes of immunoglobulin such as IgG. Another consideration may also be important: if the antigen is in a mucous membrane, once an IgA response is elicited, the presence of secretory IgA on the mucosal surface would provide a strong barrier to further penetration of inert antigen into the body. Indeed, replicating invasive mucosal pathogens would be likely natural stimuli, eliciting episodic exacerbations (synpharyngitic?) of nephritis. In contrast, IgG antibody, which is phlogogenic, is not an effective barrier to penetration of the mucosa by antigen.

The models of IgA nephropathy established so far provide insights into pathogenesis. Modifications of these models will likely result in even better understanding of pathophysiologic mechanisms operative not only in IgA nephropathy but also in glomerulonephritis in general. Further study may also provide insights into ways of modulating the immune response to permit arrest or reversal of glomerular diseases.

REFERENCES

1. Rifai A, Small PA, Teague PO, Ayoub EM: Experimental IgA nephropathy. J Exp Med 150:1161–1173, 1979.
2. Isaacs K, Miller F: Antigen size and charge in immune complex glomerulonephrits. II. Passive induction of immune deposits with dextran–anti-dextran immune complexes. Am J Pathol 111:298–306, 1983.
3. Lamm ME: Cellular aspects of immunoglobulin A. Adv Immunol 22:223–290, 1976.
4. Vaerman JP, Heremans JF: Origin and molecular size of IgA in the mesenteric lymph of the dog. Immunology 18:27–38, 1977.
5. Mostov KE, Kraehenbuhl JP, Blobel G: Receptor-mediated transcellular transport of immunoglobulin: synthesis of secretory component as multiple and larger transmembrane forms. Proc Natl Acad Sci USA 77:7257–7261, 1980.
6. Isaacs K, Miller F, Lane B: Experimental model for IgA nephropathy. Clin Immunol Immunopathol 20:419–426, 1981.
7. Isaacs K, Miller F: Role of antigen size and charge in immune complex glomerulonephritis. I. Active induction of disease with dextran and its derivatives. Lab Invest 47:198–204, 1982.

8. Emancipator SN, Gallo GR, Lamm ME: Experimental IgA nephropathy induced by oral immunization. J Exp Med 157:572–582, 1983.
9. Genin C, Sabatier JC, Berthoux FC: IgA mesangial deposits in C3H/HeJ mice after oral immunization. Proc Eur Dial Transplant Assoc 21:703–708, 1985.
10. Imai H, Nakamoto Y, Askaura K, Miki K, Yasuda T, Miura AB: Spontaneous glomerular IgA deposition in ddY mice: an animal model of IgA nephritis, Kidney Int 27:756–761, 1985.
11. Gormly AA, Smith PS, Seymour AE, Clarkson AR, Woodroffe AJ: IgA glomerular deposits in experimental cirrhosis. Am J Pathol 104:50–54, 1981.
12. Melvin T, Burke B, Michael AF, Kim Y: Experimental IgA nephropathy in bile duct ligated rats. Clin Immunol Immunopathol 27:369–377, 1983.
13. Emancipator SN, Gallo GR, Razaboni R, Lamm ME: Experimental cholestasis promotes the deposition of glomerular IgA immune complexes. Am J Pathol 113:19–26, 1983.
14. Rifai A, Millard K: Glomerular deposition of immune complexes prepared with monomeric or polymeric IgA. Clin Exp Immunol 60:363–368, 1985.
15. Emancipator SN, Gallo GR, Lamm ME: IgA nephropathy: perspectives on pathogenesis and classification. Clin Nephrol 24:161–179, 1985.
16. Lomax-Smith JD, Zaborwarny LA, Howarth GS, Seymour AE, Woodroffe AJ: The immunochemical characterisation of mesangial IgA deposits. Am J Pathol 113:359–364, 1983.
17. Monteiro RC, Halbwachs-Mecarelli L, Berger J, Lesavre P: Characteristics of eluted IgA in primary IgA nephropathy. Contrib Nephrol 40:107–111, 1984.
18. Monteiro RC, Noel LH, Halbwachs-Mecarelli L, Berger J, Lesavre P: Charge and size of mesangial IgA in IgA nephropathy. Kidney Int 28:666–671, 1985.
19. Pfaffenbach G, Lamm ME, Gigli I: Activation of the guinea pig alternative complement pathway by mouse IgA immune complexes. J Exp Med 155:231–246, 1982.
20. Emancipator SN, Lamm ME: Nephritis associated with C3 deposition in murine IgA nephropathy: a role for classical pathway activation by codeposited IgG or IgM [abstr]? In: Robinson RR (ed) Proceedings of the 9th international congress of nephrology, 1984, p 238.
21. Whitworth JA, Leibowitz S, Kennedy MC, Cameron JS, Chantler C: IgA and glomerular disease. Clin Nephrol 5:33–38, 1976.
22. Woodroffe AJ, Gormly AA, McKenzie PE, Wootton AM, Thomspon AJ, Seymour AE, Clarkson AR: Immunologic studies in IgA nephropathy. Kidney Int 18:366–374, 1980.
23. Rifai A, Mannik M: Clearance kinetics and fate of mouse IgA immune complexes prepared with monomeric or dimeric IgA. J Immunol 130:1826–1832, 1983.
24. Rifai, Mannik M: Clearance of circulating IgA immune complexes is mediated by a specific receptor on Kupffer cells in mice. J Exp Med 160:125–137, 1984.
25. Okada M, Okamura K, Ohmura N, Kitaoka T: Clinicopathologic study of IgA nephropathy in comparison with mesangial proliferative glomerulonephritis without IgA deposits [abstr]. In: Robinson RR (ed) Proceedings of the 9th international congress of nephrology, 1984, p 117.

The authors' work was supported by NIH grants CA-32582 and DK-38544 from the U.S. Public Health Service, and The John Lowey Research Grant from the Kidney Foundation of Ohio.

14. SUMMARY OF THE PATHOGENESIS OF IgA NEPHROPATHY

ANDREW J. WOODROFFE

As in so many conditions, the causes of IgA nephropathy and its close relative, Henoch-Schönlein purpura (HSP), remain obscure despite considerable efforts in human and animal experimentation. However, such efforts over the past ten years have taught us something about the mechanisms involved in mesangial IgA nephritis and this chapter reviews this knowledge, paying special tribute to those involved and emphasizing areas that may prove ultimately to be of diagnostic, prognostic, or therapeutic value to patients with IgA nephropathy.

THE NATURE OF THE DEPOSITS

All patients with IgA nephropathy have mesangial IgA deposits; this much is certain! Concomitant C3 and, in some, IgG, IgM, and fibrinogen may be present. Quantitation of the last three are of some value in the pathologic differentation of isolated IgA nephropathy, HSP, and mesangial IgA nephritis secondary to alcoholic liver disease [1]. C1q deposits are unusual in primary IgA nephropathy and this, together with the greater frequency of β1H than C4-bp glomerular deposits [2], indicates that the alternative pathway of complement activation predominates in this condition.

Recently several studies have focused on the subclasses of IgA in the glomerular deposits [3–7] (table 14–1 [6]). Most now agree that IgA1 is the predominant subclass present in patients with primary IgA nephropathy, but

Table 14-1. The nature of the mesangial deposits [6]

	No. of patients	A_1	A_2	J chain	SC
Primary					
IgA nephropathy	11	10	2	10	0
HSP	7	5	1	4	0
Mesangial IgA nephritis associated with alcoholic cirrhosis	16	15	2	13	1
SLE	5	5	3	5	0

Table 14-2. Binding of exogenous SC to the mesangial deposits in IgA nephropathy

Reference	
Egido et al. [11]	16/20
Valentijn et al. [12]	11/13
Katz et al. [7]	0/10
Lomax-Smith et al. [6]	1/10

this observation is of little value in differentiating between a mucosal or a systemic origin for the IgA since it is acknowledged that IgA1 and IgA2 are both produced in mucosae. There is general agreement that secretory component (SC) is not present in the glomerular deposits but, again, this does not preclude mucosally derived IgA from being responsible for the deposits.

J chain, independent of IgM, has been identified in the mesangia of patients with IgA nephropathy [6, 8] and this observation is in keeping with the hypothesis that the IgA deposits are polymeric [9]. This hypothesis is further supported by immunochemical characterization of the IgA eluted from renal biopsy sections [10]. Analysis of these eluates by high-performance liquid chromatography showed that approximately 70% of the IgA was of molecular weight greater than 160,000 daltons. The elution conditions used in these experiments are also known to dissociate immune complexes and so the results in no way preclude the participation of antigen–polymeric IgA complexes.

The affinity of the mesangial deposits for SC has also been used as an indication of the polymeric nature of the IgA. Some immunofluorescence studies have reported in vitro binding of SC to the mesangial areas of renal biopsy sections from patients with IgA nephropathy in a manner independent of the influence of IgM [11, 12] (table 14–2). Our studies have shown this SC-binding phenomenon to be largely restricted to patients with glomerular IgA deposits associated with alcoholic cirrhosis or systemic lupus erythematosus [6], a divergence that may reflect differences of patient selection or experimental technique.

Idiotypic analysis of the mesangial IgA has not yet been reported, but no shared idiotype was observed between serum IgA from patients with primary IgA nephropathy and the monoclonal IgA from an individual with a benign IgA monoclonal gammopathy and mesangial IgA nephritis [13]. This area deserves further attention, including a search for antiidiotypic antibodies and rheumatoid factor in the serum and the glomerular deposits of patients with IgA nephropathy.

In contrast, considerable effort has been directed to the search for antigens and for the antibody specificity of the mesangial IgA. We have been unable to identify common dietary (BSA) or gut flora (*Escherichia coli*) antigens in the deposits and have searched unsuccessfully for infectious antigens in renal biopsies from patients who had identifiable infections immediately prior to episodes of macrohematuria. With regard to antibody specificity, there has been one tentative report of the antimesangial reactivity of eluted IgA [14]. More recently, the reactivity of IgA eluted from cryostat sections of IgA nephropathy biopsies with the mesangial areas of their own and other patients' biopsies has been described [15]. Such eluates have also been shown to contain antibodies reactive with tonsillar cells obtained from patients with IgA nephropathy [16].

In conclusion, the immunochemical nature of the mesangial deposits in IgA nephropathy is consistent with antigen-polymeric IgA complexes predominantly of A1 subclass, and perhaps multispecific for ubiquitous mucosally derived antigens.

MEDIATION OF INJURY AND CLINICAL CORRELATES

There is a real quandary in this area since it appears from animal studies and clinical observations that IgA deposits can be present without signs of tissue injury. For example, mesangial deposits of IgA can be induced in mice by the oral administration of various foreign proteins [17]. However, these mice develop mesangial proliferative disease and hematuria only if given a subsequent parenteral dose of the relevant antigen. In man, mesangial IgA deposits have frequently been observed in the absence of overt renal disease, and vascular deposits of IgA are commonly found in skin biopsies from patients with IgA nephropathy without skin disease. In addition, there is no clear correlation between the amount of mesangial IgA and the severity of the glomerulonephritis [18] and one occasionally sees severe disease with only scant amounts of IgA.

Apparently, some other factor(s) is required for the initiation of injury (table 14-3). Intuitively, the complement system seems likely to play a role. Aggregated IgA is known to stimulate the alternative pathway of complement activation [19] and this could be responsible for local chemotaxis and inflammation. However, one often sees large amounts of mesangial or cutaneous C3 with no inflammation or injury. Platelet activation and

Table 14-3. Possible mediators of glomerular injury in IgA nephropathy

IgA polymers and IC
Complement
Fibrin
Platelets
Proteinases
Prostaglandins
Macrophages
Glomerular sclerosis

coagulation with fibrin deposition are also known to occur, but their contribution to glomerular injury is undefined. Other suggested mediators include proteinases and, of course, the prostaglandins, which have been shown recently to be produced by the mesangium [20]. The role of the macrophage is now well established in crescentic glomerulonephritis, but these cells have been shown to be relatively uncommon in most studies of mesangial proliferative disease [21]. The recogition of Ia-positive cells in the rat mesangium is of considerable interest and it has been suggested that such cells may act locally to regulate the immune response [22]. Finally, the mesangial deposits may alter the normal glomerular circulation with local vasodilatation and the development of glomerular sclerosis [23]. Mesangiolysis and glomerular capillary aneurysms have also been described as possible causes for the sclerotic lesions [24].

How might the above postulated mechanisms account for the frank hematuria in some patients, for the acute renal failure in others, and for the progressive glomerular sclerosis, hypertensive vascular disease, and tubulointerstitial lesions in some 20% of patients? In addition, why do some patients develop clinically overt skin, joint, and gut disease in association with nephritis (HSP), with ostensibly the same basic immunopathogenesis being operative? The answers to these questions are beyond the understanding of this author.

In conclusion, it is necessary to keep an open mind regarding the mediation of "IgA disease." This area has not been adequately studied and it may ultimately provide the major therapeutic advance that is so sorely needed.

HUMORAL ABNORMALITIES

Remote from the glomerulus, a number of abnormalities have been described that may be of central significance. The serum concentration of IgA is elevated in up to 50% of patients with IgA nephropathy [25], albeit not correlating with disease activity or prognosis. Many investigators have reported increased amounts of polymeric serum IgA [9] and some have shown

Table 14-4. IgA class circulating immune complexes in IgA nephropathy

		Ref.
Conglutinin binding assay		
Katz et al	56%	7
Coppo et al.	31%	26
Lesavre et al.	39%	27
Doi et al.	27%	28
Raji cell assay		
Edigo et al.	64%	29
Lesavre et al.	68%	27
Anti-IgA inhibition binding assay		
Valentijn et al.	78%	12

a correlation between this parameter and active disease (J. Feehally, personal communication). IgA class immune complexes (table 14-4) are also frequently detected by conglutinin binding, IgA inhibition, and Raji cell assays [7, 12, 26–29] and, in some reports, the complexed IgA is polymeric [29]. This latter observation is totally consistent with a murine model of IgA nephropathy in which the IgA must be both polymeric and complexed in order to produce mesangial deposits [30]. Some investigators have reported a correlation between the level of IgA class immune complexes and disease activity [9] and, of special interest, a significant delay in the postprandial clearance of such complexes in IgA nephropathy patients [31]. In some instances, these complexes have been shown to contain antibodies to food antigens. Studies indicate that the "macromolecular" (10–21S) IgA is of the A1 subclass [12], but, as pointed out earlier, this does not help to define the site of production of nephritogenic IgA. Potentially causative derangements in IgA production and clearance are discussed below under *Cellular immune abnormalities*.

However, one group has put forward a humoral mechanism to explain the persistence of IgA complexes in the circulation [32] and this should be recognized in the current context. The study reports a subtle defect in the ability of the sera of patients with IgA nephropathy to solubilize mesangial IgA deposits. The authors found that patients' sera are less proficient in the solubilization of IgA deposits from autologous and heterologous renal biopsy tissue than were sera from healthy controls and showed that the mechanism for this solubilization was complement dependent. Clinical trials are now being conducted to determine the efficacy of treatment with danazol [33], an agent that "stabilizes" the complement pathway.

What is known of the antibody specificity of the mesangial IgA deposits? Indirectly, serum studies shown that there is an increased titer of antibodies to BSA in patients with IgA nephropathy [34] and an increase in immune complexes containing antibodies to ovalbumin [31]. However, neither of

Table 14-5. Abnormalities in IgA production by peripheral blood mononuclear cells from patients with IgA nephropathy

	Observed			Postulated			
Reference	↑ Spontaneous production	↑ PWM-stimulated production	↓ Con-A suppression	T-cell abn.	B-cell abn.	Macrophage abn.	Serum effect
Hale et al. [42]	Yes	Yes	No	No	Yes	NT[a]	No
Egido et al. [39]	No	Yes	Yes	Yes	Yes	NT	Yes
Perl et al. [45]	Yes	No	No	NT	NT	Yes	NT

[a]NT, not tested.

these antigens has been identified in the glomerular deposits. Similar observations have been reported with respect to the prevalence of antinuclear antibodies in the sera [35] and polyethylene glycol precipitates of sera [36] from patients with IgA nephropathy.

In conclusion there is evidence for polymeric IgA class immune complexes in the mediation of IgA nephropathy, but the derivation of these complexes, and the reasons for their pathogenicity, are not understood.

CELLULAR IMMUNE ABNORMALITIES

Many studies have been undertaken to identify abnormalities in IgA production (immunoregulation) and clearance. With regard to immunoregulation, several investigators have reported elevated $OKT_{4/8}$ ratios in patients with IgA nephropathy [37–39]. Other "numerical" cellular abnormalities include an increase in IgA-bearing lumphocytes [40] and an increase in T$\propto$ cells [41]. However, "functional" cellular abnormalities seem more likely to be relevant, and there are now many studies that deal with abnormalities in Ig production by lymphocytes isolated from such patients (table 14-5). Some authors have shown increased production of IgA, IgG, and IgM by unstimulated cultures of peripheral blood mononuclear cells [42], others have reported selectively increased production of IgA by pokeweed mitogen-stimulated cultures [39], and others a defect in concanavalin-A-induced IgA-specific suppressor T-cell activity [43]. In addition, our group has recently identified an increase in IgA-specific B-cell activity in patients with IgA nephropathy [42], similar in many respects to that described in HSP and systemic lupus erythematosus (SLE) [44]. One study suggests that macrophages are required for the observed augumentation in IgA production [45]. With some exceptions, there has been no correlation between such indices and disease activity and, therefore, the relevance of these observations is still uncertain. In part, these limitations may be due to the selection of peripheral blood mononuclear cells rather than mucosally derived cells for study. In one

Table 14-6. HLA-DR typing in IgA nephropathy patients with end-stage renal failure [53]

	B12 (%)	B35 (%)	DR4 (%)
Patients (103)	3.9	13.6	30.1
Controls (134)	2.9	9.7	31.4

study employing tonsillar cells, an increase in IgA production has been reported, and this IgA has been shown to be polymeric by virtue of its affinity for free SC [46].

In attempting to determine whether such aberrations in immunoregulation play a primary or secondary role in the pathogenesis of IgA nephropathy, it seems relevant to attempt correlations of these abnormalities with HLA-DR genotypes and with other immunopathologic "markers" of disease. Several studies have pointed to a genetic basis for IgA nephropathy: namely, an increased prevalence of BW 35 and/or DR 4 in some series [47, 48], an association with a homozygous C4 null phenotype [49], instances of familial IgA nephropathy [50, 51], and racial differences in prevalence of disease [52]. In our own patients, and in an Australian survey of patients with end-stage renal failure due to IgA nephropathy (table 14-6) [53], we have been unable to find correlations with BW 12, BW 35, or DR 4, and could not detect abnormalities in IgA production by peripheral blood mononuclear cells of first-degree relatives [42]. Conversely, it is known (at least in mice) that the number of T∝ cells is positively influenced by the serum IgA concentration [54], an observation that might suggest that the abnormalities of cellular IgA immunoregulation in patients with IgA nephropathy are simply a reflection of their raised serum IgA concentrations. We have investigated this possibility by studying the effect of patients' sera on the production of IgA by control peripheral blood mononuclear cells and found no differential effect when compared with control sera [42].

A similar problem applies to the allocation of a primary or secondary pathogenic role to the defects observed in the clearance of Fc and C3b by patients with IgA nephropathy [38, 55]. As in SLE, these defective immune clearance mechanisms are probably secondary to saturation of receptors with IgA and C3 rather than causal, a possible exception being the mesangial IgA nephritis that is associated with alcoholic liver disease [56].

In conclusion, there is good evidence for increased production of IgA in patients with IgA nephropathy and this includes the production of polymeric IgA by tonsillar cells as well as peripheral blood lymphocytes. The precise mechanism responsible for the increased production is still a matter of some contention. Defective clearance of immune complexes from the circulation may also be important, but this seems more likely to be a consequence rather than the cause of the increased immune complex load.

SUMMARY

A number of generally accepted observations can be made regarding the pathogenesis of IgA nephropathy, First, the mesangial IgA deposits are dimers or polymers of the A1 subclass. Second, the IgA is probably complexed with antigen. Third, this material is derived from the circulation and is probably deposited in "showers" following mucosally presented antigen exposure. Fourth, there is increased production of IgA and its polymers by both mucosal and peripheral blood lymphocytes. This appears to be a "primary" (?genetic) abnormality, but there is no consensus yet regarding the precise level of the immunoregulatory defect.

Less is known of the mediation of tissue injury in IgA nephropathy and HSP or, for that matter, why some individuals develop the systemic condition and others have isolated renal disease. It is quite apparent that the IgA alone is not injurious and that other mediators are involved. This area needs more study, not least because it may be more amenable to new treatment strategies that the immunoregulatory disturbance that appears to make ubiquitous antigens nephritogenic in these patients.

REFERENCES

1. Woodroffe AJ, Clarkson AR, Seymour AE, Lomax-Smith JD: Mesangial IgA nephritis. Springer Semin Immunopathol 5:321–332, 1982.
2. Miyazaki R, Kuroda M, Akiyama T, Otani I, Tofuku Y, Takeda R: Glomerular deposition and serum levels of complement control proteins in patients with IgA nephropathy. Clin Nephrol 21:335–340, 1984.
3. Andre C, Berthoux FC, Andre F, Gillon J, Genin C, Sabatier J-C: Prevalence of IgA_2 deposits in IgA nephropathies. N Engl J Med 303:1343–1346, 1980.
4. Conley ME, Cooper MD, Michael AF: Selective deposition of immunoglobulin A_1 in immunoglobulin A nephropathy, anaphylactoid purpura nephritis, and systemic lupus erythematosus. J Clin Invest 66:1432–1436, 1980.
5. Tomino Y, Endoh M, Nomoto Y, Sakai H: Immunoglobulin A_1 in IgA nephropathy. N Engl J Med 305:1159–1160, 1981.
6. Lomax-Smith JD, Zabrowarny LA, Howarth GS, Seymour AE, Woodroffe AJ: The immunochemical characterization of mesangial IgA deposits. Am J Pathol 113:359–364, 1983.
7. Katz A, Nenkirk MM, Klein MH: Circulating and mesangial IgA in IgA nephropathy. Contrib Nephrol 40:74–79, 1984.
8. Tomino Y, Sakai H, Miura M, Endoh M, Nomoto Y: Detection of polymeric IgA in glomeruli from patients with IgA nephropathy. Clin Exp Immunol 49:419–425, 1982.
9. Egido J, Sancho J, Blasco R, Lozano L, Hernando L: Immunologic aspects of IgA nephropathy in humans. In: Robinson RR (ed) Proceedings of the 9th international congress on nephrology, vol 1. New York: Springer-Verlag, 1984, pp 652–664.
10. Monteiro RC, Habwachs-Mecarelli L, Berger J, Lesavre P: Characteristics of eluted IgA in priamry IgA nephropathy. Contrib Nephrol 40:107–111, 1984.
11. Egido J, Sancho J, Mampaso F, Lopez-Trascasa M, Sanchez-Crespo M, Blasco R, Hernando L: A possible common pathogenesis of the the mesangial IgA glomerulonephritis in patients with Berger's disease and Schönlein-Henoch syndrome. Proc Eur Dial Transplant Assoc 17:660–666, 1980.
12. Valentijn RM, Radl J, Haayman JJ, Vermeer BJ, Weening JJ, Kauffmann RH, Daha MR, van Es LA: Macromolecular IgA in the circulation and mesangial deposits in patients with primary IgA nephropathy. Contrib Nephrol 40:87–92, 1984.

13. Droz D, Noel LH, Barbanel C, Leibowitch J: Glomérulonéphrite à dépôts intercapillaires d'IgA lors d'une gammapathie monoclonale benigne. Nouv Presse Med 10:3652–3653, 1981.
14. Lowance DC, Mullins JD, McPhaul JJ: Immunoglobulin A (IgA) associated glomerulonephritis. Kideny Int 3:167–176, 1973.
15. Tomino Y, Endoh M, Nomoto Y, Sakai H: Specificity of eluted antibody from renal tissue of patients with IgA nephropathy. Am J Kidney Dis 1:276–280, 1982.
16. Tomino Y, Sakai H, Endoh M, Suga T, Miura M, Kaneshige H, Nomoto Y: Cross-reactivity of IgA antibodies between renal mesangial areas and nuclei of tonsillar cells in patients with IgA nephropathy. Clin Exp Immunol 51:605–610, 1983.
17. Emancipator SN, Gallo GR, Lamm ME: Experimental IgA nephropathy induced by oral immunization. J Exp Med 157:572–582, 1983.
18. Sinniah R, Ku G: Clinicopathologic correlations in IgA nephropathy. In: Robinson RR (ed) Proceedings of the 9th international congress on nephrology, vol 1. New York: Springer-Verlag, 1984, pp 665–685.
19. Pfaffenbach G, Lamm ME, Gigli I: Activation of the guinea pig alternative complement pathway by mouse IgA immune complexes. J Exp Med 155:231–247, 1982.
20. Scharschmidt LA, Dunn MJ: Prostaglandin synthesis by rat glomerular mesangial cells in culture: effect of angiotensin II and arginine vasopressin. J Clin Invest 71:1756–1764, 1983.
21. Hooke DH, Hancock WW, Gee DC, Kraft N, Atkins RC: Monoclonal antibody analysis of glomerular hypercellularity in human glomerulonephritis. Clin Nephrol 22:163–168, 1984.
22. Schreiner GF, Cotran RS: Localization of an Ia-bearing glomerular cell in the mesangium. J Cell Biol 94:483–488, 1982.
23. Couser WG: Mesangial IgA nephropathies: steady progress. West Med 140:89–91, 1984.
24. Sinniah R, Churg J: Effect of IgA deposits on the glomerular mesangium in Berger's disease. Ultrastruct Pathol 4:9–22, 1983.
25. Clarkson AR, Seymour AE, Thompson AJ, Haynes WDG, Chan Y-L, Jackson B: IgA nephropathy: a syndrome of uniform morphology diverse clinical features and uncertain prognosis. Clin Nephrol 8:457–471, 1977.
26. Coppo R, Basolo B, Martina G, Rollino C, De Marchi M, Giacchino F, Mazzucco G, Messina M, Piccoli G: Circulating immune complexes containing IgA, IgG and IgM in patients with primary IgA nephropathy and with Henoch-Schoenlein nephritis: correlation with clinical and histologic signs of activity. Clin Nephrol 18:230–239, 1982.
27. Lesavre P, Digeon M, Bach JF: Analysis of circulating IgA and detection of immune complexes in primary IgA nephropathy. Clin Exp Immunol 48:61–69, 1982.
28. Doi T, Kanatsu K, Sekita K, Yoshida H, Nagai H, Hamashima Y: Detection of IgA class circulating immune complexes bound to anti-C3d antibody in patients with IgA nephropathy. J Immunol Methods 69:95–104, 1984.
29. Egido J, Sancho J, Hernando P, Gonzalez J, Hernando L: Presence of specific IgA immune complexes in IgA nephropathy. Contrib Nephrol 40:80–86, 1984.
30. Rifai A, Small PA, Teague PO, Ayoub EM: Experimental IgA nephropathy. J Exp Med 150:1161–1173, 1979.
31. Sancho J, Egido J, Rivera F, Hernando L: Immune complexes in IgA nephropathy: presence of antibodies against diet antigens and delayed clearance of specific polymeric IgA immune complexes. Clin Exp Immunol 54:194–202, 1983.
32. Tomino Y, Sakai H, Suga T, Miura M, Kaneshige H, Endoh, M, Nomoto Y: Impaired solubilization of glomerular immune deposits by sera from patients with IgA nephropathy. Am J Kidney Dis 3:48–54, 1983.
33. Tomino Y, Sakai H, Miura M, Suga T, Endoh M, Nomoto Y: Effect of danazol in solubilization of immune deposits in patients with IgA nephropathy. Am J Kidney Dis 4:135–140, 1984.
34. Woodroffe AJ, Gormly AA, McKenzie PE, Wooton AM, Thompson AJ, Seymour AE, Clarkson AR: Immunologic studies in IgA nephropathy. Kidney Int 18:366–374, 1980.
35. Nomoto Y, Sakai H: Cold reacting antinuclear factor in sera from patients with IgA nephropathy. J Lab Clin Med 74:76–87, 1979.
36. Cohen RS, Russell MT, Dickey LE, Schwartz MM, Roberts JL: Properties of IgA isolated from serum of patients with IgA glomerulopathy. In: Robinson RR (ed) Proceedings of the 9th international congress on nephrology. (1984, p 274A. New York: Springer-Verlag).

37. Chatenoud L, Bach MA: Abnormalities of T cell subsets in glomerulonephritis and systemic lupus erythematosus. Kidney Int 20:267–274, 1981.
38. Bannister KM, Drew PA, Clarkson AR, Woodroffe AJ: Immunoregulation in glomerulonephritis, Henoch-Schönlein purpura and lupus nephritis. Clin Exp Immunol 53:384–390, 1983.
39. Egido J, Blasco R, Sancho J, Lozano L: T cell dysfunction in IgA nephropathy: specific abnormalities in the regulation of IgA synthesis. Clin Immunol Immunopathol 26:201–212, 1983.
40. Nomoto Y, Sakai H, Arimori S: Increase of IgA-bearing lymphocytes in peripheral blood from patients with IgA nephropathy. Am J Clin Pathol 71:158–160, 1979.
41. Sakai H, Endoh M, Tomino Y, Nomoto Y: Increase of IgA specific helper T cells in patients with IgA nephropathy. Clin Exp Immunol 50:77–82, 1982.
42. Hale GM, Bannister KM, Clarkson AR, Woodroffe AJ: Immunoregulatory abnormalities in IgA nephropathy. In: Robinson RR (ed) Proceedings of the 9th international congress on nephrology. New York: Springer-Verlag, 1984, p 281A.
43. Sakai H, Nomoto Y, Arimori S: Decrease of IgA-specific suppressor T cell activity in patients with IgA nephropathy. Clin Exp Immunol 38:243–248, 1979.
44. Beale MG, Nash GS, Bertovich MJ, MacDermott RP: Similar disturbances in B cell activity and regulatory T cell function in Henoch-Schönlein purpura and systemic lupus erythematosus. J Immunol 128:486–491, 1982.
45. Perl SI, Wilkinson A, Williams DG: IgA and IgG production by lymphocytes in IgA glomerulonephritis. Kidney Int 28:856, 1985.
46. Egido J, Blasco R, Lozano J, Sancho J, Garcia-Hoyo R: Immunological abnormalities in the tonsils of patients with IgA nephropathy: inversion in the ratio of IgA: IgG bearing lymphocytes and increased polymeric IgA synthesis. Clin Exp Immunol 57:101–106, 1984.
47. Berthoux FC, Gagne A, Sabatier JC, Ducret F, Le Petit JC, Marcellin M, Mercier B, Brizard CP: HLA-Bw35 and mesangial IgA glomerulonephritis. N Engl J Med 298:1034–1035, 1978.
48. Hiki Y, Kobayashi Y, Tateno S, Sada M, Kashiwagi N: Strong association of HLA-DR4 with benign IgA nephropathy. Nephron 32:222–226, 1982.
49. McLean RH, Wyatt RJ, Julian BA: Complement phenotypes in glomerulonephritis: increased frequency of homozygous null C4 phenotypes in IgA nephropathy and Hencoh-Schönlein purpura. Kidney Int 26:855–860, 1984.
50. Egido J, Blasco R, Sancho J, Lozano L, Gutierrez-Millet V: Immunologic studies in a familial IgA nephropathy. Clin Exp Immunol 54:532–538, 1983.
51. Julian BA, Quiggins PA, Thompson JS, Woodford SY, Gleason K, Wyatt RJ: Familial IgA nephropathy: evidence of an inherited mechanism of disease. N Engl J Med 312:202–208, 1985.
52. Galla JH, Kohaut EC, Alexander R, Mestecky J: Racial differences in the prevalence of IgA-associated nephropathies. Lancet 2:522, 1984.
53. Disney APS: Australian and New Zealand dialysis and transplant registry, 1984.
54. Hoover RG, Heikman S, Berger HM, Rebbe N, Lynch RG: Expansion of Fc receptor-bearing T lymphocytes in patients with immunoglobulin G and immunoglobulin A myeloma. J Clin Invest 67:308–311, 1981.
55. Nicholls K, Kincaid-Smith P: Defective in vivo Fc- and C3b-receptor function in IgA nephropathy. Am J Kidney Dis 4:128–134, 1984.
56. Woodroffe AJ: IgA, glomerulonephritis and liver disease. Aust NZ J Med 11:109–111, 1981.

15. THE TREATMENT OF IgA NEPHROPATHY

ANTHONY R. CLARKSON

Overt clinical features of IgA nephropathy frequently resolve spontaneously and the disease may remain quiescent clinically for months or years. As such, episodes of macroscopic hematuria and evanescent decline in renal function are probably not reliable indices of long-term disease activity whereby the effects of treatment may be gauged. Urinary abnormalities, particularly microscopic hematuria, persist in the majority of patients, however, and many develop gradually increasing proteinuria and hypertension. It is the policy of our unit to monitor these features and serial measurements of renal function to assess progress. It has become clear, however, from study of repeat renal biopsies, that such monitoring does not reflect accurately the changes occurring in kidney morphology. Although there is a loose association between disease progression as assessed by decline of renal function, proteinuria and hypertension with glomerular sclerosis, interstitial scarring and vascular changes, these features are often present in biopsies from patients with no symptoms. By contrast, it is not unusual to discover rather bland changes of mesangial proliferative glomerulonephritis in patients with overt symptoms.

These factors require careful consideration when formulating treatment protocols for patients with IgA nephropathy. Moreover in a condition that varies so widely in severity and rate of progression, the decision whether to treat at all is the most important. Accurate assessment of any specific or nonspecific treatment therefore requires controlled studies with large treatment and control groups well matched for such factors as age, sex, degree of hypertension, proteinuria, and renal impairment, and the presence or absence of macroscopic hematuria episodes. In addition, histologic assessment of changes induced by therapy remains a fundamental requirement of any trial as at present there is no other specific marker for the disease. Patently, an ethical problem exists here as any specific treatment should be aimed at young patients early in the course of their disease (see chapter 18).

Conceptually, the aim of treatment is cure. In IgA nephropathy cure implies prolonged remission of clinical symptoms and urinary abnormalities, stability of hypertension and renal function, resolution of histologic abnormalities, and disappearance of IgA immunofluorescence and electron-dense deposits [1].

THE SEARCH FOR SPECIFIC THERAPY

As yet, no specific treatment is known to affect positively the course of IgA nephropathy. Pathogenetic mechanisms are not clearly defined and indeed may vary in individual patients. There are many potential areas wherein therapy may produce beneficial effects, however, by interrupting the disease process. Figure 15-1 demonstrates a schema of possible pathogenetic events leading to mesangial deposition, glomerular inflammation, and scarring. Little is known of the factors that promote deposition absorption or removal of mesangial immune material, but table 15-1 lists some possibilities.

ANTIGEN EXPOSURE

Several investigators have searched carefully for antigens common to many patients with IgA nephropathy [2, 3] without success. Current opinion suggests that the nature of the antigen may not be as important as the nature of the antibody response, as causative agents implicated have included ubiquitous viruses, bacteria, and food. Nevertheless, Kincaid-Smith and Nicholls [4] have reported a decline in the rate of red cell excretion associated with long-term tetracycline therapy. This is regarded as an important observation by these workers, who relate high red cell excretion to recurrent glomerular crescent formation and disease progression.

Important in this regard also may be alcohol ingestion. Alcohol is known to enhance absorption of macromolecules from the gut [5]. In our series of over 300 patients, there are five who claim a direct relationship between excessive alcohol ingestion and episodes of macroscopic hematuria. Refraining from alcohol has caused cessation of these episodes.

LYMPHOID TISSUE

Increasingly the pathogenesis of IgA nephropathy is being linked to disorders or aberrations of mucosal immunity. In particular, exacerbations of macroscopic hematuria are related to infections of tonsils, respiratory

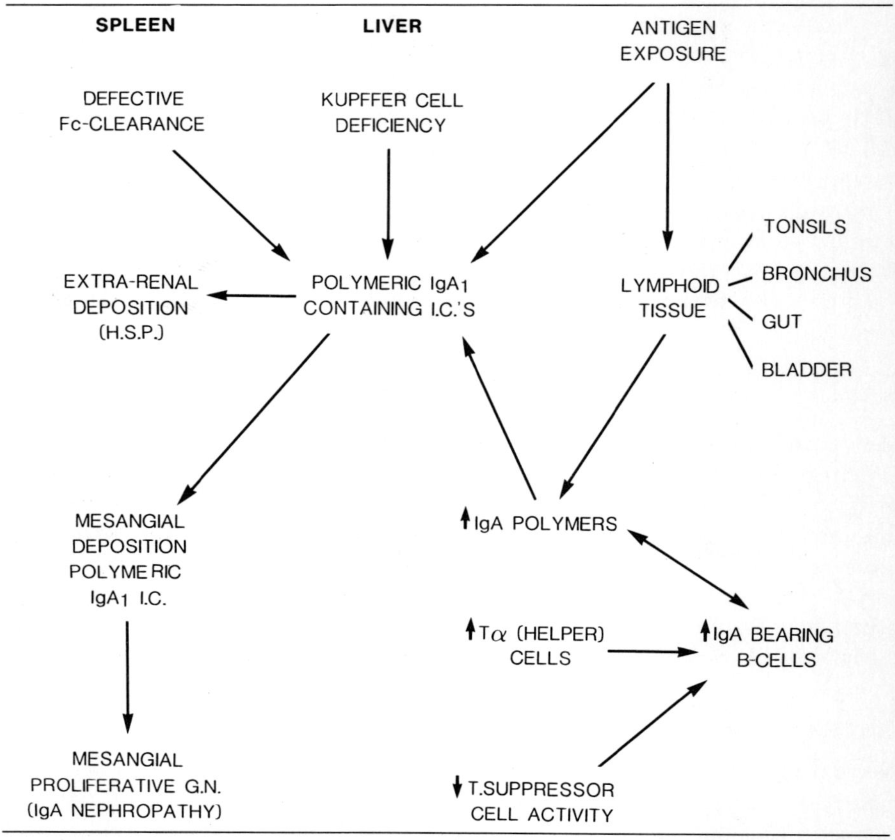

Figure 15-1. Schema of possible pathogenetic events leading to mesangial deposition of IgA.

(bronchi), gastrointestinal, and urinary tracts. If, as is postulated, antigenic stimulation of these tissues leads to increased production of dimeric IgA1 in IgA nephropathy patients, a strong case can be made for reduction in size of this lymphoid mass. Already tonsillar tissue from IgA nephritic patients has been shown to produce increased quantities of polymeric IgA1 when compared with nonnephritic patients (see chapter 11). It is not surprising, therefore, that improvement in the clinical features has been claimed following tonsillectomy [6]. Certainly, the tonsils are more amenable to removal without loss of body function than the other aforementioned tissues, but in addition they provide the site of the majority of infections leading to macroscopic hematuria (78% in our series). As suspected, however, episodes may recur following infections at other sites, as has occurred in several of our patients. It is the policy of our unit to rely on the usual otorhinolaryngologic

Table 15.1. Factors Determining Fate of Mesangial IgA Deposits

1. Rate of deposition and quantity of immune deposits
   (a) Antigen exposure
   (b) Production
   (c) R.E. clearance
2. Charge and size of deposits
3. Complement-mediated solubilization
4. Mesangial macrophage activity
5. Mediators
   (a) Complement
   (b) Coagulation
   (c) Platelets
   (d) Free oxygen radicals
6. Interruption of mesangial traffic
   (a) Angiotensin II
   (b) Prostaglandins
7. Physical factors
   (a) Hyperfiltration
   (b) Hypertension

indications for tonsillectomy in our patients. We would need to be convinced by evidence provided from a controlled study of tonsillectomy to change this policy.

IgA POLYMERS

For many years, therapy in progressive forms of glomerulonephritis was aimed at diminishing antibody production by using immunosuppressive agents. Unfortunately, during this period, immunofluorescence studies were not routinely applied to renal biopsies, although it seems certain in retrospect that many cases of IgA nephropathy were treated with such drugs as corticosteroids, azathioprine, and cyclophosphamide. Little evidence exists to suggest benefit was derived, although even now there is no recorded controlled study of a well-defined patient group.

Phenytoin

Phenytoin sodium has been shown by several groups of workers to lower serum IgA concentrations in epileptic subjects [7–12]. As serum IgA concentrations are raised in many patients with IgA nephropathy, phenytoin was used in a controlled trial of treatment by our group [13]. Despite causing significant decrease in serum IgA concentration in 74% of treated patients over a two-year period of follow-up, no clinical biochemical, serologic, or pathologic differences were observed between treatment and control groups.

Similar findings were reported by Coppo et al. [14] in a small group of patients with IgA nephropathy and Henoch-Schönlein purpura. Despite a fall in serum IgA concentrations, these authors found no significant changes in the circulating concentrations of IgA-containing immune complexes. Previously, Lopez-Trascasca et al. [15] had demonstrated a fall in the previously high polymeric serum IgA levels in patients treated with phenytoin.

Study of the affects of phenytoin on IgA polymers have been few and, despite this drug's seeming ineffectiveness when used alone, further study is perhaps warranted. Particularly, this may be the case if used in combination with agents which may influence mesangial IgA deposition.

Plasma exchange

Theoretically, plasma exchange may influence the course of IgA nephropathy by reducing circulating IgA polymers, circulating IgA immune complexes, and inflammatory mediators. Our experience [16] demonstrated that a single 2-liter exchange using a Hemonetics model 30 blood cell separator produced a mean reduction of serum IgA by 47%. While measurements of IgA polymers were not possible at that time, it is assumed these were removed. Like other authors [17, 18], we have noted resolution of acute symptoms (macroscopic hematuria, renal function impairment) associated with plasma exchange in patients with IgA nephropathy and Henoch-Schönlein purpura (HSP) [19]. Spontaneous in vitro IgA and IgG synthesis by peripheral blood mononuclear cells returned to normal from their previous high values following plasma exchange in one of our patients and corresponded with a sudden and sustained improvement in his clinical state. Unfortunately, this is an isolated observation and, while some other patients have shown a similar dramatic clinical improvement, others have not. Further controlled systematic studies are required.

Cyclosporine A

Theoretically cyclosporine A, a polypeptide derivative of fungal metabolism with a highly specific inhibitory effect on T-lymphocytes, may be of value in altering IgA metabolism. No reports of treatment of IgA nephropathy or HSP are available at present, however, although we have seen IgA nephropathy recur in a transplanted kidney at three months after grafting while the patient was receiving cyclosporine A.

IMMUNE COMPLEXES

Considerable evidence now exists to support the concept that the mesangial and extraglomerular deposits of IgA in both IgA nephropathy and HSP result from the deposition of circulating IgA-containing immune complexes. This is reviewed in chapters 4 and 11. There exist few therapeutic modalities that will alter immune complex load consistently. Of these, plasma exchange is the most tried, but not in a controlled fashion.

Plasma exchange

Despite clinical improvement observed with plasmapheresis in three patients treated by Hene and Kater [17], circulating immune complexes remained, a finding similar to that of McKenzie et al. [16] in a patient with severe HSP nephritis. By contrast Coppo et al. [20] recently noted clinical recovery in a patient with rapidly progressive IgA nephropathy treated by plasmapheresis, associated with removal of IgA-containing circulating immune complexes. By far, the largest group of patients subjected to plasma exchange therapy is that of Becker and Kincaid-Smith at the Royal Melbourne Hospital (G. Becker, personal communication). Analysis of their data suggests that this treatment may alter the course of the disease only while it is continued. All 22 patients treated showed deteriorating renal function in the three months prior to starting plasma exchange and most were receiving cyclosphosphamide, warfarin, and dypyridamole. Plasmapheresis was associated with improvement of renal function in 12, while in five patients renal function remained the same and in a further five there was deterioration. Follow-up indicated that the positive effect of plasmapheresis was temporary as five of the 12 "improvers," all of the five patients who had stable renal function, and four of the five who had deteriorating renal function during treatment are now on chronic hemodialysis. Cessation of treatment was accompanied by rapid deterioration in renal function. The preliminary results of this study are therefore tantalizing in the sense that it appears that plasma exchange therapy may influence disease progression, but seemingly does not alter significantly or permanently factors obviously important in pathogenesis.

In our experience, plasma exchange has not resulted in removal of mesangial IgA deposits, but disappearance of IgA and C3 deposits from the walls of dermal postcapillary venules was noted in four of five patients treated by Hene and Kater [17]. Increased C3b- and Fc-mediated clearance has been documented after plasmapheresis [21] whereas cyclophosphamide did not influence these functions. Whether mesangial deposits are influenced similarly is unknown.

MESANGIAL IgA DEPOSITS

Factors that potentially determine the fate of mesangial IgA deposits are shown in table 15-1. Possible means of altering the rate of deposition and quantity of immune deposits have been mentioned previously. In experimental animals, dose, size, and electrical charge are important determinants of glomerular capillary wall or mesangial deposition. As in animals, current evidence suggests that complexes of sufficient size to form lattices are prerequisites for the human disease. Thus J-chain-linked oligomeric IgA complexes, possibly of negative charge, are likely to be responsible for the mesangial deposits. Examination of physical or therapeutic means of interrupting this process is in its infancy.

Complement-mediated solubilization

On the basis of studies performed in vitro on renal biopsies from patients with IgA nephropathy, sera from the patients were shown to have a decreased capacity to solubilize the immune deposits compared with sera from healthy individuals [22]. On the basis that this deficiency was related to defective complement component activity, danazol, a testerone derviative known to increase serum complement levels in patients with complement deficiency, was administered to seven patients with IgA nephropathy [23]. Treated patients had less proteinuria and their sera demonstrated an increasing capacity for solubilization of mesangial deposits from renal biopsies in vitro, when compared with pretreatment sera. The long-term effect of such treatment is not known.

Mediators

Heparin and warfarin as anticoagulants, dipyridamole, and other agents with antiplatelet activity have been used extensively in the treatment of many forms of glomerulonephritis. Unfortunately, no controlled trials of this therapy either as single agents or in combinations with immunosuppressive drugs have been reported in IgA nephropathy. It is our impression that the disease course is not influenced by such treatment. In an interesting development, Hamazaki et al. [24] reported a preliminary trial of the use of eicosopentanoic acid (EPA) in patients with IgA nephropathy. This trial was based on the observation of Prickett et al. [25] that the mortality and incidence of severe glomerulonephritis in NZB/W mice were reduced by the addition of EPA to the diet, and the favorable effects of its use on the prevention of atherosclerosis [26].

It demonstrated that EPA appeared to prevent the deterioration of renal function in a treated group that was observed in untreated patients. Further studies are needed to confirm this observation and to determine whether changes in coagulation [27], platelet function [28], or production of oxygen-derived free radicals are responsible for this improvement. If the latter is found to be important, further refinement of diet or the introduction of inhibitors of oxy-radical production may be of advantage.

INTERRUPTION OF MESANGIAL TRAFFIC

Sequential studies of the mesangium after administration of substances such as ferritin, thorotrast, and gold to animals suggest that some of these may move toward the hilum of the glomerulus to the region of the juxtaglomerular apparatus. In addition, macromolecules may be removed from the mesangium as a result of ingestion by either mesangial cells or macrophages. It has been suggested that these substances are cleared from the mesangium to the lymphatic system or renal interstitium, or regurgitate into the glomerular capillary lumen. Factors such as size, shape, stickiness, and negative charge may favor mesangial localization. In the experimental animal, immune complexes already deposited impair the removal of aggregated IgG. Ureteric obstruction and angiotensin II have also been shown to increase mesangial deposition. Finally, mesangial cells grown in culture have been shown to produce prostaglandins [29].

In the future, it is likely that more attention will be paid, in patients with IgA nephropathy, to removal of mesangial IgA deposits. A strong candidate for therapy, alone or in combination with other drugs, is the angiotensin-converting enzyme inhibitor, Captopril. Captopril's influence on the kidney primarily reflects reduced angiotensin-II formation although reduced kinin degradation or increased prostaglandin synthesis is possible [30, 31]. Furthermore, Captopril interferes with immune regulation by inducing a suppressor circuit involving monocytes and a T8 suppressor lymphocyte [32]. Use of this drug may speed mesangial traffic and enhance removal of IgA deposits.

Physical factors

Hyperfiltration

Considerable evidence now exists that glomerular hyperfiltration leading to focal glomerulosclerosis and hyalinosis may be an integral mechanism leading to progression of renal impairment in patients with a large variety of renal diseases [33]. Certainly the morphologic features observed in cases of advanced IgA nephropathy support this point of view. We have observed dramatic improvement or stabilizing of renal function in patients with IgA nephropathy treated with reduced protein intake, although strict blood pressure control was also a feature of their management.

Hypertension

Strict blood pressure control is still considered by our unit to be the single most important factor in the effective treatment of patients with IgA nephropathy. As mentioned above, we possess circumstantial evidence strongly suggesting that adequate treatment of hypertension delays the progression of renal impairment. Perhaps the most appropriate hypotensive agent may be Captopril.

GENERAL CONSIDERATIONS

Acute renal failure

Episodes of acute renal failure, sometimes requiring dialysis, are not uncommon in IgA nephropathy [34, 35]. Treatment with corticosteroids, immunosuppressive drugs, and anticoagulants conveys no significant benefits in these situations, as results with conservative therapy are equally good [36]. These patients recover baseline renal function with dialysis and appropriate antibiotics.

Systemic symptoms

The presence of palpable purpura, particularly on the lower limbs and buttocks, polyarthritis, and gastrointestinal symptoms together with glomerulonephritis denoting Henoch-Schönlein purpura often evokes a different therapeutic response from the physician to that of primary IgA nephropathy. There is no evidence that the nephritis of HSP behaves differently from primary IgA nephropathy. Corticosteroid therapy is widely used in HSP, but does not influence the course of nephritis, rash, or arthropathy. Dramatic resolution of gastrointestinal lesions, particularly intramural hematomas, has, however, been described with both corticosteroids and plasma exchange therapy.

RENAL TRANSPLANTATION

IgA nephropathy presents no barrier to successful renal transplantation. Its recurrence in successful grafts has, however, provided insights into the nature of the primary disease. Recurrent mesangial electron-dense deposits have been reported with some regularity in patients with both IgA nephropathy [37, 38, 39, 40] and HSP [41, 42] receiving renal grafts. Recurrence is not related to HLA matching and affects approximately half the patients from three months to four years after transplantation. Clinically the recurrent disease is mild with macroscopic hematuria or cutaneous lesions (in the case of HSP) being most unusual. None of the 17 patients described by Berger et al. [43] have developed renal insufficiency after ten years although we have noted this in one case. Disease recurrence in grafts correlates well with reappearance in the circulation of IgA-containing immune complexes [44].

The other intriguing observation regarding transplantation concerns the disappearance of mesangial IgA deposits from kidneys already diseased with IgA nephropathy which inadvertently have been transplanted into patients without IgA nephropathy or HSP [45, 46]. Besides drawing attention to host factors important in the genesis of the disease, transplantation has provided, unwittingly, an opportunity to study the effects of immunosuppressive drugs on disease evolution. Unfortunately, corticosteroids, azathioprine, and cyclosporine A have not prevented disease recurrence.

SUMMARY

No satisfactory treatment exists for IgA nephropathy or HSP and indeed there has been a paucity of controlled therapeutic trials. This perhaps reflects the lack of clear clinical definition of the "syndrome of IgA nephropathy" until recently and poor understanding of its pathogenesis. In the future, more specific treatment will evolve with improved knowledge of mucosal immunity, the role of polymeric IgA and its regulation in determining mesangial deposition, and the factors determining mesangial function in health and disease.

REFERENCES

1. Clarkson AR, Woodroffe AJ: Therapeutic perspectives in mesangial IgA nephropathy. Contrib Nephrol 40:187–194, 1984.
2. Nagy J, Uj M, Szuks G, Trinn CS, Burger J: Herpes virus antigens and antibodies in kidney biopsies and sera of IgA glomerulonephritic patients. Clin Nephrol 21:259–263, 1984.
3. Woodroffe AJ, Goormly AA, McKenzie PE, Wootton AM, Thompson AJ, Seymour AE, Clarkson AR: Immunologic studies in IgA nephropathy. Kidney Int 18:366–374, 1980.
4. Kincaid-Smith PS, Nicholls K: Mesangial IgA nephropathy. Am J Kidney Dis 3:90–102, 1983.
5. Worthington BS, Meserole L, Syrotuck JA: Effects of daily ethanol ingestion on intestinal permeability to macromolecules. Dig Dis 28:23–32, 1978.
6. Lagrue G, Sadreux T, Laurent J, Hirbec G: Is there a treatment for IgA glomerulonephritis? Clin Nephrol 14:161, 1980.
7. Sorrel TC, Forbes IJ, Burness FR, Rishbieth RHC: Depression of immunological function in patients treated with phenytoin sodium (sodium diphenylhydantoin). Lancet 2:1233–1235, 1971.
8. Grob PJ, Herold, GE: Immunological abnormalities and hydantoins, Br Med J 2:561–563, 1972.
9. Sorrel TC, Forbes IJ: Depression of immune competence by phenytoin and carbemazepine: studies in vivo and in vitro. Clin Exp Immunol 20:273–279, 1975.
10. Seager J, Wilson J, Jamison DL, Hayward AR, Soothill JC: IgA deficiency, epilepsy and phenytoin treatment. Lancet 2:632–635, 1975.
11. Aarli JA, Tonder O: Effect of anti-epileptic drugs on serum and salivary IgA. Scand J Immunol 4:391–391, 1975.
12. Fontana A, Sauter R, Grob PJ, Joller H: IgA deficiency, epilepsy and hydantoin medication. Lancet 2:228–231, 1976.
13. Clarkson AR, Seymour AE, Woodroffe AJ, McKenzie PE, Chan Y-L, Wootton AM: Controlled trial of phenytoin therapy in IgA nephropathy. Clin Nephrol 13:215–218, 1980.
14. Coppo R, Basolo B, Bulzomi MR, Piccoli G: Ineffectiveness of phenytoin treatment on IgA-containing circulating immune complexes in IgA nephropathy. Nephron 36:275–276, 1984.
15. Lopez-Trascasca M, Egido J, Sancho J, Hernando L: Evidence of high polymeric IgA levels in serum of patients with Berger's disease and its modification with phenytoin treatment. Proc Eur Dial Transplant Assoc 16:513, 1979.
16. McKenzie PE, Taylor AE, Woodroffe AJ, Seymour AE, Chan Y-L, Clarkson AR: Plasmapheresis in glomerulonephritis. Clin Nephrol 12:97–108, 1979.
17. Hene RJ, Kater L: Plasmapheresis in nephritis associated with Henoch-Schönlein purpura and in primary IgA nephropathy. Plasma Ther Transfus Technol 4:165–173, 1983.
18. Kauffmann RH, Hourwert DA: Plasmapheresis in rapidly progressive Henoch-Schönlein glomerulonephritis and the effect on circulating IgA immune complexes. Clin Nephrol 16:155–160, 1981.
19. Bannister KM, Drew PA, Clarkson AR, Woodroffe AJ: Immunoregulation in glomerulonephritis, Henoch-Schönlein purpura and lupus nephritis. Clin Exp Immunol 53:384–390, 1983.
20. Coppo R, Basolo B, Giachino O, Rocatelli D, Lajola D, Mazzucco G, Amore A, Piccoli G: Plasmapheresis in a patient with rapidly progressive idiopathic IgA nephropathy: removal of IgA-containing immune complexes and clinical recovery. Nephron 40:488–490, 1985.
21. Nicholls K, Kincaid-Smith P: Defective in vivo Fc- and C3b-receptor function in IgA nephropathy. Am J Kidney Dis 4:128–134, 1984.
22. Tomino Y, Sakai H, Suga T, Kaneshige H, Endoh M, Nomoto Y: Impaired solubilization of tissue-deposited immune-complexes by sera from patients with IgA nephropathy. Am J Kidney Dis 3:48–54, 1983.
23. Tomino Y, Sakai H, Miura M, Suga T, Endoh M, Nomoto Y: Effect of Danazol on solubilization of immune deposition in patients with IgA nephropathy. Am J Kidney Dis 4:135–140, 1984.
24. Hamazaki T, Tateno S, Shishedo H: Eicosapentanoic acid and IgA nephropathy. Lancet 1:1017–1018, 1984.
25. Prickett JD, Robinson DR, Steinberg AD: Effects of dietary enrichment with eicosapenta-

noic acid upon auto-immune nephritis in female NZB/NZW F_1 mice. Arthritis Rheum 26:133–139, 1983.
26. Dyerberg J, Bang, HD: Atherogenesis and haemostasis in Eskimos: the role of the prostaglandin-3 family. Haemostasis 8:227–233, 1979.
27. Sanders TAB, Roshanai F: The influence of different types of W-3 polyunsaturated fatty acids on blood lipids and platelet function in healthy volunteers. Clin Sci 64:91–99, 1983.
28. Hay CRM, Durber AP, Saynor R: Effects of fish oil on platelet kinetics in patients with ischaemic heart disease. Lancet 1:1269–1272, 1982.
29. Michael AF: The glomerular mesangium. Contrib Nephrol 40:7–18, 1984.
30. Kreisberg JI, Karnovsky MJ, Levine L: Prostaglandin production by homogeneous cultures of rat glomerular epithelial and mesangial cells. Kidney Int 22:355–359, 1982.
31. Hollenberg NK: Angiotensin-converting enzyme inhibition: renal aspects. J Cardiovasc Pharmacol 7:540–544, 1985.
32. Deleraissy J-F, Galanaud P, Balavoine J-F, Wallon C, Dormont J: Captopril and immune regulation. Kideny Int 25:925–929, 1984.
33. Brenner BM, Meyer TW, Hotstetter TH: Dietary protein intake and the progressive nature of kidney disease: the role of haemodynamically mediated glomerular injury in the pathogenesis of progressive glomerular sclerosis in aging, renal abaltion and intrinsic renal disease. N Engl J Med 307:652–659, 1982.
34. Clarkson AR, Seymour AE, Thompson AJ, Haynes WDG, Chan Y-L, Jackson B: IgA nephropathy: a syndrome of uniform morphology, diverse clinical features and uncertain prognosis. Clin Nephrol 8:459–471, 1977.
35. Kincaid-Smith P, Bennett WM, Dowling JP, Ryan GB: Acute renal failure and tubular necrosis assoicated with haematuria due to glomerulonephritis. Clin Nephrol 19:206–210, 1983.
36. Clarkson AR, Seymour AE, Chan Y-L, Thompson AJ, Woodroffe AJ: Clinical, pathological and therapeutic aspects of IgA nephropathy. In: P. Kincaid-Smith. A. D'Apice, R. Atkins (eds) Progress in glomerulonephritis New York: John Wiley and Sons, 1979, pp 247–160.
37. Berger J, Yaneva H, Nabarra B, Barbanel C: Recurrence of mesangial deposition of IgA after renal transplantation. Kidney Int 1:232–241, 1975.
38. Mathew TH, Mathews DC, Hobbs, JB, Kincaid-Smith P: Glomerular lesions after renal transplatation. Am J Med 7:177–190, 1975.
39. Morzycka M, Croker BP, Siegler HF, Tisher CC: Evaluation of recurrent glomerulonephritis in kidney allografts. Am J Med 72:588–598, 1982.
40. Siegler HF, Ward FE, MacCoy RE, Weinerth JL, Gunnels JC, Stickel DL: Long-term results with forty-five living-related renal allograft recipients genetically identical for HLA. Surgery 81:274–283, 1977.
41. Levy M, Moussa RA, Habib R, Gagnadoux MF, Broyer M: Anaphylactoid purpura nephritis and transplantation. Kidney Int 22:326, 1982.
42. Baliah T, Kim KH, Anthone S, Anthone R, Montes M, Andres GA: Recurrence of Henoch-Schönlein purpura glomerulonephritis in transplanted kidneys. Transplantation 18:343–346, 1974.
43. Berger J, Noel LH, Nabarra B: Recurrence of mesangial IgA nephropathy after renal transplantation. Contrib Nephrol 40:195–197, 1984.
44. Le Savre P, Digeon M, Bach JF: Analysis of circulating IgA and detection of immune complexes in primary IgA nephropathy. Clin Exp Immunol 48:61–69, 1982.
45. Silva FG, Ghanda P, Priani CL, Hardy KA: Disappearance of glomerular mesangial IgA deposits after renal allograft transplantation. Transplantation 33:214–216, 1982.
46. Sanfilippo F, Croker BP, Bollinger RR: Fate of four cadaveric renal allografts with mesangial IgA deposits. Transplantation 33:370–372, 1982

16. THE FUTURE: A JAPANESE PERSPECTIVE

YASUHIKO TOMINO

IgA nephropathy is a distinct clinicopathologic entity originally described by Berger and Hinglais in 1968 [1]. IgA nephropathy (so-called Berger's disease) is a more common type of glomerulonephritis in Japan than in France, the USA, and England [2–4]. Patients with IgA nephropathy account for more than 30% of patients with primary glomerulonephritis in Japan [4]. It is still unknown whether geographic and/or genetic factors are involved in the difference in the prevalence. Although IgA nephropathy is assumed to be an immune-complex-mediated glomerulonephritis, the antigens and exacerbating factors involved in this disease have not yet been identified. Moreover, there is no specific treatment of patients with IgA nephropathy. The purposes of this chapter are: (a) to describe the approach to pathogenesis and exacerbating factors, and (b) to describe the trials in new treatments for patients with IgA nephropathy.

APPROACH TO THE PATHOGENESIS

IgA nephropathy is considered to be an immune-complex-mediated glomerulonephritis as follows [5]: (1) depositions of IgA and C3 are observed in the glomerular mesangial areas by immunofluorescence, (2) electron-dense deposits are observed in the same areas, (3) IgA and/or C3 are also deposited in the vascular walls of subcutaneous or intramuscular vessels by imunofluorescence, (4) IgA-dominant immune complexes in sera are determined using several different techniques, and (5) the recurrence of IgA nephropathy occurred in the renal grafts of transplanted patients. Histopathologically, IgA nephropathy is characterized by mesangial hypertrophy with or without mesangial cell proliferation. Therefore, IgA nephropathy is generally considered to be a proliferative glomerulonephritis induced by deposition of IgA-dominant immune complexes. It is yet to be determined whether the immune complexes detected in IgA nephropathy are circulating soluble antigen–antibody complexes or specific antibodies directed against renal tissues. There are no data regarding implanted mesangial antigens in IgA nephropathy, i.e., immune complex formation in situ. Virus-like particles and/or microtubular structures were occasionally observed in the glomerular mesangial areas by electron microscopy (T. Itoh, personal communication). It is still unknown whether such materials are antigenic substances in patients with IgA nephropathy. Lowance et al. [6] have reported that some patients with IgA nephropathy demonstrated an antimesangial antibody that reacted with mesangial areas in normal kidneys. Clarkson et al. [7] have not been able to detect antimesangial antibody activity in sera from patients with IgA nephropathy. Recently, we reported that eluted IgA antibodies obtained from renal tissues in IgA nephropathy were specifically recombined with the mesangial areas of these patients [8]. The eluted antibodies reacted with only 60% of the renal tissues from patients with IgA nephropathy. It is postulated that these antibodies show some heterogeneity among patients with IgA nephropathy. There is speculation that there are several antigenic materials in renal tissues from patients with IgA nephropathy and vice versa. We have also indicated that the antibodies obtained from IgA nephropathy did not show any antimesangial activity because they did not react with normal glomeruli or nephritic glomeruli other than those from patients with IgA nephropathy [8].

André et al. [9] reported that IgA2 was frequently observed in glomeruli from patients with IgA nephropathy and Henoch-Schönlein purpura (HSP) nephritis by immunofluorescence. On the other hand, Conley et al. [10] and the authors [11] noted that IgA1 deposition was mainly observed in glomeruli from patients with these diseases. Recently, we have also reported that IgA1-dominant immune complexes were phagocytosed by peripheral blood polymorphonuclear leukocytes in patients with IgA nephropathy [12]. The J (joining) chain was deposited in the glomerular mesangial areas from some patients with IgA nephropathy as described by Komatsu et al. [13] and the authors [14]. Although the deposition of secretory component (SC) was not observed in the glomeruli [2], SC binding capacity to glomerular mesangial areas was observed in patients with IgA nephropathy [15]. It was indicated that immune complexes deposited in glomeruli were mainly composed of IgA1 dimers or polymers in patients with IgA nephropathy [14]. Recently, Valentijn et al. [16] detected macromolecular IgA1 in the circulation and mesangial deposits in patients with IgA nephropathy. The subclass of IgA does not decisively indicate where it is produced. IgA1 is not only observed in the bone marrow, but also in the mucosal system although IgA1 is the predominant subclass of IgA in the bone marrow. In the bone marrow, 70% of IgA1 is monomer. It is generally considered that the numbers of cells containing IgA polymers and J chain are higher in the mucosal system than in the bone marrow.

The antigens involved in IgA nephropathy have not yet been identified. Since IgA is an important immunoglobulin for defense mechanisms against exogenous antigens in the mucosal system, the antigens might be located in the mucosal membranes from patients with IgA nephropathy. It is speculated that there are many kinds of antigenic substances, i.e., viruses and/or bacilli, in patients with IgA nephropathy as follows: (1) respiratory antigens, (2) intestinal antigens, (3) dietary antigens, (4) biliary antigens, and (5) dermal antigenic substances. It is still unknown whether the antigenic materials are exogenous and/or endogenous in patients with IgA nephropathy. Recently, Sinniah (17) showed the possible mechanisms for pathogenesis in IgA nephropathy. In 1980, Woodroffe et al. [18] observed a significant temporal rise in antibody titer to specific infectious antigens, i.e., gut flora or food antigens. Nagy et al. [19] indicated herpes antigens and antibodies in renal tissues and sera from patients with IgA nephropathy. Clinically, IgA nephropathy is frequently preceded by episodes of upper respiratory tract infection, which is presumed to have some viral etiology. Finlayson et al. [20] and the authors [21] reported an increase of nasal or pharyngeal IgA concentrations in some patients with IgA nephropathy.

We have recently pointed out the antigenic substances in the upper respiratory tracts from patients with IgA nephropathy as follows: first, the eluted antibodies obtained from renal tissues were labeled with iodine-125 by the chloramine-T methods. Iodine-125-labeled eluate was applied to the pharyngeal cells obtained from the same and other patients with IgA nephropathy as well as to those with other glomerular diseases using autoradiographic analysis [22]. The eluted antibodies bound with the pharyngeal cells from the same patients, but only 10% of them bound with the pharyngeal cells obtained from other patients with IgA nephropathy (figure 16-1). It is concluded that IgA antibodies deposited in renal tissues specifically bind with pharyngeal cells obtained from patients with IgA nephropathy and that these antibodies show some heterogeneity among such patients. Second, we examined the cytopathic effects (CPE) of extracts of pharyngeal cells from patients with IgA nephropathy on fibroblasts such as Vero or Hel cells [23]. Autoradiographic analysis of antigens in the fibroblasts was also performed. Briefly, freeze-and-thawed extracts of pharyngeal cells obtained from patients with IgA nephropathy, other glomerular diseases, and healthy adults were cultured with those fibroblasts at 37°C for one or two weeks. Thereafter, CPE of fibroblasts were examined with a light microscope. In addition, these fibroblasts were incubated with iodine-125-labeled eluate from the same or other patients with IgA nephropathy as described above. CPE of extracts of

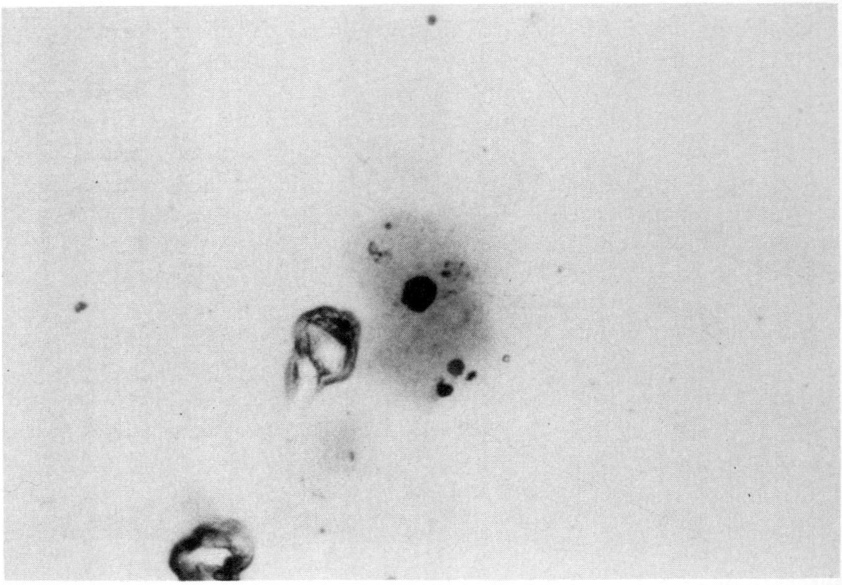

Figure 16-1. Eluted antibodies from renal tissues were bound with pharyngeal cells from the same patient with IgA nephropathy.

pharyngeal cells from patients with IgA nephropathy on Vero or Hel cells was significantly increased compared with that from patients with other glomerular diseases or healthy adults without glomerular diseases. CPE of such fibroblasts was not inhibited by a Millipore filtration of extracts of pharyngeal cells obtained from patients with IgA nephropathy (figure 16-2). It was shown that the antibodies eluted from the renal tissues of patients with IgA nephropathy specifically bound with the nuclear regions of such fibroblasts [24]. It was suggested that some antigenic substances might exist in the epithelial cells of the upper respiratory tracts of some patients with IgA nephropathy, and that such antigens could be transferred to cultured fibroblasts. The supernatants of fibroblasts previously cultured with freeze–thawed extracts of pharyngeal cells from patients with IgA nephropathy showed CPE on newly prepared fibroblasts. There might be weak pathogenic changes in the upper respiratory tracts from patients with IgA nephropathy since the degree of CPE on newly prepared fibroblasts was decreased compared with that on initially prepared fibroblasts. Third, the cultured fibroblasts described above were incubated with the serum samples from the same or other patients with IgA nephropathy [25]. These cells were stained with FITC-labeled heavy-chain-specific antihuman IgA antiserum and then examined with a fluorescent microscope. It was demonstrated that the IgA antibodies in sera obtained from patients with IgA nephropathy

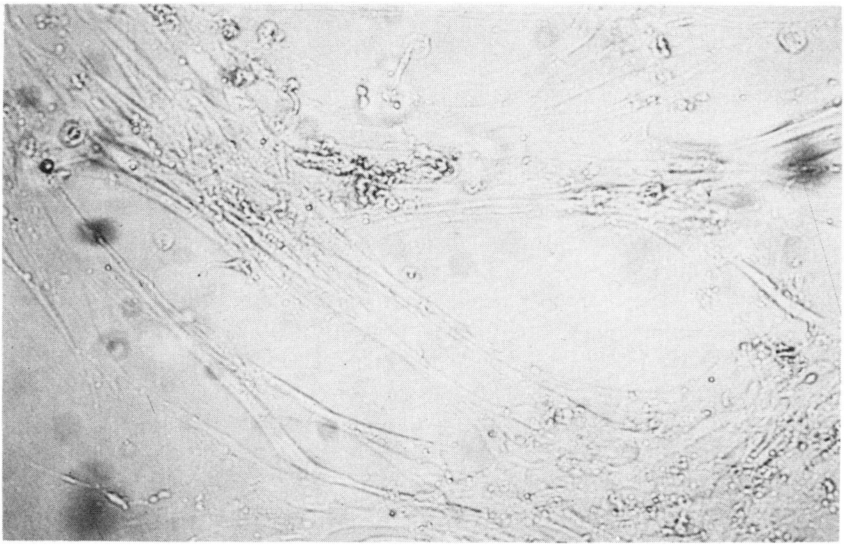

Figure 16-2. CPE of extracts of pharyngeal cells from a patient with IgA nephropathy on Hel cells.

bound with the nuclear regions of such fibroblasts. It appeared that cirulating IgA antibodies could be detected by antigenic substances that are presumably increased in the fibroblasts during the cultures with the extracts of pharyngeal cells in patients with IgA nephropathy. It was suggested that IgA antibodies in sera could be bound with some antigenic substances that were transferred from pharyngeal cells of patients with IgA nephropathy to fibroblasts in vitro and vice versa.

Some heterogeneity was observed among the patients with IgA nephropathy as described above. It appears, therefore, that some antigens such as viruses may exist in the upper respiratory tracts that provide continuous antigenic stimulation in patients with IgA nephropathy. At present, viral particles have not been observed in fibroblasts and pharyngeal cells from patients with IgA nephropathy by electron microscopy (Y. Tomino, unpublished). Further examinations are warranted to determine whether the antigenic materials in the pharyngeal cells are viral particles and/or their structural proteins in patients with IgA nephropathy. Further studies are also warranted to determine whether such antigenic materials are DNA and/or RNA viruses.

DETECTION OF EXACERBATING FACTORS

Although the clinical course of IgA nephropathy is considered to be benign, hypertension and progression to renal failure are not as rare as originally thought. Factors previously reported to be associated with disease progression have been male sex, prolonged duration, nephrotic-range proteinuria, hypertension, and glomerular sclerosis in patients with IgA nephropathy. Recently, Nicholls et al. [26] reported three cases of "malignant" IgA nephropathy. All three patients had loin pain, constantly elevated urinary erythrocyte counts, and crescents in the renal biopsy. In Japan, Yoshida and Ohno [27] indicated several progressive factors of IgA nephropathy such as severe histologic injuries, heavy proteinuria, imparied renal function, and hypertension. Several investigators indicated the development and/or exacerbating factors for patients with IgA nephropathy as follows: increasing platelet aggregation in the glomeruli, and impairment of the reticuloendothelial system (RES) including phagocytic activities of polymorphonuclear leukocytes [28, 29].

In 1980, we reported a close association between complement deposition (C3, C5, C9, and properdin) and destruction of glomerular tissues from patients with IgA nephropathy [30]. It was suggested that the analysis of complement deposition in glomeruli is useful for estimation of histopathologic alterations and thus the prognosis of patients with IgA nephropathy. Furthermore, we have reported that the solubilization of glomerular immune deposits by sera was significantly less in patients with IgA nephropathy than that by sera in healthy adults [31]. It is possible that impaired solubilization of immune complexes in vivo could lead to the accumulation of glomerular immune deposits in patients with IgA nephropathy.

Recently, Miura et al. [32], using immunofluorescence, reported the deposition of alpha-2-plasmin inhibitor (α2-PI) and/or fibrinogen in glomeruli from patients with IgA nephropathy. Glomerular injuries such as glomerular adhesion to Bowman's capsule and the celluar and/or fibrous crescent were predominantly observed in the glomeruli with α2-PI and/or fibrinogen deposits in patients with IgA nephropathy. It was suggested that the deposition of α2-PI in vivo might lead to the accumulation of glomerular fibrinogen deposits in patients with IgA nephropathy.

It is indicated that the complement systems, intraglomerular coagulation, and/or their regulating systems may play a role in the development of inflammatory changes in the glomeruli from patients with IgA nephropathy. Further examinations are warranted to determine the inhibitory and/or repair mechanisms against these major systems in patients with IgA nephropathy.

NEW TREATMENT FOR PATIENTS WITH IgA NEPHROPATHY

At present, there is no specific treatment for patients with IgA nephropathy. Previous approaches have included tonsillectomy, immunosuppressive drugs, phenytoin, and plasma exchanges [33]. In Japan, antiplatelet drugs such as dipyridamole and nonsteroidal antiinflammatory drugs were generally used for patients with chronic glomerulonephritis including IgA nephropathy [34].

Proteinuria and/or hematuria disappeared after the administration of antiplatelet drugs in some patients with IgA nephropathy.

Recently, we employed two new treatments for patients with IgA nephropathy as follows: (a) single-shot administration of urokinase for fibrinolysis in the glomeruli [35, 36], and (b) danazol administration for increasing the solubilization capacity of sera against the deposited immune complexes [37]. First, we reported the significant effects of a "single shot" administration of urokinase on fibrinolytic activities in some patients with IgA nephropathy. In 1965, urokinase was commercially produced from fresh urine in Japan. The molecular weight of urokinase is 54,000. Since urokinase is one of the activators of plasminogen in plasma, it shows defibrination capacity in vivo and in vitro. The amounts of proteinuria examined after the administration of urokinase were significantly decreased compared with those examined before the administration of urokinase in patients with IgA nephropathy. Furthermore, marked improvement of proteinuria after urokinase therapy was observed in patients without deposition of α2-PI in glomeruli from patients with IgA nephropathy as described by Miura et al. [38]. Second, we reported the significant effects of danazol on solubilization of immune deposits in patients with IgA nephropathy [37]. The solubilization capacity of sera against the glomerular immune deposits from patients with IgA nephropathy was significantly decreased as described above [31]. In 1975, Miller and Nussenzweig [39] showed that antigen–antibody aggregates were solubilized by the addition of fresh sera. It was shown that this phenomenon depends essentially on the alternative pathway of complement. The heterocyclic steroid danazol (2, 3-isoxazol derivative of 17 α-ethyl testosterone) is considered to increase the levels of serm complement in patients with complement deficiency such as hereditary angineurotic edema (HANE). It was shown that the solubilization of glomerular immune deposits by sera after the administration of danazol from patients with IgA nephropathy was significantly higher than that by sera before such treatment. The improvement of proteinuria was observed in some patients with IgA nephropathy since this was in parallel with the increase in the levels of serum C4, C3, and CH50. It was suggested that administration of danazol may be useful for the solubilization of glomerular immune deposits and for the improvement of proteinuria in some patients with IgA nephropathy.

Based on etiologic findings, further new treatment trials are warranted for patients with IgA nephropathy.

REFERENCES

1. Berger J, Hinglais N: Les dépôts intercapillarés d'IgA-IgG. J Urol Nephrol 74:694–695, 1968.
2. Shirai T, Tomino Y, Sato M, et al.: IgA nephropathy-Clinicopathology and immunopathology. Contrib Nephrol 9:88–100, 1978.
3. D'Amico G: Idiopathic mesangial IgA nephropathy. In: Glomerular injury, 300 years after Morgagni. Bertani T, Remuzzi G (eds), Milan: Wichtig Editore, pp 205–228, 1983.

4. Kitajima T, Murakami M, Sakai O: Clinicopathological features in the Japanese patients with IgA nephropathy. Jpn J Med 22:219–222, 1983.
5. McCoy RC, Abramowsky CR, Tisher CC: IgA nephropathy. Am J Pathol 76:123–144, 1974.
6. Lowance DC, Mullins JD, McPhaul JJ Jr: Immunoglobulin A (IgA) associated glomerulonephritis. Kidney Int 3:167–176, 1973.
7. Clarkson AR, Woodroffe AJ, Bannister KM, et al.: The syndrome of IgA nephropathy. Clin Nephrol 21:7–14, 1984.
8. Tomino Y, Endoh M, Nomoto Y, et al.: Specificity of eluted antibody from renal tissues of patients with IgA nephropathy. Am J Kidney Dis 1:276–280, 1982.
9. André C, Berthoux FC, André F, et al.: Prevalence of IgA2 deposits in IgA nephropathies: a clue to their pathogenesis. N Engl J Med 303:1343–1346, 1980.
10. Conley ME, Cooper MD, Michael AF: Selective deposition of immunoglobulin A1 in immunoglobulin A nephropathy, anaphylactoid purpura nephritis and systemic lupus erythematosus. J Clin Invest 66:1432–1436, 1980.
11. Tomino Y, Endoh M, Nomoto Y, et al.: Detection of immunoglobulin A1 in kidney tissues from patients with IgA nephropathy. N Engl J Med 305:1159–1160, 1981.
12. Tomino Y, Miura M, Suga T, et al.: Detection of IgA1-dominant immune complexes in peripheral blood polymorphonuclear leukocytes by double immunofluorescence in patients with IgA nephropathy. Nephron 37:137–139, 1985.
13. Komatsu N, Nagura H, Watanabe K, et al.: Mesangial deposition of J chain-linked polymeric IgA in IgA nephropathy. Nephron 33:61–64, 1983.
14. Tomino Y, Sakai H, Miura M, et al.: Detection of polymeric IgA in glomeruli from patients with IgA nephropathy. Clin Exp Immunol 49:419–425, 1982.
15. Bene M-C, Faure G, Duheille J: IgA nephropathy: characterization of the polymeric nature of mesangial deposits by in vitro binding of free secretory component. Clin Exp Immunol 47:527–534, 1982.
16. Valentijn RM, Radl J, Haayman JJ, et al.: Macromolecular IgA1 in the circulation and mesangial deposits in patients with primary IgA nephropathy. Contrib Nephrol 40:87–92, 1984.
17. Sinniah R: IgA mesangial nephropathy: Berger's disease. Am J Nephrol 5:73–83, 1985.
18. Woodroffe AJ, Gormly AA, McKenzie PE, et al.: Immunologic studies in IgA nephropathy. Kidney Int 18:366–374, 1980.
19. Nagy J, Uj M, Szucs G, et al.: Herpes virus antigens and antibodies in kidney biopsies and sera of IgA glomerulonephritis. Clin Nephrol 21:259–262, 1984.
20. Finlayson G, Alexander R, Juncos L, et al.: Immunoglobulin A glomerulonephritis: a clinicopathologic study. Lab Invest 32:140–148, 1975.
21. Tomino Y, Endoh M, Kaneshige H, et al.: Increase of IgA in pharyngeal washings from patients with IgA nephropathy. Am J Med Sci 286:15–21, 1983.
22. Tomino Y, Sakai H, Endoh M, et al.: Cross-reactivity of IgA antibodies between renal mesangial areas and nuclei of tonsillar cells in patients with IgA nephropathy. Clin Exp Immunol 51:605–610, 1983.
23. Tomino Y, Sakai H, Miura M, et al.: Cytopathic effects of antigens in patients with IgA nephropathy. Nephron 42:161–166, 1986.
24. Tomino Y, Sakai H, Miura M, et al.: Detection of antigenic substances in patients with IgA nephropathy. Contrib Nephrol 40:69–73, 1984.
25. Tomino Y, Sakai H, Miura M, et al.: Specific binding of circulating IgA antibodies in patients with IgA nephropathy. Am J Kidney Dis 6:149–153, 1986.
26. Nicholls K, Walker RG, Dowling JP, et al.: "Malignant" IgA nephropathy. Am J Kidney Dis 5:42–46, 1985.
27. Yoshida M, Ohno J: Primary glomerular diseases in internal medicine [in Japanese]. Pathol Clin Med 2:888–894, 1984.
28. Woo KT, Tan YO, Yap HK, et al.: Beta2-microglobulin in mesangial IgA nephropathy. Nephron 37:78–81, 1984.
29. Sato M, Morikawa K, Koshikawa S: Attachment of polymorphonuclear leukocytes to glomeruli in IgA nephropathy. Clin Immunol Immunopathol 29:111–118, 1983.
30. Tomino Y: Complement system in IgA nephropathy. Tokai J Exp Clin Med 5:15–22, 1980.
31. Tomino Y, Sakai H, Suga T, et al.: Impaired solubilization of glomerular immune deposits by sera from patients with IgA nephropathy. Am J Kidney Dis 3:48–53, 1983.

32. Miura M, Tomino, Endoh M, et al.: Immunofluorescent studies on alpha 2-plasmin inhibitor (α2-PI) in glomeruli from patients with IgA nephropathy. Clin Exp Immunol 62:380–386, 1985.
33. Clarkson AR, Woodroffe AJ: Therapeutic perspectives in mesangial IgA nephropathy. Contrib Nephrol 40:187–194, 1984.
34. Kurokawa K, Yoshida M, Sakai O, et al.: IgA nephropathy in Japan. Am J Nephrol 5:127–137, 1985.
35. Tomino Y, Miura M, Suga T, et al.: Defibrination of intraglomerular fibrin deposits by urokinase in patients with IgA nephropathy. Jpn J Nephrol 26:275–280, 1984.
36. Tomino Y, Miura M, Suga T, et al.: Effects of a "single shot" of urokinase on fibrinolytic activities in patients with IgA nephropathy. Tokai J Exp Clin Med 9:43–47, 1984.
37. Tomino Y, Sakai H, Miura M, et al.: Effects of danazol on solubilization activities of immune deposits in patients with IgA nephropathy. Am J Kidney Dis 4:135–140, 1984.
38. Miura M, Tomino Y, Yagame M, et al.: Significant correlation between the immunofluorescence of alpha 2-plasmin inhibitor in glomeruli and the effects of urokinase therapy in patients with IgA nephropathy. Annals Academy of Medicine 15:255–257, 1986.
39. Miller GW, Nussenzweig, V.: A new complement function: solubilization of antigen–antibody aggregates. Proc Natl Acad Sci USA 72:418–422, 1975.

17. THE FUTURE: AN AUSTRALIAN PERSPECTIVE

ANDREW J. WOODROFFE

The recognition of Berger's disease is still relatively recent and awareness of its high prevalence and true functional importance is even more so. Therefore, one of our first obligations should be to educate the profession with respect to the diagnostic importance of IgA nephropathy as a frequent cause of hematuria, proteinuria, hypertension, and renal failure. In doing so, we should stress the significance of "synpharyngitic" hematuria and of the presence of "glomerular type" red blood cells in the urine and referral for renal biopsy should be advocated as the definitive investigation in such patients. Without such promotion, the condition will continue to be underdiagnosed and its true prevalence grossly understated. In turn, we need to carry out formal epidemiologic and life-table analytic studies of IgA nephropathy, as exemplified by Sinniah et al. in Singapore [1, 2] and D'Amico in Milan [3].

Continued research into the pathogenesis of the condition is vital and it is to be hoped that research-funding bodies in Australia will see this as a high priority; data indicating that IgA nephropathy is now the most frequent type of glomerulonephritis in Australian dialysis patients [4] should help to make this point. The present chapter addresses the areas of research activity in IgA nephropathy that the author would like to pursue, given enough time and money in the future, while emphasizing that there is nothing uniquely Australian about these ideas. Indeed, the value of a multinational approach to IgA nephropathy research was most evident at the recent meetings in Milan [5] and in Los Angeles [6].

FUTURE RESEARCH AND PRIORITIES

Antigen identification

This is necessary to prove the immune complex nature of the mesangial deposits, this still being only a working hypothesis, albeit one that is strongly supported on the other grounds (see chapter 14). Techniques for the identification of antigen and the specificity of antibody have been established for both circulating and glomerular immune complexes, but their application is limited by the need to know what to look for, and a negative result means nothing. Likely antigens are common dietary and gut flora proteins or polysaccharides and, of course, specific infectious agents responsible for individual episodes of clinical disease activity. We and others have looked for such antigens in the mesangial deposits without success, but this could be due to masking by excess in vivo antibody. In theory, this problem could be overcome by preliminary partial elution of the sections or by using "antigen immunofluorescence" [7], but both approaches present additional difficulties. The recovery of IgA from microeluates of biopsy sections would allow a search for antibody specificity and this technique has already been used successfully by one group in identifying antibodies to the mesangia and to tonsillar cells obtained from patients with IgA nephropathy [8, 9]. This last approach is limited by the amount of renal tissue and is probably only practicable if open biopsies are performed. Studies with circulating immune complexes share the same kind of problems and, in addition, the relevance of serum proteins to the mesangial deposits will always be open to question. To summarize, this area of research is of academic importance, but the technical problems and interpretive difficulties may be limiting.

In vivo clearance studies

The use of Fc (splenic) or C3b (hepatic)-mediated clearance determinations in patients with IgA nephropathy has been expedient rather than optimal and it should be possible to carry out similar studies using radiolabeled polymeric IgA. Such studies have already been performed in patients with liver disease in whom a selective reduction of the fractional catabolic rate of ^{125}I-polymeric IgA was observed [10]. However, the problem in IgA nephropathy patients may still be to determine whether any observed impairment in clearance is primary or secondary to saturation of receptor sites.

Studies of IgA production

Extensive analysis of the relevant numerical and functional parameters of peripheral blood lymphocytes (PBL) has already been carried out in IgA nephropathy patients (reviewed in chapter 14). Most of these studies provide evidence of an immunoregulatory defect in these patients with an increase in the production of IgA, but there is no consensus regarding the precise nature of the defect. Further studies are required, particularly to identify specific abnormalities in T- and/or B-cell function and to look for correlates with other parameters such as serum IgA concentrations and disease activity. In addition, more PBL studies need to be carried out in the relatives of patients and these should be combined with HLA typing.

In contrast, relatively little work has been done on aspects of mucosal and secretory immunity and these areas of research are likely to be both productive and important. Currently, there are data that indicate normal numbers of intestinal IgA-bearing lymphocytes [11], increased tonsillar IgA plasma cells [12], an increased production of polymeric IgA by tonsillar cells [13], and a normal (J. Feehally, personal communication) or increased [14] IgA content of nasopharyngeal secretions. Further quantitative studies of total IgA and of the A1 and A2 subclasses in secretions are needed together with a functional evaluation of the IgA response to musosally presented antigens. This last approach could provide definitive data regarding the integrity and function of the secretory immune system in patients with IgA nephropathy.

Analysis of the mediation of glomerular injury

Very little is understood about the mediation of injury in IgA nephropathy. As indicated earlier (see chapter 14), IgA deposits alone do not appear to be responsible and, while complement, coagulation, proteinases, prostaglandins, and macrophages have all been suggested as possible mediators of injury, there are really no firm data one way or the other.

This is a critical area both for understanding why glomerular and, in some instances, skin, joint, and gut diseases develop and for planning logical new forms of treatment. Animal models of "IgA disease" are likely to help us in these respects. Perhaps the most biologically relevant model is that induced in mice by oral administration of foreign proteins [15], but others, including the passive administration of IgA immune complexes, may also be suitable for these purposes.

The development of a serum diagnosis for IgA nephropathy

In the same way that ANA and anti-DNA antibody determinations are routinely used to screen for systemic lupus erythematosus a blood test for IgA nephropathy would be of great value. There are already a number of serologic abnormalities described in IgA nephropathy patients (increased serum IgA, IgA class immune complexes, polymeric serum IgA, cold-reactive ANA, etc.—see chapter 14), but none of these is present in all patients.

A deliberate search for a specific serologic marker is most important. One suggested approach is an assay based on the recognition of neoantigens expressed on complexed IgA1 dimers in the serum of such patients. This and other appropriate assay systems are worthy of analysis.

Prognostic indices

One of the most frustrating clinical problems is the uncertainty of the long-term prognosis for renal function in an individual patient. We need to identify the early indices that can differentiate patients with progressive disease from those with a benign course.

A number of clinicopathologic features that appear to be associated with a poor prognosis have already been described (reviewed in chapters 7 and 8). Briefly, these include hypertension, proteinuria, and elevated serum creatinine; glomerular sclerosis, interstitial fibrosis, and vascular changes. The presence or absence of macrohematuria as a prognostic marker is still unresolved as is the HLA typing. With respect to the latter, we have found no HLA-DR antigen associations in IgA nephropathy and, in particular, no antigen more frequently in the poor-prognosis patients [16]. Finally, most investigators agree that the amount of mesangial IgA does not correlate with prognosis.

It is very clear that more studies are needed in this area and that these will have to include additional, perhaps as yet undefined, parameters and mediators of the disease.

Development of treatment

Existing approaches to treatment have already ben reviewed (see chapter 15). These have included antibiotics, tonsillectomy, prednisolone, cyclophosphamide, antiplatelet drugs, urokinase, phenytoin, danazol, dapsone, and plasma exchange. There have been occasional reports of success, but I think most nephrologists remain skeptical and are of the opinion that there is currently no effective treatment for the disease. The high incidence of recurrent disease in grafted kidneys is particularly disappointing, at least with conventional immunosuppressive therapy—data from cyclosporine-treated patients are not yet available.

In theory, future advances in therapy may stem from reducing antigen exposure, decreasing IgA production, increasing the clearance of IgA polymers and complexes, or blocking the mediators of glomerular injury (figure 17–1). The first approach is probably not feasible, but the others should be, at least in experimental models of disease. In subsequent application to the treatment of patients, it is absolutely essential that there be carefully designed clinical trials.

SUMMARY

The future is never easy to predict, but, with respect to IgA nephropathy, I can foresee the condition becoming accepted as an important entity in Australia, albeit with continued discussion as to the proper subcategorization of such patients, and that increased efforts will be allocated to studying the

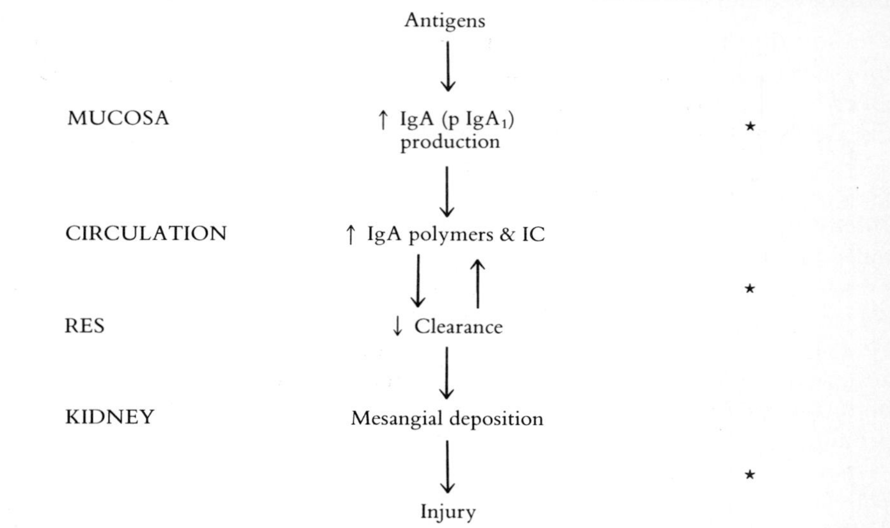

Figure 17-1. Scheme of the pathogenesis of IgA nephropathy and steps (*) at which new forms of treatment could be directed.

Table 17-1. Priorities of future research in IgA nephropathy

Clinical and epidemiologic studies	+++
Antigen identification	±
In vivo clearance studies	+
Studies of mucosal production of IgA	++
Analysis of the mediators of glomerular injury	++++
Development of a serum diagnosis	+++
Establishment of prognostic indicies	++++
Development of treatment	++++++

prevalence, epidemiology, natural history, and pathogenesis of the condition. All of these aspects are important, but I would rank them as in table 17–1, with most emphasis being placed on the development and evaluation of new and potentially effective forms of treatment. In pursuing these priorities, it may be profitable to involve people from disciplines other than nephrology, pathology, and immunology. Fresh insights are needed and these may be forthcoming in collaborative work with biochemists, physiologists, or clinical pharmacologists.

REFERENCES

1. Sinniah R, Pwee HS, Lim CH: Glomerular lesions in asymptomatic microscopic haematuria discovered on routine medical examination. Clin Nephrol 5:216–228, 1976.
2. Sinniah R, Lim CH, Pwee HS: Glomerular lesions in patients with asymptomatic persistent

and orthostatic proteinuria discovered on routine medical examination. Clin Nephrol 7:1–14, 1977.
3. D'Amico G: Natural history and treatment of idiopathic IgA nephropathy. In: Robinson RR (ed) Proceedings of the 9th international congress on nephrology, vol 1. New York: Springer-Verlag, 1984, pp 686–701.
4. Seventh Report of the Australian and New Zealand Dialysis and Transplant Registry, July 1984.
5. 1st international Milano meeting of nephrology on IgA mesangial nephropathy. Contrib Nephrol 40: – , 1983.
6. Symposium on IgA nephropathy, Los Angeles. In: Robinson RR (ed) international congress on nephrology, vol 1. New York: Springer-Verlag, 1984, pp 645–701.
7. Woodroffe AJ, Wilson CB: An evaluation of elution techniques in the study of immune complex glomerulonephritis. J Immunol 118:1788–1794, 1977.
8. Tomino Y,Endoh M, Nomoto Y, Sakai H: Specificity of eluted antibodies from renal tissues of patients with IgA nephropathy. Am J Kidney Dis 1:276–280, 1982.
9. Tomino Y, Sakai H, Endoh M, Suga T, Miura M, Kaneshige H, Nomoto Y: Cross-reactivity of IgA antibodies between renal mesangial areas and nuclei of tonsillar cells in patients with IgA nephropathy. Clin Exp Immunol 51:605–610, 1983.
10. Delacroix DL, Elkon KB, Geubel AP, Hodgson HF, Dive C, Vaerman JP: Changes in size, subclass, and metabolic properties of serum immunoglobulin A in liver diseases and in other diseases with high serum immunoglobulin A. J Clin Invest 71:358:367, 1983.
11. Westberg NG, Baklien K, Schmekel B, Gillberg R, Brandtzaeg P: Quantitation of immunoglobulin-producing cells in small intestinal mucosa of patients with IgA nephropathy. Clin Immunol Immunopathol 26:442–445, 1983.
12. Bene MC, Faure G, Hurault de Ligny B, Kessler M, Duheille J: Quantitative immunohistomorphometry of the tonsillar plasma cells evidences an inversion of the immunoglobulin A versus immunoglobulin G secreting cell balance. J Clin Invest 71:1342–1347, 1983.
13. Egido J, Blasco R, Lozano L, Sancho J: Immunological abnormalities in tonsils of patients with IgA nephropathy: inversion in the percentage of IgA verus IgG-bearing lymphocytes and increased polymeric IgA synthesis. Clin Exp Immunol 57:101–106, 1984.
14. Tomino Y, Endoh M, Kaneshige H, Nomoto Y, Sakai H: Increase of IgA in pharyngeal washings from patients with IgA nephropathy. Am J Med Sci 286:15–21, 1983.
15. Emancipator SN, Gallo GR, Lamm ME: Experimental IgA nephropathy induced by oral immunization. J Exp Med 157:572–582, 1983.
16. Disney APS: Australian and New Zealand Dialysis and Transplant Registry, 1985.

18. THE FUTURE: A PEDIATRIC PERSPECTIVE

RONALD J. HOGG, ABDALLA RIFAI, JUDY B. SPLAWSKI, and ROBERT J. WYATT

Since an unfavorable clinical outcome is now expected for a significant percentage of IgA nephropathy patients [1–9], the demonstration of factors that are associated with the development of end-stage renal disease will be an important area of investigation in the next few years. In order to understand whether risk factors that are identified in adult patients will be important for the pediatric patient, it is necessary to consider the differences in expression of clinical disease that exist between adult and pediatric patients.

An examination of European and American series of pediatric and adult patients with IgA nephropathy reveals that clinical presentations often differ between the two age groups [1–8, 10–14]. In Europe and North America, children usually present with macroscopic hematuria [5, 7, 8, 10], whereas less than half of the adult patients have macroscopic hematuria. In Asia, both children and adults with IgA nephropathy have a low incidence of macroscopic hematuria [9, 15–17]. The reasons for these disparities need to be clarified. In addition, most of these studies indicate that adult patients *without* macroscopic hematuria are *more likely* to develop chronic renal failure [1, 5, 6, 13]. In contrast, a large pediatric series from North America suggests that children with macroscopic hematuria are more likely to have severe disease [10, 18].

Another reported difference between pediatric and adult IgA nephropathy patients is a lower frequency of elevated serum IgA concentration in pediatric patients. The frequency of this finding in most adult series is about 40% [1,

3, 6], and, although published data on serum IgA concentration in pediatric patients are limited, the frequency of children with an elevated level *for age* is usually reported to be in the range of 20% [3, 8, 10]. Finally, it should be noted that few of the reported studies on IgA-related immunologic parameters, such as circulating IgA complexes, polymeric IgA, or T-cell subsets, give data on the age of the subjects. Presumably, few of these studies include a significant number of children. Thus, little is known about IgA-related immunologic parameters for children with IgA nephropathy. This area requires additional study.

In this chapter, we expand on areas of research that we believe should be explored in order to further define these apparent differences in the clinical and laboratory expressions of IgA nephropathy between children in the West compared to children in the East and adults throughout the world.

HOST FACTORS

Studies to determine children "at risk": genetic profiles

Evidence implicating an inherited component in the pathogenesis of IgA nephropathy has been provided by at least 14 reports of familial disease [15, 19–31]. A major obstacle to the future investigation of the mechanism of inheritance of IgA nephropathy is the probability that mesangial IgA deposition occurs in a vast number of individuals who never have any manifestation of clinical disease [32] and the demonstration that some individuals detected with clinical disease go into an apparent phase of remission in which the urinalysis becomes normal [5]. It will be necessary, therefore, to perform repeated urinalyses in all family members to obtain adequate phenotypic profiles.

An alternative approach to the demonstration of familial IgA nephropathy may be provided by immunologic surveillance of family members. A number of immunologic abnormalities have been demonstrated in first-degree relatives of IgA nephropathy patients. Sakai et al. showed that at least one first-degree relative of ten patients had an increased number of IgA-bearing lymphocytes [33]. Egido et al. performed studies in a father and son who both had IgA nephropathy and also in two brothers who were clinically unaffected [29]. While the father and all three sons had increased production of polymeric IgA following stimulation of their lymphocytes by pokeweed mitogen, increased serum concentrations of polymeric IgA were only demonstrated in the two individuals with IgA nephropathy. When these observations were extended to 25 first-degree relatives of seven patients, 60% demonstrated an elevated production of polymeric IgA after pokeweed mitogen stimulation [34]. These observations fit the hypothesis that a primary defect involving excess polymeric IgA production leads to clinically evident disease in only a small percentage of affected individuals.

The data from the immunologic studies in patients and their first-degree relatives, along with data from the familial case studies, are consistent with the existence of a single disease susceptibility gene for IgA nephropathy that could be inherited in an autosomal dominant fashion. Clinical disease would occur in individuals who had an additional defect(s), such as impaired clearance of IgA complexes. From a pediatric perspective, the identification of susceptible children and the observation of the clinical behavior of these children over time holds great potential for the identification of factors that are important for disease expression.

In many studies, the prognostic significance of particular HLA alleles has been examined and an association with poor outcome has been suggested for B35 in France [35], DR4 in Japan [26], and DR blanks in the Netherlands [2]. However, none of the pediatric series of IgA nephropathy patients have examined the frequency or prognostic relevance of HLA antigen frequencies. In the future, prospective studies of large numbers of patients with onset in childhood might provide new insights into the reasons for the presence or lack of HLA associations in the disease. Such studies may answer the question of whether particular alleles can be correlated with the severity of the histologic lesion and/or the prognosis of the patient.

Evaluation of the immunologic mechanisms responsible for IgA deposition in the kidneys of children with IgAN

Elevated serum IgA levels, increased numbers of IgA-bearing cells in the peripheral blood, and increased in vitro synthesis of IgA have all been described in patients with IgA nephropathy [36–38], suggesting either excessive chronic stimulation of a normal mucosa or an abnormal response to a normal stimulus. A mucosal etiology is also suggested by the typical prodromal infectious illness that is observed in most of the children with IgA nephropathy who have episodes of gross hematuria.

Abnormal chronic stimulation of a normal mucosa has been the basis for utilizing gastrointestinal immunization to develop an experimental model for IgA nephropathy [39]. The elevation of the polymeric form of IgA and circulating IgA immune complexes also supports a role for mucosal stimulation [36, 40–42]. However, definitive proof of mucosal abnormality is lacking. Although the tonsils of patients with IgA nephropathy were found to have increased numbers of IgA plasma cells—suggesting increased stimulation [43]—subsequent studies of gastrointestinal biopsies from eight patients with IgA nephropathy were found to be normal [44]. Intermittent abnormalities or more subtle defects of the mucosa remain possibilities that should be investigated further.

Another possible explanation for the IgA abnormalities found in these patients involves an abnormal response to a normal stimulus. This is consistent with the genetic studies discussed above and with the finding that asymptomatic family members may have similar immune defects [34]. Also, the fact that IgA nephropathy can occur so early in childhood and can continue to be a life-long disease suggests that an immunologic defect may contribute to the etiology. The production and secretion of IgA appear to be intact in that polymer and monomer forms of IgA are present as well as both subclasses; therefore, a defect in the regulation of IgA is possible. Recent evidence suggests, that after immunization with a specific antigen, IgA antibodies to antigens other than the immunizing antigen were also elevated, suggesting a polyclonal rather than a selective response [45]. IgA responses are highly dependent on T cells and T-cell factors. T-cell abnormalities have been noted in patients and in asymptomatic relatives [34, 46]. Determination of OKT4 to OKT8 ratios or helper/inducer versus suppressor/cytotoxic cells has led to varied results [46, 47]. Alterations of these T-cell subsets need to be verified. An elevation of T cells with receptors for the Fc portion of the IgA molecule has also been reported in patients with IgA nephropathy [48, 49]. Both augmentation and suppression of IgA responses have been attributed to these cells [50, 51]. The role of these cells in the regulation of IgA secretion needs to be defined before the clinical significance of the abnormalities in IgA nephropathy can be determined.

Very few immunologic studies have been reported in pediatric patients with IgA nephropathy. The goal of future studies should include investigation of the immunologic parameters in children. Comparisons should be made with age-matched controls to allow for developmental differences. Immunologic studies of family members should be done to detect immunologic defects that may play a role in the etiology of the disease.

ENVIRONMENT FACTORS: SEARCH FOR "THE ANTIGEN" IN CHILDREN WITH IgAN

One of the most poorly defined areas relative to the role of immune complexes in children with IgA nephropathy is precise identification of the antigen involved. The close temporal relationship between an upper respiratory tract or gastrointestinal infection and episodes of gross hematuria has been described as a frequent feature of IgA nephropathy in children [7, 8, 11, 12]. The fact that this has also been associated with circulating IgA immune complexes [52] strongly implicates infectious agents as the source of antigen.

The possible role of viral antigens has been suggested recently by studies of Tomino et al. [53], who demonstrated that IgA antibodies eluted from renal tissues of patients with IgA nephropathy specifically bound to nuclear regions of only fibroblasts cocultured with the same patients' tonsillar extracts. These eluted antibodies, however, were heterogeneous because only 10% of the cases had IgA that reacted with tonsillar cells obtained from other IgA nephropathy patients. Nagy et al. [54] reported that IgA antibodies to Epstein-Barr virus capsid antigen (EBV-VCA) were significantly more frequent in the circulation of IgA nephropathy patients. Attempts to identify a specific viral antigen in the glomerular deposits in these studies, however, were unsuccessful.

Enthusiasm for future studies to define a viral etiology for IgA nephropathy should be tempered by a potentially equivalent role for a bacterial agent. Such a role was initially suggested by Clarkson et al. [55], who referred to a group of five patients with IgA nephropathy and acute renal failure associated with bacterial infection. Collectively, these observations suggest that the antigen repertoire in IgA immune-complex-mediated nephropathy is diverse. This diversity may be reflected by the spectrum of renal histopathologic changes, by the differences in clinical manifestations of Henoch-Schönlein purpura as opposed to primary IgA nephropathy without systemic features, and by the unpredictability of disease outcome reported in IgA nephropathy. Whether the initial or a different antigen is associated with each recurrent episode remains to be examined. The likely variability in antigenic composition of IgA immune complexes during the course of IgA nephropathy will nullify the use of any single antimicrobial agent in treatment. Persistence of IgA complexes in the glomeruli or circulation requires a continuous source of antigen supply. It is unknown whether a persistent infection or antiidiotypes that possess the internal image of the antigen may serve as a reservoir.

It will be important to define in future studies how the role of differing antigens can be integrated into the total clinical picture. Studies to answer this problem in children will require a comprehensive approach and a long-term research program that combines the efforts of pediatric nephrologists, pathologists, microbiologists, and immunologists: Characterization of viral and/or bacterial isolates from the upper respiratory or gastrointestinal tract of children during periods of exacerbations and convalescence will be very important. Serologic analysis for IgA-specific antibodies to suspected or isolated microbial antigens should be conducted on paired sera. In addition, eluates of renal biopsies, when available, need to be analyzed by sensitive immunoassays for specific antibodies or suspected microbial antigens, and aliquots of patients' sera should be preserved for potential use in a future investigation. The establishment of antigenic, serologic, histopathologic, and clinical profiles for each child will aid in establishing the much searched for criteria of diagnosis, prognosis, and potential therapy for IgA nephropathy. It is very unlikely that either the scientific expertise or the necessary population of children to develop these criteria will be available in a single pediatric nephrology center. Successful achievement of the stated objectives will almost certainly demand multicenter collaboration. It should be emphasized that identification of exogenous antigens should start, if possible, with the earliest presentation during childhood. These patients are the ideal subjects for long-term prospective studies.

EFFECTOR MECHANISMS

Delineation of the IgA subtypes involved in IgAN in children: polymer vs monomer

The increased serum IgA in IgA nephropathy has been reported to be predominantly polymeric IgA [36]. However, there are also reports that suggest that monomeric IgA levels may be elevated as well [56]. In vitro studies demonstrate an increase in the secretion of polymeric IgA [38]. Deposits of IgA in the kidney have been found by some investigators to contain J chain and to bind secretory component, suggesting that it is polymeric; however, other groups have failed to confirm these findings [57, 58].

Elevation of predominantly polymer IgA would suggest increased secretion of IgA plasma cells located at mucosal surfaces. An increase in the number of IgA-containing plasma cells at the mucosal surfaces and an increase in the secretion of polymeric IgA by these cells have been described [43]. An elevation of monomeric IgA, as well as polymeric IgA, would suggest a more generalized abnormality of IgA regulation that may or may not be specifically related to mucosal immunity. Since all patients with elevations of IgA do not get IgA nephropathy, an increased level of IgA by itself would not appear to be the cause of the renal pathology. The increased serum IgA levels may, however, contribute to the glomerular injury that is induced by the formation of increased numbers of IgA-containing immune complexes.

Children have an increased polymeric to monomeric IgA ratio than that seen in adults [59–62]. Although IgA nephropathy can be seen as early as three years of age, the peak incidence of this disease in children is 8.8 years in girls and ten years in boys [63]. At the present time, there is not enough evidence to speculate on whether there is an age relationship between the normal development of the different forms of IgA and the time of onset of disease; however, further investigation of these developmental differences may be important in enhancing our understanding of the etiology of IgA nephropathy.

Most studies report deposition of the IgA1 subtype in the kidneys [64, 65]. This may be due to the fact that 80% of serum IgA is the IgA1 subclass. There are only a few reported biologic differences between the subclasses. Only IgA1 binds to the asialoglycoprotein receptors in the liver. The importance of this pathway for hepatic clearance, however, is unclear [66]. More information is needed on the antigenic restriction and regulation of the IgA subclasses to determine whether the IgA1 subclass plays a major role in the pathogenesis of this disease. Newborns have nearly equal serum levels of IgA1 and IgA2; IgA1 begins to be predominant at 3.5 months [67]. Developmental differences may again provide a mechanism whereby this issue can be probed.

Determination of the role of defective IgA clearance

The role of defective IgA clearance in the pathogenesis of IgA nephropathy remains poorly understood. This is due, in part, to the lack of information regarding the normal mechanisms that are called upon to handle IgA complexes and dispose of them where necessary. Experimentally, removal of IgA immune complexes from the circulation of rodents is mediated by a specific IgA receptor on Kupffer cells [68]. Although similar work has not been attempted in humans, indirect evidence for an analogous mechanism has been derived from the studies of Kater et al. [69], who demonstrated a direct correlation between a characteristic pattern of IgA deposits in both liver sinusoids and renal parenchyma in patients with alcoholic liver disease. These studies suggest that impairment in the removal of IgA immune complexes by a receptor on liver sinusoidal cells may result in their glomerular deposition. In this respect, the association of alcoholic liver disease and IgA nephropathy is well established [70].

Several recent reports have examined the relationship between splenic clearance of IgG-coated red blood cells and IgA nephropathy [71–73]. However, a major criticism of those studies has been the use of IgG RBC as a probe. Neither the class of antibody used nor the particulate nature of the complex bear any resemblance to IgA immune complexes. Ideally, the investigation of a defect in the elimination of circulating IgA immune complexes in IgA nephropathy requires the use of soluble IgA immune complexes, with defined size and composition, as a probe. Such probes could be used in trace amounts to measure clearance and assess function of specific IgA removal in patients with IgA nephropathy. However, the stress associated with repeated blood sampling in the pediatric patient makes this approach less desirable than the development of a different approach that would utilize this probe in vitro.

Finally, it should be noted that, in marked contrast to the large number of studies documenting circulating IgA immune complexes in adult patients, there is a paucity of similar information in children. Thus, the relevance of a defect in IgA removal to childhood IgA nephropathy must be preceded by clinical studies to determine whether high levels of IgA immune complexes are present in the circulation of pediatric patients with IgA nephropathy.

Role of complement in IgAN

A number of previous studies suggest that the alternative complement pathway has a pathogenic role in IgA nephropathy [74, 75]. This concept has been supported by other studies that indicate the ability of IgA-containing material to activate the alternative complement pathway in vitro [76–78]. Such activators include chemically aggregated myeloma IgA [76], IgA immune complexes made with mouse myeloma IgA [77], and aggregated human secretory IgA [78]. A major problem with the application of these data to human IgA nephropathy is the possibility that the IgA aggregates or complexes used are different in concentration and/or composition to the polymeric IgA or circulating IgA complexes that might be present in vivo in either children or adults.

Measurement of serum concentrations of individual complement proteins in adult IgA nephropathy patients shows that, except in the unusual instances of partial deficiency states, the levels are normal or increased [79]. However, since complement activation may be present in the face of normal levels of C3 [80], sensitive assays for breakdown fragments generated upon activation of C3 and C4 are needed to determine whether activation is occurring in an individual. The limited data on complement breakdown fragments in IgA nephropathy patients consistently show C3 activation in 50% of the patients [80, 81]. Although the above data are extremely limited, they do indicate a potential role for C3 activation in the pathogenesis of IgA nephropathy. We believe that future prospective studies of IgA nephropathy in children should include the determination of a possible correlation between complement breakdown fragment concentrations and parameters such as renal function, episodes of macroscopic hematuria, and the severity of histologic lesions. However, such studies will require a large number of pediatric patients to have serial plasmas obtained during different phases of disease activity.

CLINICAL ASPECTS

Further assessment of the prognostic importance of gross hematuria and/or severe proteinuria in children with IgAN

As indicated elsewhere in this text, there have been disparate reports of the prognostic import that should be ascribed to episodes of gross hematuria and/or severe proteinuria in children and adults with IgA nephropathy. If gross hematuria proves to be a reliable marker of further and/or progressive glomerular injury [82], reduction in the frequency of this classic and readily identifiable feature will be a useful indicator of therapetuic response in clinical trials. Hence it is important that further clarification of the meaning and significance of gross hematuria be obtained. This will require very careful assessment of studies of renal function before, during, and after periods of gross hematuria. In a small series of pediatric patients, Linné et al. [83] found that gross hematuria, occurring early in the disease course, was associated with a reversible depression of glomerular filtration rate (GFR), which they considered to be a functional response. However, the same authors also stated that patients who showed progressive irreversible deterioration of GFR had more frequent and more severe bouts of gross hematuria. Thus, the extent to which renal parenchymal damage followed the episodes of gross hematuria appeared to vary within a small number of patients. More definitive studies will require a much larger group of patients, a point recently emphasized by Robson [84].

The significance of severe proteinuria in children with IgA nephropathy has also become somewhat obscure as the result of some recent observations [85, 86]. There seems to be little doubt that, in general, children with heavy proteinuria have the most severe glomerular lesions [7, 10, 87] and the least favorable prognosis [7, 87]. However, there appears to be a significant number of children who have nephrotic-range proteinuria associated with mild glomerular lesions. Such children have usually shown excellent clinical responses to corticosteroids and/or cytotoxic agents [85, 86], suggesting a dissociation between the mild IgA-induced mesangiopathy and the heavy proteinuria in some children with this disease. Further clarification of the prognostic importance of heavy proteinuria in individual patients is therefore needed.

Future goals in the treatment of childhood IgA nephropathy

As indicated above, more information is necessary to determine whether any aspects of the pathogenesis of IgA nephropathy may be amenable to therapeutic intervention. Attention should be focused on the immunologic insult that is thought to trigger this mesangiopathy. The subsequent treatment modalities that will be developed should be oriented most specifically at patients in whom the disease process has not caused irreversible renal parenchymal damage. This should include children in whom evidence of disease, by definition, has been of relatively short duration.

When considering future pediatric treatment protocols, an issue of great importance will be the determination of the appropriate patients in whom the treatment will be evaluated. The methods that will be used to assess successful therapy will have to be sensitive since IgA nephropathy is so often an indolent disease. Levy et al. [88] have suggested that treatment protocols should be directed only toward children with diffuse proliferative glomerulonephritis since these are the patients who have been shown to be most likely to develop progressive disease in follow-up studies. This approach may be appropriate with future considerations of "invasive" measures such as tonsillectomy [89], plasmapheresis [90], or intravenous "pulses" of methylprednisolone [91], but it would seem appropriate to include children with "less severe" disease (i.e., WHO classes 1 and 2, and/or low-grade or absent proteinuria) in long-term studies when agents with relatively low toxicity [92] are used to modify the initial immunologic insult, since it has been shown by Berger that patients with "few segmental lesions" may also progress to CRF within a few years [21].

The most appropriate measures to assess the success of future treatments have not been defined, but it is essential that any study design should also include a control group since the clinical expression of IgA nephropathy fluctuates greatly in many patients. Repeat renal biopsies and serial immunologic studies should be considered since these may provide early indications of success or failure. It may be possible to conduct meaningful studies of children with IgA nephropathy within the general framework of protocols oriented toward adults. However, if this is done, it is essential that the results be expressed in terms of the specific age groups under study.

An alternative approach to prospective studies of IgA nephropathy in children will be made possible by multicenter collaborative studies. It is apparent that the large number of patients identified in 26 pediatric centers in Japan by Kitajima et al. [9] would provide an excellent patient group for prospective studies. Similarly, in US children, a large number of patients have been identified by the Southwest Pediatric Nephrology Study Group [10, 18]. Regardless of the specific collaborative arrangements, whether they be regional, national, or international, there seems little doubt that multicenter therapeutic trials of specific treatments for IgA nephropathy in children constitute one of the most important methods by which we may reduce the number of patients who are destined to develop end-stage renal failure from this disease in adult life.

It is also relevant in this section to reiterate that proteinuria has been associated with more severe histologic changes [10] and a poor prognosis in most patients with IgA nephropathy [87]. However, the extent to which the magnitude of the proteinuria per se may result in the progressive deterioration has not yet been elucidated. There is now increasing evidence that persistent passage of abnormally large quantities of protein across the glomerular filter may induce progressive renal dysfunction in a variety of renal diseases. It is likely therefore that progressive dietary restriction of protein will become an integral component of the treatment of IgA nephropathy in adults. Caution should be exercised before this approach is extended to children, however, since the overall consequences (including growth) of protein restriction in growing children with IgA nephropathy have not yet been elucidated.

Future role of school urine-screening programs to identify IgAN

In the largest series of children with IgA nephropathy yet reported [9], Kitajima et al. reported clinical and pathologic features in 500 patients from 26 Japanese departments of pediatrics. The information was collected by means of a questionnaire that was circulated throughout that nation. It is important to note that, of the 304 boys and 196 girls identified by this survey, 74.2% were diagnosed following the discovery of "chance proteinuria and/or hematuria, which is accidentally detected by annual physical checkups at schools ...." The authors also noted that "since the law obliges school children and adults to undergo urinalysis in Japan, there are rather many cases of nephritis detected as chance proteinuria." The fact that almost three out of four cases of IgA nephropathy in the Japanese children identified in this study would not have been diagnosed if the customary indications for renal biopsy in Australia, the USA, or the UK had been in effect raises a question as to the number of children with IgA nephropathy who are *not diagnosed* in these latter countries.

Should other countries adopt the Japanese approach to diagnose children with IgA nephropathy early in the disease course? At the present time, the paucity of knowledge regarding useful outcome indicators in such asymptomatic patients and the complete absence of effective therapeutic measures leads us to conclude that early diagnosis is of dubious value in the routine care of such patients. If careful follow-up studies are performed in populations that are identified, however the information that ensues may result in more definitive statements regarding prognosis and treatment. If that happens, it will be necessary to completely reevaluate the potential benefit of school screening programs in countries where they are not presently performed.

SUMMARY

The major premise on which the present chapter has been based is that IgA nephropathy is a major contributor to the end-stage renal disease population worldwide. We have reviewed the many avenues of research that may be explored to obtain a more thorough understanding of IgA nephropathy in children. It is our conviction that the origins of IgA nephropathy usually reside in childhood and that the development of successful modes of intervention during this period will offer the greatest potential for reducing the high morbidity and mortality associated with this disease in adults. The development of well-defined prospective studies to evaluate the immunogenetics of IgA nephropathy, the mechanisms of progressive disease, and the indications for treatment will require some invasive procedures and drug trials in children who otherwise might be followed conservatively. However, the lack of such studies will leave the present gaps unfilled, and the prognostic and therapeutic advice will remain anecdotal and unsatisfactory. Hopefully, this will not be the case.

REFERENCES

1. Droz D: Natural history of primary glomerulonephritis with mesangial deposits of IgA. Contrib Nephrol 2:150–157, 1976.
2. Van der Peet J, Arisz L, Brentjens JRH, Marrink J, Hoedemaeker PhJ: The clinical course of IgA nephropathy in adults. Clin Nephrol 8:335–340, 1977.
3. Clarkson AR, Seymour AE, Thompson AJ, Haynes WDG, Chan Y-L, Jackson B: IgA nephropathy: a syndrome of uniform morphology, diverse clinical features and uncertain prognosis. Clin Nephrol 8:459–471, 1977.
4. Berger J, Yaneva H, Crosnier J: La glomerulonéphrite à dépôts mésangiaux d'IgA: une cause frequente d'insuffisance renal terminale. Nouv Presse Med 9:219–21, 1980.
5. Wyatt RJ, Julian BA, Bhathena DB, Mitchell BL, Holland NH, Malluche HH: IgA nephropathy: presentation, clinical course and prognosis in children and adults. Am J Kidney Dis 4:192–200, 1984.
6. D'Amico G, Imbasciati E, Barbiano di Belgioioso G, Bertoli S, Fogazzi G, Ferrario F, Fellin

G, Ragni A, Colasanti G, Minetti L, Ponticelli C: Idiopathic IgA mesangial nephropathy: clinical and histological study of 374 patients. Medicine 64:49–60, 1985.
7. Levy M, Beaufils H, Gubler MC, Habib R: Idiopathic recurrent macroscopic hematuria and mesangial IgA-IgG deposits in children (Berger's disease). Clin Nephrol 2:63–69, 1973.
8. Michalk D, Waldherr R, Seelig HP, Weber HP, Scharer K: Idiopathic mesangial IgA-glomerulonephritis in childhood: description of 19 pediatric cases and review of the literature. Eur J Pediatr 134:13–22, 1980.
9. Kitajima T, Murakami M, Sakai O: Clinicopathological features in the Japanese patients with IgA nephropathy. Jpn J Med 22:219–222, 1983.
10. Southwest Pediatric Nephrology Study Group: A multicenter study of IgA nephropathy in children. Kidney Int 22:643–652, 1982.
11. Kerr KK, Makker SP, Moorthy B: IgA nephropathy in children (Berger's disease): a clinicopathologic study in children. Int J Pediatr Nephrol 4:11–18, 1983.
12. McEnery PT, McAdams AJ, West CD: Glomerular morphology, natural history and treatment of children with IgA nephropathy. In: Kincaid-Smith P, Mathew TH, Becker EL (eds) Glomerulonephritis. New York: John Wiley and Sons, 1973, pp 305–320.
13. Beukhof JR, Ockhuizen TH, Halie LM, Westra J, Beelen JM, Donker AJM, Hoedemaeker PhJ, Van der Hem GK: Subentities within adult primary IgA-nephropathy. Clin Nephrol 22:195–199, 1984.
14. Hood SA, Velosa JA, Holley KE, Donadio JF Jr: IgA-IgG nephropathy: predictive indices of progressive disease. Clin Nephrol 16:55–62, 1981.
15. Okada M, Tsuchida H, Yamamoto S: Familial mesangial IgA nephropathy, In: Yoshitoshi Y, Ueda Y (eds) Glomerulonephritis. Baltimore: University Park Press, 1979, pp 201–223.
16. Nakahara C, Aosai F, Hasegawa O, Ito H, Matsuo N, Hajikano H, Sakaguchi H: IgA nephropathy in children: a modified view of clinico-pathological characteristics. Pediatr Res 14:995(A), 1980.
17. Ohno J: Discussion, pp 133–134. In: Glassock RJ, Kurokawa K: IgA nephropathy in Japan. Am J Nephrol 5:127–137, 1985.
18. Hogg RJ, Silva FG: IgA nephropathy: natural history and prognostic indicators in children. Contrib Nephrol 40:214–221, 1984.
19. Tolkoff-Rubin NE, Cosimi AB, Fuller T, Rubin RH, Colvin RB: IgA nephropathy in HLA-identical siblings. Transplantation 26:430–433, 1978.
20. Sabatier JC, Genin C, Assenat H, Colon S, Ducret F, Berthoux FC: Mesangial IgA glomerulonephritis in HLA-identical brothers. Clin Nephrol 11:35–38, 1979.
21. Berger J: Idiopathic mesangial IgA, In: Hamburger J, Crosnier J, Grunfeld J-P (eds) Nephrology. New York: John Wiley and Sons, 1979, pp 535–541.
22. Katz A, Karanicolas S, Falk JA: Family study in IgA nephritis: a possible role of HLA antigens. Transplantation 29:505–506, 1980.
23. Montoliu J, Darnell A, Torras A, Ercilla G, Valles M, Revert L: Familial IgA nephropathy: report of two cases and brief review of the literature. Arch Intern Med 140:1374–1375, 1980.
24. Sinniah R, Javier AR, Ku G: The pathology of mesangial IgA nephritis with clinical correlation. Histopathology 5:469–490, 1981.
25. Rambausek M, Seelig HP, Andrassy K, Waldherr R, Kehry I, Lenhard V, Ritz E: Mesangial IgA-glomerulonephritis. Dtsch Med Wochenschr 108:125–130, 1981.
26. Kashiwabara H, Shishido H, Tomura S, Tuchida H, Miyama T: Strong association between IgA nephropathy and HLA-DR4 antigen. Kidney Int 22:377–382, 1982.
27. Wyatt RJ, Julian BA, Weinstein A, Rothfield NF, McLean RH: Partial H (B1H) deficiency and glomerulonephritis in two families. J Clin Immunol 2:110–117, 1982.
28. Hene RJ, De Glas-Vos JW, Valentijn R, Gmelig Mayling FC, Krediet RT, Kater L: Aspects serologiques et genetiques dans deux families atteintes de néphropathie primitive à IgA. Nephrologie 3:94A, 1982.
29. Egido J, Balsco R, Sancho J, Lozano L, Gutierrez-Millet V: Immunological studies in a familial IgA nephropathy. Clin Exp Immunol 54:532–538, 1983.
30. Feehally J, Dyer PA, Davidson JA, Harris R, Mallick NP: Immunogenetics of IgA nephropathy: experience in a UK centre. Dis Markers 2:493–500, 1984.
31. Julian BA, Quiggins PA, Thompson JS, Woodford SY, Gleason K, Wyatt RJ: Familial IgA nephropathy: evidence of an inherited mechanism of disease. N Engl J Med 312:202–208, 1985.

32. Sinniah R: Occurrence of mesangial IgA and IgM deposits in a control necropsy population. J Clin Pathol 36:276–279, 1983.
33. Sakai H, Nomoto Y, Arimori S, Komori K, Inouye H, Tsuji K: Increase of IgA-bearing peripheral blood lymphocytes in families of patients with IgA nephropathy. Am J Clin Pathol 72:452–456, 1979.
34. Egido J, Blasco RA, Sancho J, Hernando L: Immunological abnormalities in healthy relatives of patients with IgA nephropathy. Am J Nephrol 5:14–20, 1985.
35. Berthoux FC, Genin C, Gagne A, Le Petit JC, Sabatier JC: HLA B35 antigen and mesangial IgA glomerulonephritis: a poor prognosis marker? Proc Eur Dial Transplant Assoc 16:551–555, 1979.
36. Lopez Trascasa M, Egido J, Sancho J, Hernando L: IgA glomerulonephritis (Berger's disease): evidence of high serum levels of polymeric IgA. Clin Exp Immunol 42:247–254, 1980.
37. Nomoto Y, Sakai H, Arimori S: Increase of IgA-bearing lymphocytes in peripheral blood from patients with IgA nephropathy. Am J Clin Pathol 71:158–160, 1979.
38. Egido J, Blasco R, Sancho J, Lozano L, Sanchez-Crespo M, Hernando L: Increased rates of polymeric IgA synthesis by circulating lymphoid cells in IgA mesangial glomerulonephritis. Clin Exp Immunol 47:309–316, 1982.
39. Emancipator SN, Gallo GR, Lamm ME: Experimental IgA nephropathy induced by oral immunization. J Exp Med 157:572–582, 1983.
40. Valentijn RM, Kauffmann R, Brutel de la Riviere G, Daha M, Vanes LA: Presence of circulating macromolecular IgA in patients with hematuria due to primary IgA nephropathy. Am J Med 74:375–381, 1983.
41. Lesavre PH, Pigeon M, Bach JF: Analysis of circulating IgA and detection of immune complexes in primary IgA nephropathy. Clin Exp Immunol 48:61–69, 1983.
42. Hall RP, Stachura I, Cason J, Whiteside TL, Lawley TJ: IgA-containing circulating immune complexes in patients with IgA nephropathy. Am J Med 74:56–63, 1983.
43. Egido J, Blasco R, Lozano L, Sancho J, Garcia-hoyo R: Immunological abnormalities in tonsils of patients with IgA nephropathy: inversion of the ratio of IgA:IgG bearing lymphocytes and increased polymeric IgA synthesis. Clin Exp Immunol 57:101–106, 1984.
44. Westberg NG, Baklien K, Schmekel B, Gillberg R, Brandtzaeg P: Quantitation of immunoglobulin-producing cells in small intestinal mucosa of patients with IgA nephropathy. Clin Immunol Immunopathal 26:442–445, 1983.
45. Endoh M, Suga T, Miura M, Tomino Y, Nomoto Y, Sakai H: In vivo alteration of antibody production in patients with IgA nephropathy. Clin Exp Immunol 57:564–570, 1984.
46. Egido J, Blasco R, Sancho J, Lozano L: T-cell dysfunctions in IgA nephropathy: specific abnormalities in the regulation of IgA synthesis. Clin Immunol Immunopathal 26:201–212, 1983.
47. Rothschild E, Chatenoud L: T cell subset modulation of immunoglobulin production in IgA nephropathy and membranous glomerulonephritis. Kidney Int 25:557–564, 1984.
48. Sakai H, Endoh M, Tomino Y, Nomoto Y: Increase of IgA-specific helper Tα cells in patients with IgA nephropathy. Clin Exp Immunol 50:77–82, 1982.
49. Adachi M, Yodoi J, Masuda T, Takatsuki K, Uchino H: Altered expression of lymphocyte Fcα receptor in selective IgA deficiency and IgA nephropathy. J Immunol 131:1246–1251, 1985.
50. Endoh M, Sakai H, Nomoto Y, Tomino Y, Kaneshige H: IgA-specific helper activity of Tα cells in human peripheral blood. J Immunol 127:2612–2613, 1981.
51. Sakai H, Nomoto Y, Arimori S: Decrease of IgA-specific suppressor T cell activity in patients with IgA nephropathy. Clin Exp Immunol 38:243–248, 1979.
52. Valentijn RM, Kauffmann RH, De la Reviere M, Daha MR, Van Es LA: Presence of circulating macromolecular IgA in patients with hematuria due to primary IgA nephropathy. Am J Med 74:375–381, 1983.
53. Tomino Y, Sakai H, Miura M, Nomoto Y, Umehara K, Hashimoto K: Detection of antigenic substances in patients with IgA nephropathy. Contrib Nephrol 40:69–73, 1984.
54. Nagy J, Uj M, Szucs G, Trinn C, Burger T: Herpes virus antigens and antibodies in kidney biopsies and sera of IgA glomerulonephritic patients. Clin Nephrol 21:259–262, 1984.
55. Clarkson AR, Seymour AE, Chan YL, Thompson AJ, Woodroffe AJ: Clinical, pathological

and therapeutic aspects of IgA nephropathy. In: Kincaid-Smith P, D'Apice AJF, Atkins RC (eds) Progress in glomerulonephritis. New York: John Wiley, 1977, pp 283–309.
56. Newkirk MM, Klein MH, Katz A, Fisher MM, Underdown BJ: Estimation of polymeric IgA in human serum: an assay based on binding of radiolabeled human secretory component with applications in the study of IgA nephropathy, IgA monoclonal gammopathy and liver disease. J Immunol 130:1176–1181, 1983.
57. Bene MC, Faure G, Duheille J: IgA nephropathy: characterization of the polymeric nature of mesangial deposits by in vitro binding of free secretory component. Clin Exp Immunol 47:527–534, 1982.
58. Katz A, Newkirk MM, Klein MH: Circulating and mesangial IgA in IgA nephropathy. In: D'Amico G, Minnetti L, Ponticelli C (eds) IgA mesangial nephropathy. Basel: Karger, 1984, pp 74–79.
59. Splawski JB, Woodard CS, Denney RM, Goldblum RM: Rapid development of polymeric IgA in the serum of infants. Clin Res 31:902A, 1983.
60. Savilahti E: Immunoglobulin-containing cells in the intestinal mucosa and immunoglobulins in the intestinal juice in children. Clin Exp Immunol 11:415–425, 1972.
61. Haworth JC, Dilling L: Concentration of A globulin in serum, saliva and nasopharyngeal secretions of infants and children. J Lab Clin Med 67:922–933, 1966.
62. Delacroix DL, Liroux E, Vaerman JP: High proportion of polymeric IgA in young infants' sera and independence between IgA size and IgA subclass distributions. J Clin Immunol 3:51–55, 1983.
63. Hogg RJ, Silva FG: IgA nephropathy: natural history and prognostic indices in children. In: D'Amico G, Minnetti L, Ponticelli C (eds) IgA mesangial nephropathy. Basel: Karger, 1984, pp 214–221.
64. Valentijn RM, Radl J, Haaijman JJ, Vermeer BJ, Weening JJ, Kauffmann RH, Daha MR, Van Es LA: Circulating and mesangial secretory component-binding IgA-1 in primary IgA nephropathy. Kidney Int 26:760–766, 1984.
65. Conley ME, Cooper MD, Michael AF: Selective deposition of immunoglobulin A1 in immunoglobulin A nephropathy, anaphylactoid purpura nephritis and systemic lupus erythematosus. J Clin Invest 66:1432–1436, 1980.
66. Stockert RJ, Kressner MS, Collins JC, Sternlieb I, Morell AG: IgA interaction with the asialoglycoprotein receptor. Proc Natl Acad Sci USA 79:6229–6231, 1982.
67. Conley ME, Arbeter A, Douglas SD: Serum levels of IgA1 and IgA2 in children and in patients with IgA deficiency. Mol Immunol 20:977–981, 1983.
68. Rifai A, Mannik M: Clearance of circulating IgA immune complexes is mediated by a specific receptor on Kupffer cells in mice. J Exp Med 160:125–137, 1984.
69. Kater L, Jobsis AC, Baart de la Faille-Kuyper EH, Vogten AJM, Grijm R: Alcoholic hepatic disease: specificity of IgA deposits in liver. Am J Clin Pathol 71:51–57, 1979.
70. Berger J, Yaneva H, Nabarra B: Glomerular changes in patients with cirrohsis of the liver. Adv Nephrol 7:3–32, 1978.
71. Lawrence S, Pussel BA, Charlesworth JA: Mesangial IgA nephropathy: detection of defective reticulophagocytic function in vivo. Clin Nephrol 16:280–283, 1983.
72. Nicholls K, Kincaid-Smith P: Defective in vivo Fc- and C3b-receptor function in IgA nephropathy. Am J Kidney Dis 4:128–134, 1984.
73. Roccatello D, Coppo R, Piccoli G: Monocyte–macrophage system function in IgA nephropathy. Contrib Nephrol 40:130–136, 1984.
74. Evans DJ, Gwyn Williams D, Peters DK, Sissons JGP, Boulton-Jones JM, Ogg CS, Cameron JS, Hoffbrand BI: Glomerular deposition of properdin in Henoch-Schönlein syndrome and idiopathic focal nephritis. Br Med J 3:326–328, 1973.
75. Tomino Y: Complement system in IgA nephropathy. Tokai J Exp Clin Med 5:14–22, 1980.
76. Gotze O, Muller-Eberhard HJ: The C3-activation system: an alternative pathway of complement activation. J Exp Med 134:905–1085, 1971.
77. Pfaffenbach G, Lamm ME, Gigli I: Activation of guinea pig alternative complement pathway by mouse IgA immune complexes. J Exp Med 155:231–247, 1982.
78. Boakle RJ, Pruitt KM, Mestecky J: The interactions of human complement with interfacially aggregated preparations of human secretory IgA. Immunochemistry 11:543–548, 1974.
79. Julian BA, Wyatt RJ, McMorrow RG, Galla JH: Serum complement proteins in IgA nephropathy. Clin Nephrol 20:251–258, 1983.

80. Lagrue G, Branellec A, Intrator L, Moisy M, Sobel A: Evaluation du C3d dans les néphropathies glomérulaires chroniques primitives. Nouv Presse Med 8:1153–1156, 1979.
81. Wyatt RJ, Kanayama Y, Julian BA, Sugimoto S, Curd JG: C3 activation in IgA nephropathy. Kidney Int 27:226A, 1985.
82. Kincaid-Smith P, Nicholls K: Mesangial IgA nephropathy. Am J Kidney Dis 3:90–102, 1983.
83. Linné T, Aperia A, Broberger O, Bergstrand A, Bohman S-O, Rekola S: Course of renal function in IgA glomerulonephritis in children and adolescents. Acta Paediatr Scand 71:735–743, 1982.
84. Robson A: Pediatric perspectives. Am J Kidney Dis 2:566–567, 1983.
85. Southwest Pediatric Nephrology Study Group: Association of IgA nephropathy with steriod-responsive nephrotic syndrome. Am J Kidney Dis 5:157–164, 1985.
86. Mustonen J, Pasternack A, Rantala I: The nephrotic syndrome in IgA glomerulonephritis: response to corticosteriod therapy. Clin Nephrol 20:172–176, 1983.
87. Andreoli SP, Yum MN, Bergstein JM: IgA nephropathy in children: significance of glomerula basement membrane deposition of IgA. Am J Nephrol 6:28–33, 1986.
88. Levy M, Gonzales-Burchard S, Broyer M, Dommergues J-P, Foulard M, Sorez J-P, Habib R: Outcome of Berger disease in children. Medicine 64:157–180, 1985.
89. Lagrue G, Sadreux T, Laurent J, Hirbec G: Is there a treatment of mesangial IgA glomerulonephritis [letter to the editor]. Clin Nephrol 16:161, 1981.
90. Hene RJ, Valentijn RM, Kater L: Plasmapheresis in nephropathy of Henoch-Schönlein purpura and primary IgA nephropathy. Kidney Int 22:409A, 1982.
91. Bergstein J: IgA nephropathy [letter to the editor]. Clin Nephrol 9:258–259, 1978.
92. Hamazaki T, Tateno S, Shishido H: Eicosapentaenoic acid and IgA nephropathy. Lancet 1:1017–1018, 1984.

INDEX